AF765197

Allergens and respiratory pollutants

Published by Woodhead Publishing Limited

Woodhead Publishing Series in Biomedicine

1 Practical leadership for biopharmaceutical executives
J. Y. Chin

2 Outsourcing biopharma R&D to India
P. R. Chowdhury

3 Matlab® in bioscience and biotechnology
L. Burstein

4 Allergens and respiratory pollutants
Edited by M. A. Williams

5 Concepts and techniques in genomics and proteomics
N. Saraswathy and P. Ramalingam

6 An introduction to pharmaceutical sciences
J. Roy

7 Patently innovative: How pharmaceutical firms use emerging patent law to extend monopolies on blockbuster drugs
R. A. Bouchard

8 Therapeutic protein drug products: Practical approaches to formulation in the laboratory, manufacturing and the clinic
Edited by B. K. Meyer

9 A biotech manager's handbook: A practical guide
Edited by M. O'Neill and M. H. Hopkins

10 Clinical research in Asia: Opportunities and challenges
U. Sahoo

11 Therapeutic antibody engineering: Current and future advances driving the strongest growth area in the pharma industry
W. R. Strohl and L. M. Strohl

12 Commercialising the stem cell sciences
O. Harvey

13

Published by Woodhead Publishing Limited

14 **Human papillomavirus infections: From the laboratory to clinical practice**
F. Cobo
15 **Annotating new genes: From *in silico* to validations by experiments**
S. Uchida
16 **Open-source software in life science research: Practical solutions in the pharmaceutical industry and beyond**
Edited by L. Harland and M. Forster
17 **Nanoparticulate drug delivery: A perspective on the transition from laboratory to market**
V. Patravale, P. Dandekar and R. Jain
18 **Bacterial cellular metabolic systems: Metabolic regulation of a cell system with ^{13}C-metabolic flux analysis**
K. Shimizu
19 **Contract research and manufacturing services (CRAMS) in India**
M. Antani, G. Gokhale and K. Baxi
20 **Bioinformatics for biomedical science and clinical applications**
K-H. Liang
21 **Deterministic versus stochastic modelling in biochemistry and systems biology**
P. Lecca, I. Laurenzi and F. Jordan
22 **Protein folding *in silico*: Protein folding versus protein structure prediction**
I. Roterman-Konieczna
23 **Computer-aided vaccine design**
T. J. Chuan and S. Ranganathan
24 **An introduction to biotechnology**
W. T. Godbey
25 **RNA interference: Therapeutic developments**
T. Novobrantseva, P. Ge and G. Hinkle
26 **Patent litigation in the pharmaceutical and biotechnology industries**
G. Morgan
27 **Clinical research in paediatric psychopharmacology: A practical guide**
P. Auby
28 **The application of SPC in the pharmaceutical and biotechnology industries**
T. Cochrane
29 **Ultrafiltration for bioprocessing**
H. Lutz
30 **Therapeutic risk management of medicines**
A. K. Banerjee and S. Mayall

31 21st century quality management and good management practices: Value added compliance for the pharmaceutical and biotechnology industry
S. Williams

32

33 CAPA in the pharmaceutical and biotech industries
J. Rodriguez

34 Process validation for the production of biopharmaceuticals: Principles and best practice.
A. R. Newcombe and P. Thillaivinayagalingam

35 Clinical trial management: An overview
U. Sahoo and D. Sawant

36 Impact of regulation on drug development
H. Guenter Hennings

37 Lean biomanufacturing
N. J. Smart

38 Marine enzymes for biocatalysis
Edited by A. Trincone

39 Ocular transporters and receptors in the eye: Their role in drug delivery
A. K. Mitra

40 Stem cell bioprocessing: For cellular therapy, diagnostics and drug development
T. G. Fernandes, M. M. Diogo and J. M. S. Cabral

41

42 Fed-batch fermentation: A practical guide to scalable recombinant protein production in *Escherichia coli*
G. G. Moulton and T. Vedvick

43 The funding of biopharmaceutical research and development
D. R. Williams

44 Formulation tools for pharmaceutical development
Edited by J. E. A. Diaz

45 Drug-biomembrane interaction studies: The application of calorimetric techniques
R. Pignatello

46 Orphan drugs: Understanding the rare drugs market
E. Hernberg-Ståhl

47 Nanoparticle-based approaches to targeting drugs for severe diseases
J. L. A. Mediano

48 **Successful biopharmaceutical operations**
C. Driscoll
49 **Electroporation-based therapies for cancer**
Edited by R. Sundarajan
50 **Transporters in drug discovery and development**
Y. Lai
51 **The life-cycle of pharmaceuticals in the environment**
R. Braund and B. Peake
52 **Computer-aided applications in pharmaceutical technology**
Edited by J. Petrović
53 **From plant genomics to plant biotechnology**
Edited by P. Poltronieri, N. Burbulis and C. Fogher
54 **Bioprocess engineering: An introductory engineering and life science approach**
K. G. Clarke
55 **Quality assurance problem solving and training strategies for success in the pharmaceutical and life science industries**
G. Welty
56 **Nanomedicine: Prognostic and curative approaches to cancer**
K. Scarberry
57 **Gene therapy: Potential applications of nanotechnology**
S. Nimesh
58 **Controlled drug delivery: The role of self-assembling multi-task excipients**
M. Mateescu
59 ***In silico* protein design**
C. M. Frenz
60 **Bioinformatics for computer science: Foundations in modern biology**
K. Revett
61 **Gene expression analysis in the RNA world**
J. Q. Clement
62 **Computational methods for finding inferential bases in molecular genetics**
Q-N. Tran
63 **NMR metabolomics in cancer research**
M. Čuperlović-Culf
64 **Virtual worlds for medical education, training and care delivery**
K. Kahol

Woodhead Publishing Series in Biomedicine: Number 4

Allergens and respiratory pollutants

The role of innate immunity

edited by
Marc A. Williams

Oxford Cambridge Philadelphia New Delhi

Published by Woodhead Publishing Limited

Woodhead Publishing Limited, 80 High Street, Sawston, Cambridge, CB22 3HJ, UK
www.woodheadpublishing.com
www.woodheadpublishingonline.com

Woodhead Publishing, 1518 Walnut Street, Suite 1100, Philadelphia, PA 19102-3406, USA

Woodhead Publishing India Private Limited, G-2, Vardaan House, 7/28 Ansari Road, Daryaganj, New Delhi – 110002, India
www.woodheadpublishingindia.com

First published in 2011 by Biohealthcare Publishing (Oxford) Limited; republished in 2012 by Woodhead Publishing Limited
ISBN: 978-0-08-101716-6 (print) and ISBN 978-1-908818-06-5 (online)
Woodhead Publishing Series in Biomedicine ISSN 2050-0289 (print); ISSN 2050-2097 (online)

© The editor, contributors and the Publishers, 2011

The right of Marc A. Williams to be identified as the author of the editorial material in this Work has been asserted by him in accordance with sections 77 and 78 of the Copyright, Designs and Patents Act 1988.

British Library Cataloguing-in-Publication Data: A catalogue record for this book is available from the British Library.

All rights reserved. No part of this publication may be reproduced, stored in or introduced into a retrieval system, or transmitted, in any form, or by any means (electronic, mechanical, photocopying, recording or otherwise) without the prior written permission of the Publishers. This publication may not be lent, resold, hired out or otherwise disposed of by way of trade in any form of binding or cover other than that in which it is published without the prior consent of the Publishers. Any person who does any unauthorised act in relation to this publication may be liable to criminal prosecution and civil claims for damages.

Permissions may be sought from the Publishers at the above address.

The use in this publication of trade names, trademarks, service marks, and similar terms, even if they are not identified as such, is not to be taken as an expression of opinion as to whether or not they are subject to proprietary rights. The Publishers are not associated with any product or vendor mentioned in this publication.

The Publishers, editor(s) and contributors have attempted to trace the copyright holders of all material reproduced in this publication and apologise to any copyright holders if permission to publish in this form has not been obtained. If any copyright material has not been acknowledged, please write and let us know so we may rectify in any future reprint. Any screenshots in this publication are the copyright of the website owner(s), unless indicated otherwise.

Limit of Liability/Disclaimer of Warranty
The Publishers, editor(s) and contributors make no representations or warranties with respect to the accuracy or completeness of the contents of this publication and specifically disclaim all warranties, including without limitation warranties of fitness of a particular purpose. No warranty may be created or extended by sales of promotional materials. The advice and strategies contained herein may not be suitable for every situation. This publication is sold with the understanding that the Publishers are not rendering legal, accounting or other professional services. If professional assistance is required, the services of a competent professional person should be sought. No responsibility is assumed by the Publishers, editor(s) or contributors for any loss of profit or any other commercial damages, injury and/or damage to persons or property as a matter of products liability, negligence or otherwise, or from any use or operation of any methods, products, instructions or ideas contained in the material herein. The fact that an organisation or website is referred to in this publication as a citation and/or potential source of further information does not mean that the Publishers nor the editors(s) and contributors endorse the information the organisation or website may provide or recommendations it may make. Further, readers should be aware that internet websites listed in this work may have changed or disappeared between when this publication was written and when it is read. Because of rapid advances in medical sciences, in particular, independent verification of diagnoses and drug dosages should be made.

Typeset by RefineCatch Limited, Bungay, Suffolk
Printed in the UK and USA

Published by Woodhead Publishing Limited

Contents

List of illustrations

Figures

Tables

Editor's note

This book, and all chapters contained within it, is not a product of the United States Environmental Protection Agency (US EPA) and should not be interpreted as such. The views expressed of any of the authors do not necessarily represent the views of the US EPA or the US Federal Government. Materials, products or services described in any of the chapters do not represent any endorsement of said facts by the US EPA or the US Federal Government.

Published by Woodhead Publishing Limited

About the editor and contributors

Marc A. Williams is a Biologist with the US Environmental Protection Agency, Research Triangle Park, USA and was an Assistant Professor of Medicine and Environmental Medicine at The University of Rochester School of Medicine and Dentistry, NY, USA (2006 to 2009) and Instructor of Medicine at the Johns Hopkins University School of Medicine (2004 to 2006). He has a long-standing interest and program of research in the field of immunotoxicology and innate immunity with a vested interest in understanding how environmental "danger signals" trigger innate immune signalling in dendritic cells, macrophages and basophils and in determining the health effects of environmental pollutants in host immune dysfunction and pulmonary allergic diseases such as asthma. He is currently studying the cell-mediated and molecular mechanisms involved in the dysfunction of the pulmonary immune system and the roles played by respirable "dangerous triggers" including ambient pollutants like diesel exhaust and airborne particulate matter. Dr Williams has enjoyed a distinguished career in basic and translational research, especially as applied to the mechanisms of human disease in the fields of hematology, infectious diseases and immunology. He serves on several national leadership committees including those of the American Thoracic Society (ATS) and The American Academy of Asthma, Allergy and Immunology (AAAAI) of which he is a Fellow (FAAAAI). Dr Williams serves as Associate Editor of *Stem Cells and Development* and Section Editor of the *Journal of Innate Immunity.* He also serves on the editorial boards of several other leading biomedical journals, including *Biomarker Insights, Journal of Receptor, Ligand and Channel Research* and *Scientific World Journal (Immunology and Inflammation Domain).* Dr Williams is listed in *Marquis Who's Who in America* and *Cambridge Who's Who of Professionals.* He has also been instated into the Faculty of 1000 (Immunology – Section on Innate Immunity) and is the author of more than 60 original research papers, invited review articles, expert commentaries and editorials.

Timothy D. Bigby, MD, is Chief of Pulmonary and Critical Care Section of the VA San Diego Healthcare System and Professor of Medicine at the University of California, San Diego. He graduated from Baylor College of Medicine and completed his internal medicine residency at the University of Colorado. He was a research fellow at the National Jewish Hospital and the University of Colorado and completed his pulmonary and critical care fellowship at the University of California, San Francisco. He also completed a research fellowship at the Cardiovascular Research Institute at UCSF. He was an Instructor and Assistant Professor at the University of California, San Francisco until moving to the University of California, San Diego and the VA San Diego in 1989. His laboratory has focused on inflammatory cell biology and innate immunity as it relates to disorders of the airways and lungs.

Bertram Bleck, PhD, is Senior Investigator at New York University School of Medicine. He earned his PhD in Chemistry at the Westfälische Wilhelms-Universität Münster (Germany) on research into the role of fatty acid binding proteins in lipid metabolism and signal transduction. His research focus now is the immunbiology of mucosal interfaces, especially the interplay of dendritic cells with epithelial cells in the airway.

Karine Botturi completed a Master's in Immunology at the Centre d'Immunologie Marseille Luminy (CIML), Marseille, France. Dr Botturi trained in clinical research (2004) and then joined the team of Professor Magnan to complete a PhD (2004–7) training program in the field of respiratory diseases, in a project entitled "Modulation of T cell activation in asthma and chronic lung transplant rejection". She is currently Project Manager in the field of Pulmonology at the Centre d'Investigation Clinique Thorax of L'institut du thorax, Nantes, France. Currently, Dr Botturi coordinates multicenter institutional trials and pharmaceutical clinical trials in the field of severe asthma, cystic fibrosis, pulmonary hypertension, COPD and lung transplantation. In research, Dr Botturi is part of INSERM team "Bronchial diseases and allergies", integrated in the UMR 915 L'institut du thorax, Nantes, France. Dr Botturi also develops clinical research in a translational approach in the general field of T cell activation in asthma and lung transplantation (the COLT program).

Arnaud Cavaillès is a Doctor of Respiratory Medicine in the Service de Pneumologie within L'institut du thorax, Nantes, France. His clinical activity is devoted to acute respiratory care, with a specific orientation on Chronic Obstructive Pulmonary Disease. In research, Dr Cavaillès is involved in clinical research as investigator for institutional and pharmaceutical clinical trials in the field of asthma and COPD.

Michael H. Chi, MD, is currently a student at Vanderbilt University School of Medicine in Nashville, TN pursuing a Doctor of Medicine degree. Prior to entering medical school, he graduated summa cum laude in 2008 from Vanderbilt University School of Engineering with a Bachelor of Engineering degree in biomedical engineering. During his time at Vanderbilt, he has accumulated extensive lab-based research experience in the field of respiratory syncytial virus (RSV) pathogenesis. He has also co-authored a number of articles and abstracts and has given podium presentations on the topic.

Kian Fan Chung, MD, DSc, FRCP (London), is Professor of Respiratory Medicine and Head of the Experimental Studies Unit at the National Heart and Lung Institute, Imperial College London, UK. Professor Chung obtained MD and DSc degrees from the University of London. He is an Investigator of the Medical Research Council/Environmental Protection Agency UK Centre for Environment and Health and a Senior Investigator of the NHS National Institute of Health Research UK. His research interests include the mechanisms of airway inflammation and repair, and airway smooth muscle biology in relation to chronic airways diseases. He has published more than 500 scientific articles, reviews and book chapters.

Donald N. Cook, PhD, is Head of the Immunogenetics Group at the National Institute of Environmental Health Sciences (NIEHS), National Institutes of Health (NIH), USA. He earned his PhD in microbiology and immunology at McGill University in Montreal, Canada. He served as a principal scientist at Schering-Plough Research Institute and as an assistant professor in the Division of Pulmonary and Critical Care Medicine at Duke University before joining NIEHS in 2005. His laboratory studies the initiation and regulation of allergic responses to inhaled allergens. He has published more than 50 peer-reviewed articles in leading biomedical journals and has written several book chapters.

Maria A. Curotto de Lafaille, PhD, is a Principal Investigator at the Singapore Immunology Network and an Adjunct Assistant Professor at New York University School of Medicine. She received her PhD in Immunology from the University of São Paulo, Brazil, and did her post-doctoral training at the Harvard School of Public Health. She is interested in mechanisms of sensitization and tolerance to allergens and the regulation of the IgE response.

Patricia W. Finn, MD, is Director of the Division of Pulmonary and Critical Care Medicine at the University of California, San Diego. She graduated from Albert Einstein College of Medicine and completed internal medicine residency at Montefiore Hospital, fellowship in pulmonary and critical care medicine at Massachusetts General Hospital, and post-doctoral fellowship at Harvard University. She served as Instructor in Immunology and Medicine, Assistant, and Associate Professor of Medicine at Harvard Medical School before moving to University of California, San Diego in 2005. Her laboratory focuses on investigation of immune mediated pulmonary disorders, including asthma, acute lung injury, and lung transplantation.

Mark W. Frampton, MD, is Professor of Medicine and Medicine at the University of Rochester Medical Center, NY. Dr Frampton received his MD from NewYork University School of Medicine and completed post-doctoral fellowships in Pulmonary and Critical Care at Strong Memorial Hospital from 1985 to 1988. Dr Frampton has been a Fellow of the American College of Physicians since 1974 and is Board Certified in Pulmonary Disease and Internal Medicine. Dr Frampton has served on numerous committees of the American Thoracic Society.

Stavros Garantziotis, MD, is a Principal Investigator and leader of the Matrix Biology Group within the Laboratory of Respiratory Biology, National Institute of Environmental Health Sciences, Research Triangle Park, North Carolina. He is the Staff Clinician for the new Clinical Research Unit at NIEHS and remains clinically active in the field of lung transplantation and pulmonary fibrosis. His research program is focused on the role of hyaluronan in the pulmonary response to environmental injury, IαI-hyaluronan binding in models of inflammation and lung injury, and ECM participation in angiogenesis and epithelial cell survival. He is currently on the editorial board of the *American Journal of Respiratory Cell and Molecular Biology*.

Steve N. Georas, MD, is Professor of Medicine and Environmental Medicine at the University of Rochester Medical Center. From 1994 to 2006, Dr Georas was a faculty member at Johns Hopkins University, Baltimore, in the Pulmonary Division with joint appointments in Allergy/Immunology and Environmental Health Sciences. Dr Georas directs a research group investigating mechanisms of dendritic cell and T cell activation in allergic diseases. He has published numerous peer-reviewed articles in this area, is a past recipient of a Career Investigator Award from the American Lung Association, and is supported by research grants from the NIH. Dr Georas is active in peer review at the NIH, Wellcome Turst, and other funding agencies, and is a member of the American Society for Clinical Investigation.

Jonathan Grigg, MD, MRCP, FRCPCH, is Professor of Paediatric Respiratory and Environmental Medicine at Barts and the London School of Medicine, Queen Mary University London. He trained in medicine at the Royal London Hospital (UK). After a three-year clinical fellowship at the Royal Postgraduate Medical School (London), and a one-year fellowship in the Department of Pediatric Leukocyte Biology, Texas Children's Hospital, he finished his paediatric respiratory training at the Royal Children's Hospital, Melbourne (Australia). On his return to the UK, he was appointed as a Senior Lecturer in Paediatric Respiratory Medicine at the University of Leicester. His current research interests include the effects of particulate matter air pollution on vulnerability to pulmonary bacterial infection.

John W. Hollingsworth, MD, is Associate Professor in the Departments of Medicine and Immunology at Duke University Medical Center, Durham, North Carolina. Dr Hollingsworth is a physician scientist with an active research program investigating the role of genes of innate immunity in environmental lung disease. His research program is supported by the National Institute of Environmental Health Sciences (NIEHS). In addition, Dr Hollingsworth currently serves on the editorial boards of both the *American Journal of Respiratory Cell and Molecular Biology* and *Inhalation Toxicology*.

Yannick Lacoeuille is an Engineer within L'institut du thorax, Nantes, France. The clinical activity of the department is devoted to acute respiratory care, with a specific orientation on severe asthma and allergy, cystic fibrosis, pulmonary hypertension and lung transplantation. The hospital is recognized as National Center for Rare Diseases, Cystic Fibrosis. In research, Yannick Lacoeuille's main field of activity is bronchial diseases and allergies and specialized in cytometry for technical aspect. This includes the investigation of T cell activation in asthma and lung transplant recipients, both in humans and in murine models. He obtained his BSc in Biotechnology and Microscopy at the University of Nice. He joined Dr Magnan's (q.v.) team in 2005 in Marseille and is currently an integral part of the research program in Nantes where he has been since 2008. The team develops both clinical and basic research in a translational approach and

Yannick Lacoeuille participates actively in the COLT (COhort in Lung Transplantation) program.

Marie Langelot is a French Pneumonologist. She studied respiratory medicine at the Faculté de Médecine de Nantes, Université de Nantes, France. She works in the service de pneumologie, Nantes, France. At the same time, she has been a PhD student in Dr Magnan's (q.v.) INSERM team for two years. She focuses mainly on the role of T lymphocytes in murine models of allergic asthma.

Zhuowei Li, MD, is a Senior Research Associate in the Department of Medicine, Division of Pulmonary, Allergy and Critical Care Medicine at Duke University Medical Center, Durham, North Carolina. Her previous work at the Environmental Protection Agency and the University of North Carolina at Chapel Hill was focused on the pulmonary vascular effects of the criteria air pollutant, particulate matter. Her current research interests are focused on the role of pulmonary innate immunity in response to inhaled environmental toxicants including both ozone and lipopolysaccharide. She has co-authored 26 peer-reviewed original publications. She was a reviewer for *Clinical and Experimental Allergy, Journal of Molecular and Cellular Cardiology, Clinical and Molecular Allergy, Pan American Journal of Public Health,* and is a current editorial board member of *World Journal of Biological Chemistry*.

Antoine Magnan is Professor of Respiratory Medicine at Faculté de Médecine de Nantes, Université de Nantes, France and is the head of the Service de Pneumologie within L'institut du thorax, Nantes, France. The clinical activity of the department is devoted to acute respiratory care, with a specific orientation on severe asthma and allergy, cystic fibrosis, pulmonary hypertension and lung transplantation. In research, Dr Magnan's main field of activity is bronchial diseases and allergies. This includes the investigation of T cell activation in asthma and lung transplant recipients, both in humans and in murine models. He leads an INSERM team in the frame of the AVENIR program, integrated in the UMR 915 L'institut du thorax. The team develops both clinical and basic research in a translational approach. Dr Magnan leads the COLT (COhort in Lung Transplantation) program among the ten French lung transplantation centers as principal investigator. Dr Magnan is a former research fellow of the Centre d'Immunology Marseille Luminy (CIML), Marseille, France. He has published about 100 peer-reviewed articles in English.

Martin L. Moore, MD, PhD, is an Assistant Professor of Pediatric Infectious Diseases at Emory University School of Medicine. After receiving his PhD in

Genetics from the University of Georgia in 2003, he joined the laboratory of Stokes Peebles, MD (q.v.) at Vanderbilt University School of Medicine as a post-doctoral fellow. Dr Moore studied respiratory syncytial virus (RSV) in Dr Peebles's lab from 2004 to 2008 and co-authored several scientific articles on RSV pathogenesis and allergic airway inflammation. Dr Moore's expertise is in virology and mouse models of viral pathogenesis. His laboratory continues to study RSV, focusing on molecular pathogenesis, viral entry, and vaccine strategies.

Hideki Nakano, PhD, obtained his PhD degree at the University of Tokyo in Japan in 1998. He completed a post-doctoral fellowship at Duke University Medical Center in 2002 and was an Assistant Research Professor at Duke before joining NIEHS in 2007 as a Research Fellow. His interest is to understand dendritic cell-mediated immune responses. He has identified mouse plasmacytoid dendritic cells producing type 1 interferon, and demonstrated the mechanisms of chemokine-dependent dendritic cell migration, and the migratory pathway of inflammatory dendritic cells inducing T helper (Th)1 cells. He is currently studying the molecular pathways underlying the induction of effector cells such as Th2 cells in allergic asthma, as well as the signals that negatively regulate their actions once allergic pulmonary inflammation has been established. He has published more than 50 peer-reviewed articles and review articles and has written ten book chapters.

Paul W. Noble, MD, FCCP, is a Professor of Medicine and Chief of the Division of Pulmonary, Allergy and Critical Care Medicine at Duke University Medical Center, Durham, North Carolina. Dr Noble is a physician scientist with an active research laboratory focused on elucidating the basic mechanisms of lung injury, inflammation, and fibrosis. His research laboratory is funded by the National Institutes of Health. He continues to have an active clinical practice in ILD and is involved in clinical trials evaluating new therapies in IPF. Dr Noble is an elected member of the American Society of Clinical Investigation and the American Association of Physicians. He serves on the editorial boards for the *American Journal of Respiratory Cell and Molecular Biology* and the *American Journal of Respiratory and Critical Care Medicine.*

R. Stokes Peebles, Jr., MD, is Associate Professor of Medicine at Vanderbilt University Medical School, Nashville, Tennessee. He graduated with an MD degree from Vanderbilt, was a resident in Internal Medicine at Vanderbilt, and was elected to the Alpha Omega Alpha Honor Medical Society. He completed a four-year fellowship in Allergy/Clinical Immunology at Johns Hopkins School of Medicine, Baltimore, and a three-year fellowship in Pulmonary/Critical Care Medicine at Vanderbilt University. He is Board Certified in Internal Medicine, Allergy/Immunology, Pulmonary, and Critical Care. Dr Peebles has a very active research program investigating the role of eicosanoids in viral-induced and allergic lung inflammation.

Raymond Pieters, PhD, is Head of the Immunotoxicology Group and associate professor at the Institute for Risk Assessment Sciences (IRAS) of Utrecht University, Netherlands, and professor at the Institute for Life Sciences and Chemistry of the Utrecht University of Applied Sciences (UAS). He earned his PhD in Biology for research into the immunotoxic effects of organotin compounds at Utrecht University. Now the focus of his research group is on mechanistic evaluation of allergenic effects of drugs, food proteins and particulate matter, and on the development of translational assays for the assessment of safety and efficacy of compounds. Dr Pieters is involved in an international project on the evaluation of risk assessment of particulate matter, RAPTES (Risk of Airborne Particles, Toxicological and Epidemiological Studies), funded by the Netherlands Institute of Public Health (RIVM).

Anaïs Pipet is a Hospital Practitioner at the Pneumology Department (Service de Pneumologie) directed by Dr Antoine Magnan (q.v.). The latter department is part of the "Thorax Institute" (L'institut du thorax). As a pneumologist and allergologist, Dr Pipet's activities focus particularly on asthma and drug allergies. In the field of research, she takes part in the clinical research protocols as a co-investigator concerning asthma and allergies within the pneumology department.

Damien Reboulleau is an Engineer in Dr Antoine Magnan's (q.v.) team within L'institut du thorax, Nantes, France. The clinical activity of the department is devoted to acute respiratory care, with a specific focus on severe asthma and allergy, cystic fibrosis, pulmonary hypertension and lung transplantation. In research, Damien Reboulleau's main field of activity is bronchial diseases and allergies, with specialization in technical aspects of flow cytometry. He did his research Master's, directed by Dr Magnan, at The University of Nantes, studying and developing an asthma HDM-sensitive murine model. He continued with a professional Master's in platform engineering and worked in UMR 945 "immunité et infections" directed by Dr P. Debré in Paris, before returning to Dr Magnan's team in 2011. The team develops both clinical and basic research in a translational approach and Damien Reboulleau participates actively in the COLT (COhort in Lung Transplantation) program.

Joan Reibman, MD, is an Associate Professor at New York University School of Medicine and Medical Director of the NYU/Bellevue Hospital Asthma Center and the World Trade Center Environmental Health Center. She is a graduate of the Johns Hopkins University School of Medicine, Baltimore, and completed her medical residency and pulmonary training at New York University. The focus of her research group is on ambient pollutants and asthma with a focus on mucosal responses and genetic susceptibility.

Doris B. Tse, PhD, is an Associate Professor at New York University School of Medicine. She is a first generation American who graduated from Vassar College and the Graduate School of Arts and Sciences at Columbia University. She served as Associate Research Scientist at the College of Physicians and Surgeons of Columbia University and Assistant Professor at Weill Cornell Medical College before joining the faculty of New York University in 1994. A major focus of her research is studying T cell-mediated immunopathology of airway disorders which include atopic asthma, tuberculosis, and HIV-associated pulmonary infections.

John W. Upham, MD, PhD, is a Clinical Scientist working at the University of Queensland in Brisbane, Australia. He undertook specialist clinical training in pulmonology and internal medicine before completing a PhD in immunology at the University of Western Australia and a post-doctoral fellowship at McMaster University in Canada. He was appointed as a Professor of Respiratory Medicine in 2007. His research interests include the pathogenesis of allergic sensitisation and asthma, with particular emphasis on dendritic cell function and the interplay between allergy and respiratory viral infections.

Alison S. Williams, PhD, is a Research Fellow in the Molecular and Integrative Physiological Sciences program at the Harvard School of Public Health. She earned her PhD in Respiratory Pharmacology with a focus on mouse models of asthma and chronic obstructive pulmonary disease, from the National Heart and Lung Institute at Imperial College, University of London, UK. Dr Williams' current work investigates the mechanistic basis for the relationship between obesity and asthma, using mouse models to study whole-animal physiological processes and their molecular determinants. She has published 13 original research articles in leading physiological and respiratory journals.

Stephanie T. Yerkovich, PhD, is Chief Scientist at the Queensland Centre for Pulmonary Transplantation and Vascular Disease at the Prince Charles Hospital, Brisbane, Australia. Since obtaining her PhD in 2003 from the

University of Western Australia, Stephanie has been investigating immune development and immunity associated with respiratory diseases such as asthma and allergies. The focus of these studies has been the role of dendritic cells and how the response to allergens such as house dust mite is altered in atopic individuals. More recently her focus has been extended to investigate immune-mediated mechanisms occurring within the transplanted lung to better understand how these contribute to allograft dysfunction. She has published over 25 peer-reviewed journal articles.

1

An introduction to allergic inflammation and the innate immune sensing of dangerous ambient pollutants by the dendritic cell

Marc A. Williams

Abstract. Hematopoiesis is a process of cellular development and differentiation that, in adults at least, originates in the bone marrow and in the case of the myeloid cellular system continues in the peripheral blood and many of the organs to which such cells migrate. Through a series of differentiation pathways, subsets of myeloid cells are generated. Among them are professional antigen-presenting cells, termed dendritic cells or DC, that are derived from a common myeloid progenitor and constitute the most important specialized cell of the innate immune system. In the airway, DC are ideally located to rapidly sense and respond to exogenous triggers of pulmonary inflammation including such diverse environmental stimuli as aeroallergens, respirable particulate pollutants or other xenobiotics. Though the airway wall is a biologically complex cellular barrier and provides a major component of the innate immune system, interdigitated throughout the bronchial epithelium and parenchyma are several DC subsets that collectively sense and respond not only to infectious microorganisms that traffic to the lung, but also respirable environmental pollutant particles. Thus communication between the pulmonary epithelia and the interdigitating DC contributes to the maintenance of the lung as an immune-privileged organ. However, exposure of the lung to environmental airborne pollutant particles may provoke allergic inflammation. Moreover, airway inflammation in allergic asthma reflects an aberrant immune response against otherwise harmless inhaled allergens. The association between particulate air pollution and allergic asthma has been identified by epidemiological evidence, yet the biological effects of particulate air pollution in host immunity remain poorly studied. Given the escalating global burden of an increasingly prevalent and complex mixture of ambient airborne pollutants, it is no surprise that such anthropogenic triggers of allergic immune responsiveness are contributing to a variety of disease states, including allergic asthma and cardiovascular disease, enhanced susceptibility to pulmonary viral or bacterial infections and exacerbations of pre-existing airway diseases like chronic obstructive pulmonary disease (COPD). In this chapter, an overview of innate and adaptive immunology is provided that places in context the important role that the host innate immune system plays in sensing and responding to exogenous danger signals such as respirable particulate pollutants as well as an overview of some of the mechanisms that may be responsible for activating the innate allergic responses of DC. Collectively, respirable ambient pollutant particles can be considered "danger signals" of immune reactivity and the activated allergic inflammatory response sensed by dendritic cells as the "enemy within."

Keywords: innate immunity, dendritic cell, inflammation, asthma, Hygiene Hypothesis, toll-like receptor, pollution, airborne particulate matter, immunotoxicology

1.1 Introduction

In scientific research, particularly in the life sciences, history tells us that the only thing we are certain of is being certain of nothing at all, hence the importance of hypothesis-driven research. At the Battle of Waterloo of 1815, the Duke of Wellington famously stated after defeating the French armies of Napoleon: "All the business of war, and indeed all the business of life, is to endeavour to find out what you don't know by what you do; that's what I call 'guessing what was at the other side of the hill.' " In other words, one can consider this quote in the context of delineating the relative roles of the dendritic cell in allergic immunity and inflammation by hypothesis-driven research and experimentation. There have been several seminal works, including work of our own, [1–13] that have hypothesized an important role for the dendritic cell in driving allergic immune responses and contributing to the health effects associated with trafficking of respirable ambient pollutants to the lower airways.

Ambient air pollution, including coarse, fine and ultrafine particulate matter, ozone, nitrogen dioxide, sulfur dioxide, carbon monoxide, mercury, semi-volatile organic pollutants and a host of others emitted into the atmospheric air that we breathe presents serious challenges to human health. Sources of ambient airborne pollutants include diesel engine vehicles and trucks, shipping, aircraft, light and heavy industrial smoke-stacks, wood- and fossil-burning heating and cooking stoves, wild-fires, pesticides from agricultural sources, coal-burning power-plants and many other small fossil-fuel powered devices or machines. Sophisticated atmospheric and climatological research has shown that airborne pollutants in the lower atmosphere can be propelled to higher altitudes which are then shifted to geographically distant sites far from the source of the emitted pollutants by prevailing winds and other meteorological influences. This means of course that airborne pollutants can breach state lines in the continental US, traverse oceans and seas and even cross entire continents.

Moreover, the realization that the problem of geographically migratory ambient airborne pollutants and the issue of degrading air quality may worsen in the decades ahead is a cause for concern. This is particularly relevant when one considers the improving standards of living in developing countries, and thus enhanced demands for power and public transportation and with it escalating anthropogenic emissions associated with increased demands for transport and industry. As important as these considerations are, they will not be a major focus of this chapter and the reader is guided towards several publically available documents published by the US Environmental Protection Agency, the National Research Council, the National Oceanic and Atmospheric Administration, The National Aeronautics and Space Administration, and the National Science Foundation.

Studying dendritic cells (DC) in pulmonary immune responses to environmental particulate matter (PM) exposures stems from our knowledge that DC are uniquely positioned through peripheral tissues such as the lung and lymphoid or non-lymphoid organs where they are specialized for the rapid uptake, endogenous processing and presentation of antigens to naïve helper CD4+ and cytotoxic CD8+ T cells. Previously published work by us suggests a non-classic and pro-inflammatory-mediated differentiation of DC on activation by PM and aeroallergens such as ragweed extract.[1–6] It is hypothesized that ambient PM or diesel exhaust particles (DEP) exhibit immune adjuvant properties.[1–9] Ambient PM (APM) also induces epithelial cells to produce amphiregulin, GM-CSF and MIP-3α,[10–13] agents that are known to induce recruitment and survival of DC.

It seems likely, therefore, that DC will be among the first cells to sense and respond to inhaled PM. We are beginning to appreciate the potential consequences of the interaction between cells of the innate immune system and exposure to particulate matter species in driving pulmonary inflammation and Th2-mediated pro-allergic diseases. However, before discussing the complex architecture of an allergic pulmonary immune response orchestrated by airway dendritic cells, it would be remiss not to consider the history of discovery of the myeloid mononuclear cell system as well as to critically survey the scope of the global burden presented to each and every one of us by the complex ambient pollutants present in the air we breathe as well as the associated health effects and economic detriments of air pollutant particle exposure.

1.2 The mononuclear phagocyte system: key players in innate immunity

In vertebrates and mammals in particular, the immune system has evolved to provide host protection from invading pathogens. However, a pathogen is confronted by a number of immunological mechanisms evolutionarily designed to respond to infection and ideally prevent disease. Should an invading pathogen breach physical (physiological) and/or chemical (soluble) barriers, an immune response is mounted to that pathogen, a state of inflammation is invoked and the activated immune system is charged with preventing disease.

Two main arms of host immunity are defined as adaptive immune responsiveness – which is somewhat lethargic, taking days to weeks to fully respond, taking days to weeks to fully respond to the "danger" of an infection – and innate immune responsiveness – which is far more rapid, taking minutes to hours to provide a first line of immunological attack against the invading pathogen. While the adaptive or specific arm of host immunity enables the host to prepare for subsequent immunological challenges by recalling prior exposures to an infectious agent and to mount amplified responses to such agents upon each re-exposure, the innate immune system responds to such infectious agents or other exogenous "danger signals" in a less specific though much broader fashion. This is accomplished by the active engagement and/or recruitment of highly specialized cells that possess antigen uptake and microbial uptake mechanisms. Once internalized inside the cell, the microbial pathogen is either destroyed by cytolytic mechanisms or is at least constrained inside the cell until such a point that the much slower adaptive immune response has been mobilized and enters the fray.

Thus there is cooperation between the strictly antigen-specific adaptive and antigen non-specific innate immune responses. Cells that constitute the innate immune system, such as professional antigen-presenting mononuclear phagocytes, are said to synapse with and promote activation of T cells that are crucial components of the adaptive immune response. However, the innate immune system plays a dominant role in the elimination of most exogenous infectious or non-infectious agents that challenge the host. While mononuclear phagocytes play key roles in innate immune defense, in vertebrates at least, there are anatomical and physiological barriers in place that provide innate immune defense against, for example, respirable ambient pollutants, small particles or pathogenic viruses that may traffic to the conducting upper and lower airways, as well as the inflammatory responses provoked by such exogenous challenges.

The innate immune system has been evolutionarily devised to provide sequential lines of defense against potential environmental pathogens. Physiological barriers, for example as provided by the epithelial cells lining the lung, the skin, mucous membranes and complement in the blood benefit from the collaboration of the cell-mediated phagocytic and endocytic uptake mechanisms that collectively provide a first line of defense that is always present and rapid in its response. Soluble factors and other physiological barriers that precede the recruitment of the adaptive immune response provide a second line of defense, which is not always constitutively present. Such second lines of defense include secreted acute phase proteins, cytolytic enzymes, metabolic inhibitors, cytokines and chemokines and microbicidal peptides including beta-defensins and cathelicidins that collectively constitute the acute inflammatory response. However, this chapter is concerned with the role played by the mononuclear phagocyte system, and in particular myeloid dendritic cells responding to respirable exogenous ambient pollutant particles.

The mononuclear phagocyte system was recognized as an important network of cells capable of ingesting and killing bacteria in 1882 by the seminal work of Ilya Metchnikoff (1845–1916). Foremost among those cells was the antigen-presenting monocyte/macrophage system that displayed broad effector and accessory cell functions. Metchnikoff was awarded the Nobel Prize in Medicine and Physiology in 1908 for his work on phagocytosis theory (14, 15) – a prize that was jointly awarded to Paul Ehrlich for his pioneering work on the "side-chain theory" of antibody formation. (15, 16) It was previously noted that micro-organisms as well as other foreign agents were present in leukocytes. Thus Metchnikoff soon realized the importance of phagocytosis in the general context of inflammation. (17) Though the work of Metchnikoff was largely focused on the immunological basis of infectious diseases and the cell-mediated immune response, he demonstrated that mononuclear phagocytes moved toward and rapidly ingested bacteria and foreign agents – he had witnessed both a chemotactic and phagocytic immunological response. (18)

The work of Metchnikoff and his phagocytosis theory was the first experimentally-based theory in immunology that alerted the biomedical community to the importance of this process that although initially derided, eventually garnered widespread acceptance. (15, 17–20) The awarding of the Nobel Prize to Ehrlich and Metchnikoff was in part responsible for an acceleration of research in the emerging field of innate immunity that advanced the theories of humoral as well as cell-mediated immunity, particularly in defining innate as opposed to acquired/adaptive immunity. [15, 17, 20] It is interesting, then, that subsequently, Ehrlich and Metchnikoff succeeded in postulating a consensus on the "theory of immunity" – this was essentially the birth of immunology. [15, 20]

Though the monocyte/macrophage system provides important effector functions in the cell-mediated immune response to infection and malignancy, there are other mononuclear phagocytes that provide important functions in host innate immune defense and replenishment of those effector mononuclear phagocytes that provide direct anti-microbial or tumoricidal functions. [21–26] Among those cells are circulating myeloid progenitors including committed CD34+ expressing peripheral blood progenitor cells, circulating precursor monocytes, tissue-resident macrophages and a highly specialized, professional antigen-presenting cell termed the dendritic cell (Figure 1.1). An interesting facet of mononuclear cell development is that precursor myeloid progenitors in the peripheral blood and lymphatic circulation are able to replenish lymphoid or non-lymphoid tissues with newly differentiating monocytes, macrophages and DC where they acquire professional effector functions.

Mature effector cells tend to exhibit only a limited lifespan in the circulation. Consequently, there is a persistent demand for continued renewal and replacement of relatively large numbers of myeloid and lymphoid progeny during a lifetime. In a normal healthy individual, the rate of mature cell loss is balanced against the *de novo* differentiation and proliferation of lineage-committed progenitor cells. However, in a situation that presents the immune and hematologic systems with "danger signals" such as those provided by infection, acute inflammation, malignancy, trauma or severe blood loss, then the rate of precursor output of mature myeloid and lymphoid cells is increased. Whether this would also occur under conditions of allergic inflammation, chronic allergic conditions or perhaps autoimmune diseases is less clear.

Circulating monocytes have recently been shown to provide a prominent role as pre-DC precursors that when cultured in vitro with the recombinant human cytokines granulocyte-macrophage colony-stimulating factor (GM-CSF) and interleukin-4 (IL-4) differentiate to immature DC that take up, process and present antigen to naïve CD4+ T cells in lymphoid organs, thereby activating a primary immune response to the MHC-class II presented antigen. [27, 28] The striking aspect of DC immune function is their highly efficient and prolific ability to capture soluble as well as particulate antigens, to efficiently respond to exogenous or endogenous microbial and inflammatory stimuli and present antigen to helper CD4+ or cytotoxic CD8+ T cells. [29, 30] For DC to potently stimulate and shape an appropriate

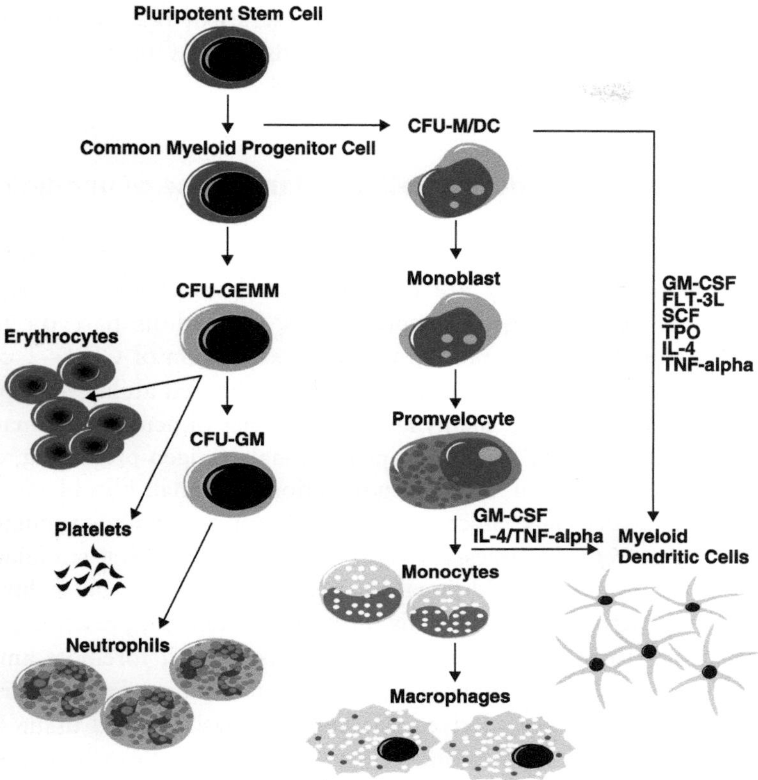

Figure 1.1 Hematopoietic development of myeloid precursors and dendritic cells. In the scheme shown, pluripotent progenitor cells undergo a series of cellular differentiation pathways such that cells of the myeloid lineage give rise to erythrocytes and platelets from the CFU-GEMM compartment (colony forming unit-granulocyte/erythrocute/monocyte/megakaryocyte). The CFU-GEMM compartment gives rise to CFU-GM (colony-forming unit granulocyte-macrophage) that under cytokine instruction gives rise to cells of the neutrophil lineage. More recent evidence suggests that the CFU-M/DC (or colony-forming unit monocyte/dendritic cell) not only differentiates to cells of the monocyte and macrophage lineage but also of the myeloid or conventional dendritic cell lineage. In the laboratory (and likely in vivo as well), the cytokines GM-CSF and IL-4 (with or without low dose TNF-alpha) drive myeloid DC development from CD14+ monocytes. In addition, access to highly pure CD34+ peripheral blood progenitor cells can be differentiated in vitro to the CFU-M/DC compartment and direcrtly to cells of the myeloid DC lineage using combinations of the cytokines GM-CSF, FLT-3L, TPO, SCF, IL-4 and TNF-alpha – conditions that have permitted expansion of DC in vitro for laboratory investigations and the immunotherapeutic targeting of human malignancies in vivo.

response by CD4+ helper T cells, a unique series of receptor-mediated, contact-dependent and soluble signals needs to be in place at the immunological synapse of DC and CD4+ T cell.

1.3 The enigmatic dendritic cell: the Janus face of immunity

There are many cells that serve important roles as antigen-presenting cells. For convenience, they are crudely defined as a) non-professional and b) professional antigen-presenting cells, defined in part on their potency to stimulate clonal proliferation and expansion of CD4+ T cells. Non-professional antigen-presenting cells have a limited ability to express cell-surface MHC class II, usually as a consequence of acute inflammation and exposure to IFNγ. Such non-professional antigen-presenting cells include various epithelial cell sub-populations, dermal fibroblasts and pancreatic beta-islet cells. Since such cells do not express co-stimulatory molecules or secrete the necessary repertoire of CD4+ T cell stimulatory cytokines (see below for additional details), they possess only a limited ability to fully activate CD4+ T cells. Professional antigen-presenting cells include among their membership many subsets of DC, foremost among which are epidermal Langerhans cells, conventional or interdigitating tissue DC (e.g. circulatory blood-derived DC and lymphatic-derived tissue DC) and thymic DC. Other professional antigen-presenting cells include B cells, endothelial cells, and epithelial cells of the thymus and of course monocytes and macrophages as briefly discussed above. Though there are many subsets of DC in the lung, peripheral circulation and throughout other major organs in the body, this issue will not be discussed in this chapter since it is critically discussed in other chapters found in this volume. The reader is thus guided to Chapters 6, 7 and 8.

Dendritic cells are by far the most prolific professional antigen-presenting cell endowed with highly potent immune stimulatory functions in the settings of infectious disease,[26, 31–35] human cancer,[36–38] autoimmune disease[39, 40] and allergic inflammatory conditions including allergic asthma[1–9, 41–46] – an adverse pulmonary inflammatory disease that will be discussed in detail below. Dendritic cells are anatomically ideally located to sense and respond to the exogenous "respirable" environment. Though there are many other structural and immune cells distributed throughout the lung architecture, cells that constitute the pulmonary innate immune system including basophils, mast cells, neutrophils, natural killer (NK) cells, NKT cells, airway epithelial cells in addition to specialized DC subsets all play key roles in protective host immune responses and allergic inflammation. Airway DC have been identified throughout the conducting airways, including the peribronchial and mediastinal lymph nodes, pulmonary vascular system, pleural fluid and pulmonary interstitial cells, where DC are interdigitated to rapidly respond to, sense, take up and process environmental aeroallergens, particulate agonists and microbial pathogens.

A critical feature of pulmonary DC as a professional antigen-presenting cell is their prolific ability to take up exogenous antigens/allergens where they are considered expert at phagocytosing soluble or particulate material and making efficient use of other uptake mechanisms including macropinocytosis and receptor-mediated endocytosis.

Once an antigen is captured by any one or combination of these uptake pathways, the antigen is degraded or processed and the derived linear peptides are presented to helper CD4+ T cells in the context of cell-surface displayed MHC class II complexes. However, DC serve many other immune functions in addition to their primary role in antigen uptake, processing and presentation. It is now recognized that DC play key roles in central tolerance where thymic sub-populations of DC process and present self antigen to T cells, resulting in negative selection and deletion of potentially autoreactive CD4+ T cells.

DC are also important in peripheral tolerance, where the potential for autoreactivity is kept in check by the ability of DC to present self-peptides in the absence of co-stimulatory molecules such as CD40-ligand (CD40L), CD80 (B7-1) and CD86 (B7-2) among others, that are otherwise necessary for optimal activation and expansion of CD4+ T cells. Following antigen uptake by Fcγ receptor-mediated phagocytosis of immunoglobulin-opsonized proteins, macropinocytosis of particulate antigens and receptor-mediated (e.g. by the macrophage mannose receptor or CD206 pathway) endocytosis of soluble antigen, the consumed antigens are degraded and presented typically via Class II major histocompatibility receptors (e.g. HLA-DR, HLA-DQ and HLA-DP) to the appropriate CD4+ T helper (Th) cell, which upon DC-mediated activation undergoes clonal expansion.

The CD4+ Th cell is thus licensed to differentiate to either a Th1 subgroup that is functionally responsible for predominantly cell-mediated immune and antibody-specific responses that provides protection against intracellular pathogens or a Th2 subgroup that predominantly facilitates protection against extracellular infections like parasitic infections as well as promoting humoral-mediated immune responses. In their broadest sense, the use of "Th1" and "Th2" to describe the polarized immunological reactivity of such T helper CD4+ subsets has come into its own as the standard definitions to account for the types of phenotypic and activation-induced immune responses displayed by those T cell sub-populations. Such reactivity is defined in part on the elaboration of particular cytokine profiles and as such defined as either Th1- or Th2-skewed immune responses (47, 48). However, the nature of the environmental "danger" triggers seen by immature DC defines the nature of T helper cell differentiation and response. This is usually considered as a three-phase response. First, naïve CD4+ Th cells are antigen-specifically activated to a so-called Th0 precursor population of undifferentiated Th cells. Second, Th0 cells are stimulated to proliferate and differentiate to either a Th1 or Th2 effector T cell populations and in the third phase of CD4+ T helper cell differentiation, Th1 and Th2 cells are fine-tuned to provide the appropriate helper effector functions necessary for antigen specific B cell populations to provide a humoral response as well as for the coordinate activation of CD8+ cytotoxic T cells.

For DC to adequately stimulate CD4+ T cell differentiation to either Th1 or Th2, the antigen-presenting DC is required to provide three signals necessary for the first phase of CD4+ T helper cell differentiation to proceed. We have already considered Signal 1 above. A mature DC that has engulfed, processed and presented antigen as linear peptides displayed in the context of cell surface-expressed MHC class II molecules provides this signal. The MHC Class II-antigen complex signals naïve CD4+ T cells via the occupation of a threshold number of T cell receptors that are specific to that presented antigen. Additionally, DC provide Signal 2 – a co-stimulatory signal provided by cell surface receptors and molecules such as CD54 (ICAM-1) CD58 (LFA-3), CD40-L, CD80 and CD86 that occupy cognate ligands or counter-receptors present on TCR-engaged CD4+ T cells. For optimal stimulation of CD4+ Th cell activation, Signal 3 is required, which is provided by a distinct pattern of cytokines secreted by mature DC. Depending on the precise repertoire of cytokines secreted by activated DC, CD4+ Th cells will commit to either a Th1 or Th2 pattern of T cell differentiation, activation and clonal expansion. The DC-derived cytokines serve to direct new expression or augment pre-existing expression of adhesion molecules, accessory and effector molecules on the CD4+ T helper cell.

It is generally thought that for Th1 cell development, co-stimulation is provided by interaction of CD28 and CD40 on T cells with CD80 and CD40L expressed on the cell surface of DC respectively and the provision of stimulatory cytokines such as IL-12p70, IL-27 and IFNγ. This in turn provokes signal transduction in CD4+ Th cells via the signaling molecule STAT4 (signal transducer and activator of transcription-4) that switches on the transcription factors T-bet (T-box transcription factor-21) responsible for the regulation of the Th1-associated cytokine IFN-γ, IRF-1

(Interferon regulatory factor-1) and ERM, an Ets-family transcription factor that is induced by IL-12 and whose expression is dependent on Stat4 activation.(49, 50) This suggests a role for ERM in initiating Th1 lineage development from naive Th precursor cells.(49–52) By contrast, for Th2 development, co-stimulation is provided by the interaction of cell surface-expressed CD28 and ICOS on T cells with CD86 and ICOS-Ligand expressed on the cell surface of DC respectively as well as the predominant interaction of IL-4 and IL-6 that modulate the differentiation of CD4+ helper T cells to a Th2 phenotype. This in turn is absolutely dependent on the activation of Stat6 in T cells to transduce IL-4-specific differentiating signals and the activation of the transcription factors GATA-3 and c-maf. (53–55) The Stat6-dependent augmentation of GATA-3 in Th2 development is important since it not only dampens T-bet activity but also suppresses IFN-γ secretion by CD4+ Th2 cells. The converse to this situation is that during the differentiation of Th1 cells, GATA-3 activity is quenched by the IL-12-mediated Stat4 signal transduction pathway and enhanced expression of T-bet. With regard the role of the transcription factor c-maf, this is thought to be expressed only in terminally differentiating and effector populations of CD4+ Th2 cells serving to enhance transcriptional and protein expression of IL-4 while dampening expression of IFN-γ.(56–58)

While DC are considered the professional antigen-presenting cell, endowed with highly specialized functions to promote either Th1 or Th2 development from naïve CD4+ Th0 cells, other antigen-presenting cells like macrophages and B cells are licensed with the ability to drive antigen-specific CD4+ Th cell differentiation. For example, since macrophages present exogenous antigen highly efficiently to effector CD4+ Th1 cells, and nominally at lower threshold levels of MHC class II antigen presentation, T cell receptor occupation and co-stimulation that is required for activation of naïve CD4+ T cells, it is reasonable to expect them to be the predominant antigen-presenting cell at the outset of an infection since they express the necessary components of signal 2 and 3 required for optimal proliferation of Th1 cells. Following this macrophage-mediated "innate immune response" to an infection and a favored Th1 adaptive response, antigen-specific B-cell activation and proliferation has occurred and B cells will contribute to the antigen presentation pathway of CD4+ T cell activation. However, B cell-dependent activation of CD4+ T helper cells more efficiently promotes a Th2-type pathway of differentiation.

Thus, during the previous discussions, one can appreciate the specialized cells and complex signals required for driving a normal or immune-protective Th1 or Th2-type immune response. Several studies referred to above, as well as by others,(59–61) have informed us that following naïve CD4+ T cell activation, specialized Th1 or Th2 effector T cells are generated that express repertoires of cytokines whose sole purpose is to promote the elimination of infectious pathogens and parasites or to support the immunological activation of CD8+ cytotoxic T cells or antibody-producing B cells. In the context of allergic or Th2-type inflammation, naïve CD4+ T cells stimulated by an IL-4-dominant repertoire of cytokines that also includes the participation of IL-6, differentiate to Th2-type effector CD4+ T cells. These are characterized by secretion of IL-4, IL-5, IL-10 and IL-13 that collectively dampen inflammation and favor immunoglobulin isotypic class-switching to IgE and IgG1 secretion in mice or IgE and IgG4 in humans. The question then is what immunological factors and which immune cells play critical roles in the promotion of an allergic immune response? The answer to this question is in part addressed by several studies that inform us of the Janus face of the enigmatic dendritic cell, where specific subsets of DC may preferentially drive Th1 or Th2 differentiation – a function of DC that is also in part influenced by the nature of the exogenous environmental trigger or "danger signal" that is sensed by and activates the DC.

1.4 Atopic inflammation

Allergy or atopy (from the Greek meaning "out of place" or "atypical disease") is a type I (immediate) hypersensitivity disorder exemplified by such conditions as asthma, rhinositis, eczema or hay fever. The classic interpretation of type I hypersensitivity is the presence of immunoglobulins of the IgE isotype directed against commonly encountered and "otherwise harmless" exogenous envirionmental antigens. Antigens that provoke atopy are usually soluble proteins derived from animal dander from cats or dogs, pollen, house dust mite or cockroach fecal particles or complexes of those protein-rich species coalesced with ambient indoor or outdoor particulate matter that is respirable and migratory to the upper and lower airways of those individuals that are exposed to such material.

A major local allergic disease is asthma. Atopic or allergic asthma is a severe pulmonary disease affecting predominantly urban industrialized Western populations with well over 300 million individuals globally affected by the disease. Atopic asthma is often considered a disease of developed countries. Clinically, asthma is largely characterized by airway inflammation coupled with transient narrowing of the airways (bronchoconstriction), secretion and deposition of mucus in the airways, resulting in extreme difficulty in breathing, wheezing, repetitive cough and, in the severest form, coma and death.

There is no cure for asthma, although the disease can be clinically managed. In the US alone an ever-increasing number of individuals are presenting with asthma and seasonal allergies such that well over 20 million people have asthma in the US and more than 50 percent of those with asthma present with the atopic or allergic form of the disease. [(59)] The morbidity, mortality and economic costs as a direct consequence of asthma are alarming. For example, one quarter of emergency room visits in the US each year are as a consequence of the exacerbations and/or complications of asthma, culminating in over two million visits to the emergency room (60). In addition, children and African Americans are of increased risk for developing and presenting with allergic asthma. [(61, 62)] Paradoxically, and for reasons that are beyond the scope of this chapter, asthma appears more prevalent among adult women than adult men, yet in children asthma is more common among males than females. [(63)] The annual cost of asthma to the US economy has been estimated to be over $18 billion. [(64)]

The genetic and familial factors that are thought to contribute to the incidence and severity of asthma are complex and only partly worked out. It is thought, for example, that should one parent have asthma then there is a roughly 33 percent chance that each child will present with asthma too. By contrast, should both parents be asthmatic, then the risk that each child will present with asthma increases to more than 70 percent. Other factors other than family history contribute to allergic asthmatic risk, such as lifestyle and socio-economic factors including rural versus urban living environments, cigarette smoking habits of the asthmatic individual, prior history of viral and/or bacterial lung infections, aeroallergen or indoor allergen exposure levels, occupational allergen exposures and environmental pollution exposure levels from vehicle emissions or high ambient pollutant particles in urban or suburban districts. [(65–67)] Indeed, there is a substantial body of literature supporting the association between increased mortality in the human population and exposures to ambient air pollution. [(68–75)]

Under normal physiological responses, individuals exposed to such triggers of immediate hypersensitivity like particulate matter or airborne allergens secrete IgA, IgM or IgG to clear those otherwise harmless antigens that are neither by themselves disease-causing microorganisms nor indeed pathogenically "dangerous" in otherwise healthy individuals. However, in atopic individuals, exposure to such "innocuous" antigen challenges directs the production of IgE for reasons that are less than transparent. In such IgE-producing hosts, reactivity to allergy-inducing antigens (allergens) can provoke severe difficulties including respiratory distress, anaphylactic shock and death. Indeed, anaphylactic shock is by itself a systemic atopic response where the hypersensitivity response affects the whole body. By contrast, a local atopic response is one which is specific to the site or specific organ of exposure to an allergen. In those individuals predisposed to allergic asthma by an unfortunate combination of genetic risk factors and environmental pressures, high levels of serum IgE and the characteristic Th2-cytokine profile of IL-4, IL-5, IL-9 and IL-13 with dampened IL-12 and IFNγ are prevalent.[76, 77] Asthma is an inflammatory disease of the upper and lower airways including the lungs. In atopic asthma, respirable allergens and indeed respirable ambient airborne pollutants provoke airway inflammation that is in part mediated by hyper-production of IgE in response to a triggering allergen that is inhaled by a susceptible individual.

The onset or severity of allergic diseases like atopic asthma are influenced not only by the time and dose of exposure to a triggering allergen as discussed above, but also as a function of the variable interactions of "susceptibility genes" with an ever-changing and variable environment. Thus, while genetic factors play an important role in the pathogenesis of asthma, exposure of individuals to a myriad of ambient or occupational environmental exposures may dictate the relative susceptibility of individuals to atopic asthma, at least in part, and as we have learned above, by the modulation of the immune response by a host of environmental triggers. These environmental cues interact with unique genetic patterns in individuals at heightened or lowered risk of developing an atopic disease. Several studies have uncovered putative genetic susceptibility factors that may predispose individuals to the development of allergic asthma as well as perhaps other allergic diseases in the lung.

A number of candidate genes have been identified as possessing a contributory role in the development of allergic diseases. Foremost among these are those genes located in the chomosomal region 5q31–33, including IL-3, IL-4, IL-5, IL-9, IL-13, TGFβ and GM-CSF, that are collectively thought to program immune responsiveness from Th1 to Th2, isotytpe switching to IgE (as opposed to IgG) and activation of mast cells, basophils and eosinophils that contribute to many of the hallmarks of the immediate hypersensitivity response in allergic or atopic inflammation. In all, more than 13 chromosomal regions and 100 candidate genes may collectively enhance the likelihood of allergic diseases such as asthma in susceptible individuals.[78–81] Many of the genes identified from such studies include cell surface receptors that play important roles in sensing and responding to microbial "danger signals" like TLRs, the LPS co-receptor CD14 and CARD15, genes involved in airway epithelial barrier integrity and innate immunity including FLG and DEFB1, and candidate genes thought to play a major role in environmental exposures and oxidative stress such as GSTM1, GSTP1 and GSTT1,[82–86] among many more others.

Indeed, in late 2007, the first genome-wide asssociation study (GWAS) that focused on asthma was published by Moffatt et al. (87). This study identified several candidate genetic biomarkers located to chromsome 17q21 that were associated with the onset of childhood asthma – findings that were reproduced in British and German studies and several other studies in subjects with diverse ethnic backgrounds (88–92). Those individuals with polymorphisms in the 5q31–33 chromosomal region often present with an exaggerated frequency in the proportion of Th2-type cells (eosinophils, basophils and so on) in allergic disease tissues in, for example, the lung as compared with non-allergic individuals. In addition, the secretion of pro-allergic cytokines like IL-4, IL-5 and IL-13 is often increased in those individuals too. Similarly, polymorphisms in the IL-4R-alpha chain on chromsome 16p have also been associated with enhanced secretion of IgE in the sera of those individuals presenting with allergic asthma.

An added level of complexity to the issue of genetic susceptibility to allergic disease posits that certain alleles in the HLA-D locus of chromosome 6p21, and particularly acquisition of HLA-DR4 and HLA-DR7, may predispose individuals to atopic diseases. Of particular note are several studies that have identified novel asthma susceptibility genes by linkage analysis and positional cloning approaches which have uncovered the following putative genes – HLA-G,[(93)] CYFIP2,[(94)] PHF11[(95)] and the enigmatic gene ADAM33 (a disintegrin and metaloproteinase domain-containing protein 33) – with putative roles in asthma and other allergic airway diseases.[(96)]

In appreciating that certain genes may predispose or enhance the susceptibility of individuals to develop an allergic disease, it is becoming increasingly clear that the environment that one is exposed to may augment disease. For example, in the case of allergic asthma, the risk of developing this disease may increase severely, as shown by studies linking early life exposures to tobacco smoke[(97, 98)] or by contrast may afford protection from the risk of developing asthma, as has been found for individuals that have either been raised on or near farms early in life[(99–101)] or exposed to bacterial or viral communicable infections. Thus exposure to various microorganisms, either prenatally or in infant life, decreases, by as yet largely unclear mechanisms, the risk for developing atopic asthma.

1.5 The hygiene hypothesis

In an attempt to assert some reasonable scientific models to help us understand how allergic asthma has increased in prevalence at the same time that our quality of life has improved an interesting concept was proposed and termed the "hygiene hypothesis".[102] At the time that this hypothesis was first published in 1989, it had already been largely acknowledged that early life exposures to viral (and likely bacterial) infections dampened the likelihood of the onset of an allergic disease like asthma later on in life. In this novel yet controversial hypothesis, Strachan [102] was the first to suggest that common allergic diseases found in children were less frequent in those that had many siblings, where presumably they were exposed to a "less sterile" environment than those children who were the only child. Presumably, exposure to viral and bacterial infections in early childhood provided protection from developing the pro-allergic Th2-mediated immune responses that may develop in children from families with only one child since the constant challenge of the immune system by disease-causing viruses and bacteria would provoke cell-mediated pro-Th1-mediated immune responses. [102]

This is an attractive (yet ultimately over-simplistic) hypothesis since pathogenic microorganisms usually elicit a protective Th1-mediated immune response and the hygiene hypothesis postulated that dampened or insufficient Th1-mediated inflammatory responses may actually subvert host immunity to a more dominant and inappropriately hyperactive Th2-mediated and pro-allergic immune response. Thus the bias would switch from one of a predominantly cell-mediated immune response to one of an antibody-mediated response coupled with immunoglobulin isotype switching, for example enhanced production of IgE.

The hygiene hypothesis particularly applicable to Western or industrialized parts of the world where there are socio-economic and quality of life pressures to adhere to overt hygiene routines as well as clinical or therapeutic practices in the use (or indeed misuse) of antibiotics to treat bacterial infections, vaccinations strategies and so forth. Under such situations, childhood infections are efficiently resolved through vaccination and use of antibiotics. Of course, the immune system is inadvertently interrupted from mounting the Th1 immune responses necessary to target intracellular pathogenic microorganisms. The immune system is therefore biased toward a Th2 pattern of T cell differentiation and augmenting the potential for that individual to an atopic allergic condition.

There is compelling evidence in support of the hygiene hypothesis. For example, many studies have shown that allergic inflammatory and autoimmune diseases are more frequent in the industrialized parts of the world than in less developed or Third World countries.[103–105] By contrast, epidemiological and population-based studies have shown that in those countries gaining in socio-economic wealth – and presumably adopting a more Westernized adherence to greater hygiene and levels of near "clinical cleanliness" in their homes, occupational environment and so forth – the development and incidence of such allergic or autoimmune disorders increases.[106, 107]

However, the hygiene hypothesis is somewhat simplistic in the assumptions made and there is evidence that weighs heavily against it. An imbalance in the Th1/Th2 cytokine paradigm would of course mean that under circumstances of a Th2-prevalence, Th1-mediated autoimmune diseases should be on the decline. Sadly, the converse is true and autoimmune diseases such as insulin-dependent or Type I diabetes and gastrointestinal disorders such as Crohn's disease are steadily increasing too. The incidence of these diseases is also more prevalent in developed and heavily urbanized nations, in much the same way as those communities that see dramatic incidences of atopic allergic diseases. Although the reasons for this are unclear, several groups have suggested diet and obesity play an important role as risk factors in the pathogenesis of asthma and indeed chronic obstructive pulmonary disease (COPD). Foremost among these considerations is the lack of vitamin D in the diet, disruption of neuro-endocrine circuits as well as the protective effect of breastfeeding against the development or incidence of both allergic asthma and diabetes.

Although these concepts are beyond the scope of this chapter, the issue of vitamin D is particularly interesting. Epidemiological and population-based studies have indicated a cause-and-effect relationship with vitamin D deficiency and the increased incidence of asthma observed in developed countries. The reason for this is that vitamin D deficiency is associated with increased airway hyper-responsiveness as well as dampened pulmonary function and difficulty in managing the symptoms of asthma by both the clinician and patient. Vitamin D deficiency is also more commonly associated with obesity in already developed or developing countries – this in turn reflects higher-risk populations for asthma, especially in those with African American ethnicity.

The immunomodulatory functions of vitamin D are particularly relevant since it is capable of not only affecting the functional differentiation and maturation of myeloid precursors but also may modulate the functional behavior of pulmonary DC.[108–114] Others have found that vitamin D dampens the synthesis of the Th1-associated cytokine IFNγ by phytohemagglutinin-stimulated human peripheral blood lymphocytes and dose-dependently attenuates the transcriptional expression of IFNγ in activated peripheral blood lymphocytes.[115] This function of vitamin D to dampen Th1-cytokine production may influence the outcome of an inflammatory response to a more pronounced Th2-type immune response by particulate matter-exposed DC. Not only are myelo-monocytic cells targets of Vitamin D (108–114), but monocyte-derived DC (which are the immediate precursors of pulmonary DC), for example, are also capable of synthesizing the precursor of vitamin D or 1, $25(OH)_2D_3$ in vitro.[111]

It is tempting to speculate that under special circumstances of an environmental pro-allergic exposure, Vitamin D production by DC in a "pro-allergic cytokine milieu" may serve to promote a Th2-mediated response by naïve CD4+ T cells. Such a situation may occur following exposure to respirable ambient particulate matter, and interaction of naïve CD4+ T cells with DC that had taken up and been stimulated by those environmental pollutant particles. This will of course require empirical determination. Nonetheless, many other studies have shown that vitamin D functionally dampens the maturation of DC, as evidenced by down-modulated expression of co-stimulatory molecules, dampened secretion of IL-12p70 and augmented IL-10 secretion.[116–119] It is possible, though highly speculative, that under such conditions, environmental particulate matter-stimulated lung DC could be conditioned to behave in a non-canonical but pro-allergic fashion, mediated in part by vitamin D and the "pro-allergic" pattern of DC maturation as we have proposed in several animal and human model studies of particulate matter exposure and non-classical differentiation and function of conventional DC.[1–4, 6]

1.6 Pulmonary dendritic cells sense the enemy within

We and others have shown that ambient pollutants, including diesel emission-source particulate matter, do not drive Th1-mediated immune responses as one might expect from their pro-oxidative and pro-inflammatory properties, but instead have been shown to promote a Th2-like pattern of allergic inflammation in many animal and human model studies. This has led to the proposal that such respirable particulate pollutants behave as immune adjuvants capable of augmenting the host response to allergen exposure or exacerbating pre-existing allergic airways diseases[1–4, 6, 7, 11, 13, 120–126] and provoking serious health effects in susceptible human subjects, particularly children with pre-existing asthma exposed to outdoor air pollutants.[127–132] These studies inform us that exposure to outdoor air pollutants can enhance the incidence of asthma, exacerbate pre-existing disease and compromise lung function.

In the context of pro-allergic inflammation in asthma and the proposed association of exposure to outdoor pollutant particles and the development of allergic asthma, there are several features of ambient pollutant particles that are seen as "dangerous" by the innate immune system. This is particularly relevant in terms of the responsiveness of pulmonary DC to environmental ambient pollutant particles. Ambient particulate matter (APM) is a complex bioorganic and biophysical mixture of heavy and transition elements, semi-volatile and non-volatile organic and inorganic compounds, allergens, endotoxins, and other biologically active components that collectively provoke a pro-inflammatory and pro-oxidative response in the lung following exposure to such material.[1–4, 6, 7, 11–13]

This complex array of "dangerous signals" provides the pulmonary DC a multi-faceted opportunity to sense and respond to such material that breaches the physiological barriers that otherwise provide a formidable mucosal immune system. Since DC are ideally positioned in the lungs, interdigitated below the substrata and between/within the tight junctions of the airway epithelium as well as throughout the parenchyma of the lung, they are uniquely positioned in space and time for the efficient sensing and uptake of particulate pollutants that traffic to the lung from the external environment. As such, DC reside in this tissue (as well as other mucosal immune sites) in an immature state of "primed" functional activation. Dendritic cells in this state of readiness are extremely efficient at taking up exogenous soluble and particulate materials by endocytic, phagocytic and macropinocytic uptake mechanisms.

Additionally, since DC display an evolutionary conserved repertoire of microbial pattern-recognition receptors termed toll-like receptors (TLRs) on their cell surface as well as TLRs that are found in the cytoplasm and associated with early and late endosomal compartments, they are armed with an impressive array of information-management and rapid-response pathways. Such rapid antigen sensing and processing pathways endow the DC with an impressive ability to process and present non-self antigen to naïve CD4+ T cells. The reader is guided to Chapters 3, 6 and 7 for additional detailed discussions of this fascinating area of mucosal and innate immunity fulfilled by sub-populations of pulmonary DC.

What is being increasingly realized is that TLRs may play a critical role in sensing and responding to respirable "non-self danger signals" during, for example, challenge of the respiratory mucosal immune system by the complex constituents of APM that freely traffic to the upper and lower conducting airways. The reader is guided to Chapters 3 and 7 for a more detailed critical discussion of these concepts. Suffice it to say here that the repertoire of exogenous and endogenous ligands recognized by cell membrane-associated and cytoplasmic or endosomal compartment-associated TLRs is expanding dramatically.[133–137]

We have shown that the interaction of APM and diesel PM with both murine and human DC is complex and the ultimate response is likely dependent, at least in part, on the coordinate activation of pattern-recognition receptor signaling, including TLRs as briefly described above and the nucleotide-binding and oligomerization domain (NOD) like receptors (NLRs). In the lung, the DC is confronted with a multitude of pathogen-associated molecular patterns (PAMPs) and "damage-associated" molecular-patterns (DAMPs) representing infection-initiated and noninfectious inflammatory responses respectively – both of which can be recognized by and promote downstream signaling from TLRs. While PAMPs are largely derived from proteins, nucleic acids or highly glycosylated proteins of bacteria, viruses or fungi, DAMPs are interesting in that they are largely derived from nuclear or cytoplasmic proteins released to the extra-cytosolic spaces following cell death, oxidative-stress induced damage or other cellular membrane-perturbing traumas. Some examples of DAMPs include structural scaffold proteins like hyaluronan derivatives or intracellular proteins such as heat-shock proteins (e.g. Hsp70. The cell stress protein Hsp70 is a particularly interesting example of an extracellular and membrane-bound heat-shock protein that is capable of associating with other proteins and activating the immune system and like its cousin Hsp60 is capable of activating DC and other innate immune cells in a TLR2 and TLR4-dependent manner.

Since DC are responsive to endogenous proteins and other ligands like DNA or RNA released from damaged or necrotic cells, it is thus not the infectious non-self or foreign invader that often is sensed and activates DC, but the "danger" signal, hence the gradual acceptance and growing interest in the concept of the "danger hypothesis".[(138–142)] Prior work by others has identified Hsp60 and Hsp70 as powerful endogenous ligands and activators of DC.[(143–145)] On exposure to various PM species, we have shown dependence on both the TLR4 and TLR2 pathways of cellular activation and the adaptor protein MyD88 using targeted gene knockout mouse models.[(2)] The adaptor protein MyD88 is important for cell membrane-associated TLR signaling and transduces its signals via the p38MAPK and p40/p42MAPK (ERK I/II) group of mitogen-activated protein kinase-dependent signaling pathways. We have previously studied the effects of APM on MyD88 gene knockout DC derived from mouse bone marrow (BM-DC) as compared their wild-type counterparts.[(2)] We found that deletion of MyD88 almost completely abolished the APM stimulated and dose-dependent secretion of IL-12p70 and IL-6 while the secretion of TNF-α was only marginally dampened in MyD88 knockout DC on stimulation by APM.[(2)] These data were interesting as they implied an MyD88-independent pathway of enhanced TNF-α secretion in response to APM. By contrast, the cell surface expression of the co-stimulatory molecule CD80 as well as MHC class II expression were actually enhanced in MyD88 knockouts on activation by APM. [2] This crucially suggested an MyD88-independent pathway was involved in the expression of those function-associated molecules and strengthens the notion that APM (as well as LPS from a separate series of experiments described in (2)), activate DC via distinct mechanisms.

We have previously found in human CD14+ monocyte-derived and CD34+ peripheral blood progenitor cell-derived DC, exposure to ambient and diesel-enriched environmental PM directed a dramatic loss in TLR2 and TLR4 expression. [3] In subsequent work we found that this phenomenon occurred within 4 hours and was still evident 24 hours after the initial PM exposure. As we have learnt above, the transmembrane expression of both TLR2 (CD282) and TLR4 (CD284) serves important functions in linking innate and adaptive immunity. TLR2 is important in the recognition of microbial products including lipoproteins, lipoteichoic acids, lipomannans and beta-glucans as well as the endogenous danger agonist Hsp60, while TLR4 serves equally crucial roles in the recognition of microbial products and predominantly transduced signals on activation by LPS. Since exacerbations of allergic asthma are often driven by airway viral and/or bacterial infections, our studies [3] suggest that one link between environmental PM exposure and the exacerbations of pulmonary allergic conditions is a relative state of immune suppression and predisposition to infections as a consequence of down-regulated TLR2 and TLR4 cell surface expression.

One could also postulate that the diminution in TLR expression in response to PM could represent an inherent mechanism to dampen the potential of pro-inflammatory airway hyperactivity and cellular damage. Nonetheless, down-regulation of TLR expression would compromise the function of DC and render them hyporesponsive upon subsequent exposure to infectious agents. Though the mechanism for our observations of temporal down-regulation of TLR2 and TLR4 expression by APM-exposed DC is a matter of further study in our lab, we have considered three possible mechanisms as perhaps being involved (Figure 1.2).

In the first mechanism, we have postulated that TLR2 and TLR4 may be sequestered from the cell surface to cytoplasmic endosomal units and recycling of the TLRs to the cell membrane. In the second most likely scenario, we are exploring the notion that TLRs are internalized, poly-ubiquitinylated and targeted for lysomal and/or proteosomal degradation. In the third equally likely scenario, we are exploring the time-dependent

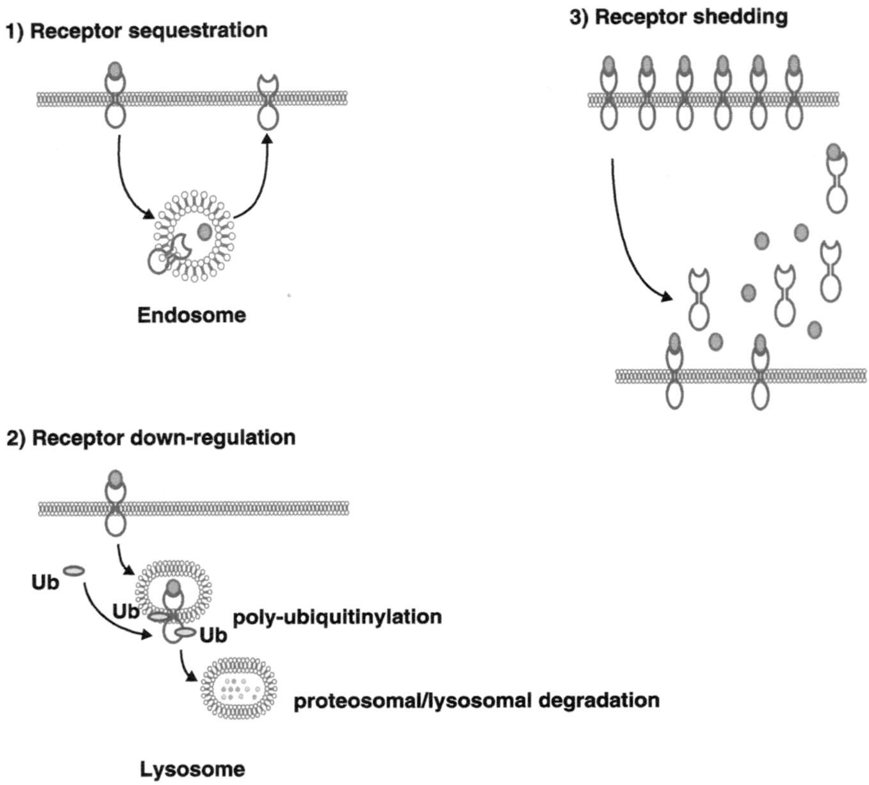

Figure 1.2 Proposed mechanisms for the down-regulation of cell-surface TLR2 and TLR4 expression on activation of human myeloid DC by ambient PM. The proposed mechanisms are hypothetical though our laboratory has shown preliminary evidence that mechanisms 2 and 3 (above) may partly account for the temporal loss of TLR2 and TLR4 by DC.

shedding of TLRs to the extracellular spaces where enzymatrically shed full-length or cleaved subunits of TLR2 and TLR4 can be detected. In preliminary experiments of co-immunoprecipitation and western immunoblotting (unpublished observations), we suspect TLR2 and TLR4 may likely be down-regulated by a combined proteosomal degradative pathway and receptor shedding mechanism (see Figure 1.2).

Thus, since DC are recognized as a key conduit of communication management between sensing of the external environment and instructing the adaptive arm of T-helper cell-mediated immunity, we have previously submitted that exposure of DC to particulate pollution may not only alter the expression of TLRs but shift the expected paradigm from one of protective immunity to one of enhanced disease severity and a quenched ability to respond to subsequent challenge by microbial danger signals. [1–3, 6]

We can thus appreciate that on each inspiration of air, the immune system, and particularly antigen-sensing sentinels of innate immunity such as DC, is constantly challenged by both harmless and potentially "dangerous" antigens such as those provided by pathogenic microorganisms. Pulmonary DC therefore are licensed with "executive decisions" with regard to mounting an appropriate protective immune response to pathogenic viruses or bacteria, or to ignore otherwise harmless exposures – a system that is compromised and ultimately fails in those individuals presenting with allergic asthma. As discussed briefly above, pulmonary DC are distributed throughout the lung and possess the unique ability to interdigitate the pulmonary epithelium, where they are able to extend cellular processes through or between the tight junctions of epithelial cells and sample the "external" environment present in the lumen of the conducting and lower airways. [146–150] In very elegant in vitro culture studies, it has been clearly shown by confocal laser scanning, conventional transmission electron microscopy and other visualization approaches, that DC come into intimate contact with deposited particles in the lung. [148–150]

Although the conducting airways and alveoli provide an otherwise intact physiological, structural and functional barrier through which micro- and nano-sized particulate matter cannot usually breach, it has been shown that such deposited particles are displaced and directly sampled by DC that gain access to the apical side of the epithelium by two separate mechanisms. The first was by extending their dendritic processes between the tight junctions of epithelial cells and the second was by transmigration through the epithelium to the luminal space where DC could then take up the microparticles. [149–150] These studies nicely demonstrated that DC and macrophages communicated to form what the authors of this work termed "a trans-epithelial interacting cellular network". [149] In this network, DC interacted with microparticle-loaded alveolar macrophages such that they sampled the particles directly from them or took up microparticles directly from the apical as well as luminal side of a three-cell culture matrix as described above. [149–150]

Our observations partly support these important studies in that we have shown exquisite sensitivity of DC to direct stimulation by APM, source-specific environmental diesel particulate matter and engineered nano-particulate matter. In addition, in differential cellular cytospin preparations and visual inspection by light microscopy, we have found particles to be present in the cytoplasm of macrophages present in bronchoalveolar fluid (BALF) samples taken from mice following acute exposure to various particulate matter species.[1, 2, 4, 6] Additionally, we expanded on previously published studies where the direct in vitro effects of ambient PM were further explored by studying the in vivo effects of PM in a naïve mouse model of a single acute exposure to APM, diesel-enriched particulate matter and silver nanoparticles.[6]

This work essentially extended our previous in vitro studies that suggested ambient PM and environmental PM do not behave as conventional immune adjuvants since both were immune-stimulatory both in vitro[1–4] and in vivo.[6] This would be expected since ambient PM is a complex mixture of bioorganic and inorganic compounds, elemental and organic carbon, heavy metals and transition elements, aeroallergens, microbial components including low levels of TLR-active agents like LPS, and other bioorganics such as aryl hydrocarbons that collectively would provoke pro-inflammatory and pro-oxidative activation of DC. It is thus likely that given the complex mixture of challenges brought to the DC and the innate immune system in more general terms on exposure to ambient PM, that environmental pollutant particles behave both as a priming and secondary stimulus. Since virtually nothing is known of the acute inflammatory effects of PM exposure in naïve mouse models in vivo, we studied the in vivo effects of ambient PM and diesel-enriched PM in mouse models 24 hours following oro-pharyngeal exposure to PM species.[6] We found that APM and diesel PM activated myeloid as well as plasmacytoid subsets of lung DC in vivo.[6] Of particular importance was our observation that on acute exposure to ambient PM (but not any of the other particles tested including diesel PM, carbon black particles or silver nanoparticles) there was marked infiltration of the lung by eosinophils. In addition, we found enhanced secretion of IL-5 in ConA expanded primary bronchial lymph node cultures and in co-cultures of primary naïve CD4+ T cells that had been exposed to highly purified lung DC in mice exposed to ambient PM in vivo. Since IL-5 plays a crucial role in eosinophil activation, survival and recruitment, the accumulation of eosinophils in the lung of ambient PM-exposed mice may be partly associated with IL-5 secretion in vivo.

1.7 Concluding remarks

We are beginning to appreciate that the environmental air, particularly highly polluted air found in urban environments as well as in developing and industrialized countries, is highly immuno-stimulatory, pro-inflammatory and pro-oxidative in potential. We are also beginning to understand the consequences of the interaction of the cells that constitute the pulmonary and peripheral innate immune system and exposure to environmental respirable particulate pollutants. Seminal studies from our work and that of others discussed in this chapter clearly implicate PM exposure and direct activation of lung DC, thus contributing to their translocation to the resident peribronchial lymph nodes and provocation of a pro-allergic pattern of Th2-like cytokine responsiveness. Our work has supported the growing concept that environmental PM species may drive allergic immunity and possibly either promote or exacerbate pre-existing allergic asthma. Though we have not empirically determined the notion of exposure to particulate pollutants and pro-allergic immunity, one of the central tenets of allergic respiratory diseases like asthma is a dominant Th2-biased immune response.

We have also appreciated in this chapter that dendritic cells are the key sentinels of the innate immune system that evolved to rapidly translate diverse environmental cues into signals that activate adaptive immunity following their interactions with pathogenic microorganisms or environmental particulates at the mucosal interface. Moreover, the identification and characterization of different DC subsets in the lung indicates to us their importance as key antigen-presenting cells in an appropriate anatomical setting to respond to inhaled particulate matter. Since respiratory tract DC are rapidly derived from circulating precursors, previous work done by our group provides a rational approximation of how DC and ambient environmental pollution particulates interact in vivo. DC are densely distributed throughout the conducting lower and upper airways as well as the respiratory epithelium, and may even directly sample the bronchial lumen as discussed above. Therefore, one might expect that DC would be among the first cells to interact with and respond to inhaled particulate pollution. Previous work done by our group as well as that from others, strongly suggests that pulmonary myeloid DC are key sentinels of pro-allergic and pro-inflammatory responses in the lung on exposure to ambient pollutants,[(1–4, 6, 7, 120–130, 147–150)] with potentially important roles in the pathogenesis of allergic asthma and other airway diseases like COPD. In both human and murine systems, we have found that particulate matter-exposed DC exhibit a non-classical or non-canonical mode of activation and differentiation that is phenotypically and functionally distinct from DC activated by other classical stimuli such as LPS or CD40L.

Moreover, we have learnt that cells of the innate immune system, such as DC and macrophages, express germ line-encoded cell surface and endosomal-associated receptors that enable them to recognize unique structural patterns that have been evolutionarily conserved in diverse species of pathogenic and non-pathogenic microbes. In this chapter, it was discussed that the TLR-mediated recognition of PAMPs and DAMPs satisfied two important directives. Firstly that occupation of TLRs by microbial or other dangerous patterns alerts the immune system to the presence of pathogens or damaged host tissues in such a way that the innate immune system can rapidly respond to and contain either the infection or the inflammatory consequences of damaged self-tissues and cells. Secondly, during the instruction of the acquired response by DC, pattern recognition by TLRs not only enables the immune system to interpret the type of invading pathogenic microorganism or nature of the "dangerous signal" but the "deciphered" signals will instruct the appropriate expansion and differentiation of CD4+ T-helper cells to either Th1 or Th2 immune responsiveness. We have also learnt that the DC additionally provide three levels of signaling on synapsing with CD4+ T cells where the first was MHC class II-presented antigen, the second was co-stimulation (CD40, CD54, CD80, CD86 and so forth) and the third, and perhaps most crucial, were cytokines secreted by DC (or other antigen-presenting cells) such as IL-12p70 that drive Th1 differentiation, or under conditions of high IL-4 and dampened IL-12 as well as IFN-γ secretion, differentiation to the Th2 pathway of CD4+ lineage commitment. We also learnt that exposure to environmental PM species including diesel particulate matter can rapidly and powerfully influence naïve CD4+ T cell lineage commitment to the pro-allergic or Th2-type of immune development.

It is anticipated that future work in the field will focus on the molecular and cellular mechanisms of action of particulate matter at the level of DC activation. Such work will likely confirm the importance of measuring alterations in the expression of TLR2 and TLR4 by DC as biomarkers of APM exposure and effect and may open the way for targeted pharmacological therapy to interrupt the detrimental effects of particulate matter on normal host innate immunity. In addition, future work in this area will enable a greater appreciation of the immune pathogenesis of allergic diseases like asthma and most importantly future research must strive to provide important tools for the management of these debilitating pulmonary diseases.

References

1 Porter M, Karp M, Killedar S, Bauer SM, Guo J, Williams D, Breysse P, Georas SN and Williams MA. (2007). Diesel-enriched particulate matter functionally activates human dendritic cells. *Am J Respir Cell Mol Biol* 37: 706–19.

2 Williams MA, Porter M, Horton M, Guo J, Roman J, Williams D, Breysse P and Georas SN. (2007). Ambient particulate matter directs nonclassic dendritic cell activation and a mixed T(H)1/T(H)2-like cytokine response by naive CD4(+) T cells. *J Allergy Clin Immunol* 119: 488–97.
3 Williams MA, Cheadle C, Watkins T, Tailor A, Killedar SY, Breysse P, Barnes K and Georas SN. (2007). TLR2 and TLR4 as potential biomarkers of environmental particulate matter exposed human myeloid dendritic cells. *Biomarker Insights* 2: 225–39.
4 Williams MA, Rangasamy T, Bauer SM, Killedar S, Karp M, Kensler TW, Yamamoto M, Breysse P, Biswal S and Georas SN. (2008). Disruption of the transcription factor Nrf2 promotes pro-oxidative dendritic cells that stimulate Th2-like immunoresponsiveness upon activation by ambient particulate matter. *J Immunol* 181: 4545–59.
5 Rangasamy T, Williams MA, Bauer S, Trush MA, Emo J, Georas SN and Biswal S. (2010). Nrf2 inhibits the maturation of murine dendritic cells by ragweed extract. *Am J Respir Cell Mol Biol* 43: 276–85.
6 Bezemer GF, Bauer SM, Oberdörster G, Breysse PN, Pieters RH, Georas SN, Williams MA. (2010). Activation of pulmonary dendritic cells and Th2-type inflammatory responses on instillation of engineered, environmental diesel emission source or ambient air pollutant particles in vivo. *J Innate Immun* 2010 Nov 23. [Epub ahead of print].
7 de Haar C., Hassing I, Bol M, Bleumink R and Pieters R. (2005). Ultrafine carbon black particles cause early airway inflammation and have adjuvant activity in a mouse allergic airway disease model. *Tox Sci* 87: 409–18.
8 Hammad H, and Lambrecht BN. (2006). Recent progress in the biology of airway dendritic cells and implications for understanding the regulation of asthmatic inflammation. *J Allergy Clin Immunol* 118: 331–6.
9 van Rijt LS, Jung S, Kleinjan A, Vos N, Willart M, Duez C, Hoogsteden HC and Lambrecht BN. (2005). In vivo depletion of lung CD11c (+) dendritic cells during allergen challenge abrogates the characteristic features of asthma. *J Exp Med* 201: 981–91.
10 Baulig A, Singh S, Marchand A, Schins R, Barouki R, Garlatti M, Marano F and Baeza-squiban A. (2009). Role of Paris PM (2.5) components in the pro-inflammatory response induced in airway epithelial cells. *Toxicology* 261: 126–35.
11 Blanchet S, Ramgolam K, Baulig A, Marano F and Baeza-Squiban A. (2004). Fine particulate matter induces amphiregulin secretion by bronchial epithelial cells. *Am J Respir Cell Mol Biol* 30: 421–7.
12 Reibman J, Hsu Y, Chen LC, Bleck B and Gordon T. (2003). Airway epithelial cells release MIP-3alpha/CCL20 in response to cytokines and ambient particulate matter. *Am J Respir Cell Mol Biol* 28: 648–54.
13 Rumelhard M, Ramgolam K, Auger F, Dazy AC, Blanchet S, Marano F and Baeza-Squiban A. (2007). Effects of PM2.5 components in the release of amphiregulin by human airway epithelial cells. *Toxicol Lett* 168: 155–64.
14 Karnovsky ML. (1981). Metchnikoff in Messina: a century of studies on phagocytosis. *N Engl J Med* 304: 1178–80.
15 Tauber AI. (1992). The birth of immunology. III. The fate of the phagocytosis theory. *Cell Immunol* 139: 505–30.

16 Kasten FH. (1996). Paul Ehrlich: Pathfinder in cell biology. 1. Chronicle of his life and accomplishments in immunology, cancer research, and chemotherapy. *Biotech Histochem* 71: 2–37.
17 Chernyak L, Tauber AI. (1988). The birth of immunology. Metchnikoff, the embryologist. *Cell Immunol* 117: 218–33.
18 Heifets L. (1982). Centennial of Metchnikoff's discovery. *J Reticuloendothel Soc* 31: 381–91.
19 Imhof BA, Dunon D. (1997). Basic mechanisms of leukocyte migration. *Horm Metab Res* 29: 614–21.
20 Tauber AI. (1990). Metchnikoff, the modern immunologist. *J Leukoc Biol* 47: 561–67.
21 Williams MA, Kouromoussis I, Syndercombe-Court D, Hendry L, Newland AC, Kelsey SM. (1995). Administration of recombinant human granulocyte-macrophage colony-stimulating factor after chemotherapy regulates the expression and secretion of monocyte tumor necrosis factor (TNF) and TNF receptors p55 and p75. *Blood* 86: 4234–42.
22 Williams MA, Kelsey SM, Collins PW, Gutteridge CN, Newland AC. (1995). Administration of rHuGM-CSF activates monocyte reactive oxygen species secretion and adhesion molecule expression in vivo inpatients following high-dose chemotherapy. *Brit J Haemat* 90: 31–40.
23 Williams MA, White SA, Miller JJ, Toner C, Withington S, Newland AC, Kelsey SM. (1998). Granulocyte-macrophage colony-stimulating factor induces activation and restores respiratory burst activity in monocytes from septic patients. *J Infect Dis* 177: 107–15.
24 Williams MA, Withington S, Newland AC, Kelsey SM. (1998). Monocyte anergy in septic shock is associated with a predilection to apoptosis and is reversed by granulocyte-macrophage colony-stimulating factor ex vivo. *J Infect Dis* 178: 1921–33.
25 Williams MA, Newland AC, Kelsey SM. (2000). Cytokine modulated transmembrane tumor necrosis factor expression is associated with enhanced monocyte-mediated killing of human leukemic targets. *Leukemia Res* 24: 317–30.
26 Williams MA, Trout R, Spector SA. (2002). HIV-1 gp120 modulates the immunological function and expression of accessory and co-stimulatory molecules of monocyte-derived dendritic cells. *J Hematother Stem Cell Res* 11: 829–47.
27 Cheong C, Matos I, Choi J-H, Danamundi DB, Shrestha E, Longhi MP, Jeffrey KL, Anthony RM, Kluger C, Nchinda G, et al. (2010). Microbial stimulation fully differentiates monocytes to DC-SIGN/CD209+ dendritic cells for immune T cell areas. *Cell* 143: 416–29.
28 Sallusto F and Lanzavecchia A. (1994). Efficient presentation of soluble antigen by cultured human dendritic cells is maintained by granulocyte/macrophage colony-stimulating factor plus interleukin 4 and downregulated by tumor necrosis factor alpha. *J Exp Med* 179: 1763–71.
29 Melman I and Steinman RM. (2001). Dendritic cells: specialized and regulated antigen processing machines. *Cell* 106: 225–58.
30 Lanzavecchia A and Sallusto F. (2001). The instructive role of dendritic cells on T cell responses: lineages, plasticity and kinetics. *Curr Opin Immunol* 13: 291–98.

31 Soloff AC and Barratt-Boyes SM. (2010). Enemy at the gates: dendritic cells and immunity to mucosal pathogens. *Cell* res 20: 872–85.
32 Grainger JR, Hall JA, Bouladoux N, Oldenhove G, Belkaid Y. (2010). Microbe-dendritic cell dialog controls regulatory T cell fate. *Immunol Rev* 234: 305–16.
33 McGill J, Heusel JW, Legge KL. (2009). Innate immune control and regulation of influenza virus infections. *J Leukoc Biol* 86: 803–12.
34 Heath WR and Carbone FR. (2009). Dendritic cell subsets in primary and secondary T cell responses at body surfaces. *Nat Immunol* 10: 1237–44.
35 Osterholzer JJ, Chen GH, Olszewski MA, Curtis JL, Huffnagle GB, Toews GB. (2009). Accumulation of CD11b+ lung dendritic cells in response to fungal infection results from the CCR2-mediated recruitment and differentiation of Ly-6Chigh monocytes. *J Immunol* 183: 8044–53.
36 Palucka K, Ueno H, Zurawski G, Fay J, Banchereau J. (2010). Building on dendritic cell subsets to improve cancer vaccines. *Curr Opin Immunol* 22: 258–63.
37 Melief CJ. (2008). Cancer immunotherapy by dendritic cells. *Immunity* 29: 372–83.
38 Alvarez D, Vollmann EH, von Andrian UH. (2008). Mechanisms and consequences of dendtritic cell migration. *Immunity* 29: 325–42.
39 Jensen SS, Gad M. (2010). Differential induction of inflammatory cytokines by dendritic cells treated with novel TLR-agonist and cytokine based cocktails: targeting dendritic cells in autoimmunity. *J Inflamm (Lond)* 7: 37.
40 Jahrsdörfer B, Vollmer A, Blackwell SE, Maier J, Sontheimer K, Beyer T, Mandel B, Lunov O, Tron K, Nienhaus G, Simmet T, Debatin K, Weiner G, Fabricius D. (2010). Granzyme B produced by human plasmacytoid dendritic cells suppresses T-cell expansion. *Blood* 115: 1156–65.
41 Lambrecht BN, Hammad H. (2010). The role of dendritic and epithelial cells as master regulators of allergic airway inflammation. *Lancet* 376: 835–43.
42 Hammad H, Chieppa M, Perros F, Willart MA, Germain RN, Lambrecht BN. (2009). House dust mite allergen induces asthma via Toll-like receptor 4 triggering of airway structural cells. *Nat Med* 15: 410–16.
43 Yerkovich ST, Roponen M, Smith ME, McKenna K, Bosco A, Subrata LS, Mamessier E, Wikström ME, Le Souef P, Sly PD, Holt PG, Upham JW. (2009). Allergen-enhanced thrombomodulin (blood dendritic cell antigen 3, CD141) expression on dendritic cells is associated with a TH2-skewed immune response. *J Allergy Clin Immunol* 123: 209–16.
44 Rate A, Upham JW, Bosco A, McKenna KL, Holt PG. (2009). Airway epithelial cells regulate the functional phenotype of locally differentiating dendritic cells: implications for the pathogenesis of infectious and allergic airway disease. *J Immunol* 182: 72–83.
45 Hammad H, Plantinga M, Deswarte K, Pouliot P, Willart MA, Kool M, Muskens F, Lambrecht BN. (2010). Inflammatory dendritic cells – not basophils – are necessary and sufficient for induction of Th2 immunity to inhaled house dust mite allergen. *J Exp Med* 207: 2097–111.
46 Dua B, Watson RM, Gauvreau GM, O'Byrne PM. (2010). Myeloid and plasmacytoid dendritic cells in induced sputum after allergen inhalation in subjects with asthma. *J Allergy Clin Immunol* 12: 133–9.

47 Mosmann TR, Cherwinski H, Bond MW, Giedlin MA, Coffman RL. (1986). Two types of murine helper T cell clone. I. Definition according to profiles of lymphokine activities and secreted proteins. *J Immunol* 136: 2348–57.

48 Mosmann TR, Coffman RL. (1989). TH1 and TH2 cells: different patterns of lymphokine secretion lead to different functional properties. *Annu Rev Immunol* 7: 145–73.

49 Ouyang W, Jacobson NG, Bhattacharya D, Gorham JD, Fenoglio D, Sha WC, Murphy TL, Murphy KM. (1999). The Ets transcription factor ERM is Th1-speciifc and induced by IL-12 through a Stat4-dependent pathway. *Proc Natl Acad Sci (USA)* 96: 3888–93.

50 Glimcher L and Singh H. (2001). Transcription factors in lymphocyte development – T and B cells get together. *Cell* 96: 13–23.

51 Staal FJ, Weerkamp F, Langerak AW, Hendriks RW, Clevers HC. (2001). Transcriptional control of T lymphocyte differentiation. *Stem Cells* 19: 165–179.

52 Hwang ES, White IA, Ho IC. (2002). An IL-4-independent and CD25-mediated function of c-maf in promoting the production of Th2 cytokines. *Proc Natl Acad Sci (USA)* 99: 13026–30.

53 Zheng W and Flavell RA. (1997). The transcription factor GATA-3 is necessary and sufficient for Th2 cytokine gene expression in CD4 T cells. *Cell* 89: 587–596.

54 Ouyang W, Ranganath SH, Weindel K, Bhattacharya D, Murphy TL, Sha WC, Murphy KM. (1998). Inhibition of Th1 development mediated by GATA-3 through an IL-4-independent mechanism. *Immunity* 9: 745–55.

55 Tanaka Y, So T, Lebedeva S, Croft M, Altman A. (2005). Impaired IL-4 and c-Maf expression and enhanced Th1-cell development in Vav1-deficient mice. *Blood* 106: 1286–95.

56 Usui T, Preiss JC, Kanno Y, Yao ZJ, Bream JH, O'Shea JJ, Strober W. (2006). T-bet regulates Th1 responses through essential effects on GATA-3 function rather than on IFNG gene acetylation and transcription. *J Exp Med* 203: 755–66.

57 Usui T, Nishikomori R, Kitani A, Strober W. (2003). GATA-3 suppresses Th1 development by downregulation of Stat4 and not through effects on IL-12Rbeta2 chain or T-bet. *Immunity* 18: 415–28.

58 Yang Y, Ochando J, Yopp A, Bromberg JS, Ding Y. (2005). IL-6 plays a unique role in initiating c-Maf expression during early stage of CD4 T cell activation. *J Immunol* 174: 3484–92.

59 "Asthma at a Glance," National Center for Environmental Health (NCEH), US CDC, 1999.

60 "New Asthma Estimates: Tracking Prevalence, Health Care and Mortality," NCHS, US CDC, 2001.

61 "Chronic Conditions: A Challenge for the 21st Century," National Academy on an Aging Society, 2000.

62 "Asthma: A Concern for Minority Populations," NIAID, NIH 2001.

63 "Morbidity and Mortality Report," NCHS, US CDC, 2003.

64 "The Costs of Asthma," Asthma and Allergy Foundation 1992 and 1998 Study, 2000 Update.

65 Pope CA, Ezzati M, Dockery DW. (2009). Fine-particulate air pollution and life expectancy in the United States. *N Engl J Med* 2009 360(4): 376–86.

66 Umetsu DT, McIntire JJ, Akbari O, Macaubas C, DeKruyff RH. (2002). Asthma: An epidemic of dysregulated immunity. *Nat Immunol* 3: 715–20.
67 Krewski D. (2009). Evaluating the effects of ambient air pollution on life expectancy. *N Engl J Med* 360: 413–15.
68 Chow JC, Watson JG, Mauderly JL, Costa DL, Wyzga RE, Vedal S, Hidy GM, Altshuler SL, Marrack D, Heuss JM, Wolff GT, Pope CA 3rd, Dockery DW. (2006). Health effects of fine particulate air pollution: lines that connect. *Air Waste Manag Assoc* 56: 1368–80.
69 Pope CA, Thun MJ, Namboodiri MM, Dockery DW, Evans JS, Speizer FE, Heath CW Jr. (1995). Particulate air pollution as a predictor of mortality in a prospective study of U.S. adults. *Am J Respir Crit Care Med* 1995 Mar; 151(3 Pt 1): 669–74.
70 Dockery DW, Pope CA 3rd, Xu X, Spengler JD, Ware JH, Fay ME, Ferris BG Jr, Speizer FE. (1993). An association between air pollution and mortality in six U.S. cities. *N Engl J Med* 329: 1753–9.
71 Katsouyanni K, Samet JM, Anderson HR, Atkinson R, Le Tertre A, Medina S, Samoli E, Touloumi G, Burnett RT, Krewski D, Ramsay T, Dominici F, Peng RD, Schwartz J, Zanobetti A; HEI Health Review Committee. (2009). Air pollution and health: a European and North American approach (APHENA). *Res Rep Health Eff Inst* 142: 5–90.
72 Eftim SE, Samet JM, Janes H, McDermott A, Dominici F. (2008). Fine particulate matter and mortality: a comparison of the six cities and American Cancer Society cohorts with a medicare cohort. *Epidemiology* 19: 209–16.
73 Abbey DE, Nishino N, McDonnell WF, Burchette RJ, Knutsen SF, Lawrence Beeson W, Yang JX. (1999). Long-term inhalable particles and other air pollutants related to mortality in nonsmokers. *Am J Respir Crit Care Med* 159: 373–82.
74 Filleul L, Rondeau V, Vandentorren S, Le Moual N, Cantagrel A, Annesi-Maesano I, Charpin D, Declercq C, Neukirch F, Paris C, Vervloet D, Brochard P, Tessier JF, Kauffmann F, Baldi I. (2005). Twenty-five year mortality and air pollution: results from the French PAARC survey. *Occup Environ Med* 62: 453–60.
75 Ostro B, Lipsett M, Reynolds P, Goldberg D, Hertz A, Garcia C, Henderson KD, Bernstein L. (2010). Long-term exposure to constituents of fine particulate air pollution and mortality: results from the California teachers study. *Environ Health Perspect* 118: 363–9.
76 Frieri M. (2007). Advances in the understanding of allergic asthma. *Allergy Asthma Proc* 28: 614–19.
77 Willart MA, Lambrecht BN. (2009). The danger within: endogenous danger signals, atopy and asthma. *Clin Exp Allergy* 39: 12–19.
78 Zhang J, Paré PD, Sandford AJ. (2008). Recent advances in asthma genetics. *Respir Res* 9: 4–4.
79 Deichmann KA, Starke B, Schlenther S, Heinzmann A, Sparholt SS, Forster J, Kuehr J. (1999). Linkage and association studies of atopy and the chromosome 11q13 region. *J Med Genet* 36(5): 379–82.
80 Ober C, Hoffjan S. (2006) Asthma genetics 2006: the long and winding road to gene discovery. *Genes Immun* 7: 95–100.
81 Vercelli D. (2008) Discovering susceptibility genes for asthma and allergy. *Nat Rev Immunol* 8: 169–82.

82 Palmer CN, Ismail T, Lee SP, Terron-Kwiatkowski A, Zhao Y, Liao H, Smith FJ, McLean WH, Mukhopadhyay S. (2007). Filaggrin null mutations are associated with increased asthma severity in children and young adults. *J Allergy Clin Immunol* 120: 64–8.
83 Levy H, Raby BA, Lake S, Tantisira KG, Kwiatkowski D, Lazarus R, Silverman EK, Richter B, Klimecki WT, Vercelli D, Martinez FD, Weiss ST. (2005). Association of defensin beta-1 gene polymorphisms with asthma. *J Allergy Clin Immunol* 115: 252–8.
84 Hoffjan S, Nicolae D, Ober C. (2003). Association studies for asthma and atopic diseases: a comprehensive review of the literature. *Respir Res* 4: 14–14.
85 Kabesch M. (2005). Candidate gene association studies and evidence for gene-by-gene interactions. *Immunol Allergy Clin North Am* 25: 681–708.
86 Halapi E, Hakonarson H. (2004). Recent development in genomic and proteomic research for asthma. *Curr Opin Pulm Med* 10: 22–30.
87 Moffatt MF, Kabesch M, Liang L, Dixon AL, Strachan D, Heath S, Depner M, von Berg A, Bufe A, Rietschel E, Heinzmann A, Simma B, Frischer T, Willis-Owen SA, Wong KC, Illig T, Vogelberg C, Weiland SK, von Mutius E, Abecasis GR, et al. (2007). Genetic variants regulating ORMDL3 expression contribute to the risk of childhood asthma. *Nature* 448: 470–3.
88 Galanter J, Choudhry S, Eng C, Nazario S, Rodríguez-Santana JR, Casal J, Torres-Palacios A, Salas J, Chapela R, Watson HG, Meade K, Lenoir M, Rodríguez-Cintrón W, Avila PC, Burchard EG. (2008). ORMDL3 gene is associated with asthma in three ethnically diverse populations. *Am J Respir Crit Care Med* 177: 1194–200.
89 Sleiman PM, Flory J, Imielinski M, Bradfield JP, Annaiah K, Willis-Owen SA, Wang K, Rafaels NM, Michel S, Bonnelykke K, Zhang H, Kim CE, Frackelton EC, Glessner JT, Hou C, Otieno FG, Santa E, Thomas K, Smith RM, Glaberson WR, et al. (2010). Variants of DENND1B associated with asthma in children. *N Engl J Med* 362: 36–44.
90 Sleiman PM, Annaiah K, Imielinski M, Bradfield JP, Kim CE, Frackelton EC, Glessner JT, Eckert AW, Otieno FG, Santa E, Thomas K, Smith RM, Glaberson W, Garris M, Gunnlaugsson S, Chiavacci RM, Allen J, Spergel J, Grundmeier R, Grunstein MM, et al. (2008). ORMDL3 variants associated with asthma susceptibility in North Americans of European ancestry. *J Allergy Clin Immunol* 122: 1225–7.
91 Bisgaard H, Bønnelykke K, Sleiman PM, Brasholt M, Chawes B, Kreiner-Møller E, Stage M, Kim C, Tavendale R, Baty F, Pipper CB, Palmer CN, Hakonarsson H. Chromosome 17q21 gene variants are associated with asthma and exacerbations but not atopy in early childhood. (2009). *Am J Respir Crit Care Med* 179: 179–85.
92 Leung TF, Sy HY, Ng MC, Chan IH, Wong GW, Tang NL, Waye MM, Lam CW. (2009). Asthma and atopy are associated with chromosome 17q21 markers in Chinese children. *Allergy* 64: 621–8.
93 Nicolae D, Cox NJ, Lester LA, Schneider D, Tan Z, Billstrand C, Kuldanek S, Donfack J, Kogut P, Patel NM, Goodenbour J, Howard T, Wolf R, Koppelman GH, White SR, Parry R, Postma DS, Meyers D, Bleecker ER, Hunt JS, et al. (2005). Fine mapping and positional candidate studies identify HLA-G as an asthma susceptibility gene on chromosome 6p21. *Am J Hum Genet* 76: 349–57.

94 Noguchi E, Yokouchi Y, Zhang J, Shibuya K, Shibuya A, Bannai M, Tokunaga K, Doi H, Tamari M, Shimizu M, Shirakawa T, Shibasaki M, Ichikawa K, Arinami T. (2005). Positional identification of an asthma susceptibility gene on human chromosome 5q33. *Am J respir Crit Care Med* 172: 183–8.

95 Zhang Y, Leaves NI, Anderson GG, Ponting CP, Broxholme J, Holt R, Edser P, Bhattacharyya S, Dunham A, Adcock IM, Pulleyn L, Barnes PJ, Harper JI, Abecasis G, Cardon L, White M, Burton J, Matthews L, Mott R, Ross M, et al. (2003). Positional cloning of a quantitative trait locus on chromosome 13q14 that influences immunoglobulin E levels and asthma. *Nat Genet* 34: 181–6.

96 Laitinen T, Polvi A, Rydman P, Vendelin J, Pulkkinen V, Salmikangas P, Mäkelä S, Rehn M, Pirskanen A, Rautanen A, Zucchelli M, Gullstén H, Leino M, Alenius H, Petäys T, Haahtela T, Laitinen A, Laprise C, Hudson TJ, Laitinen LA, Kere J. (2004). Characterization of a common susceptibility locus for asthma-related traits. *Science* 304: 300–4.

97 Alati R, Al Mamun A, O'Callaghan M, Najman JM, Williams GM. (2006) In utero and postnatal maternal smoking and asthma in adolescence. *Epidemiology* 17: 138–44.

98 Kumar R. (2008). Prenatal factors and the development of asthma. *Curr Opin Pediatr* 20: 682–7.

99 Braun-Fahrländer C, Lauener R. (2003). Farming and protective agents against allergy and asthma. *Clin Exp Allergy* 33: 409–11.

100 Riedler J, Braun-Fahrländer C, Eder W, Schreuer M, Waser M, Maisch S, et al. (2001). Exposure to farming in early life and development of asthma and allergy: a cross-sectional survey. *Lancet* 358: 1129–33.

101 Braun-Fahrländer C, Riedler J, Herz U, Eder W, Waser M, Grize L, et al. (2002). Environmental exposure to endotoxin and its relation to asthma in school-age children. *N Engl J Med* 347: 869–77.

102 Strachan DP. Hay fever, hygiene, and household size. (1989). *BMJ* 299: 1259–60.

103 Schwartz R. (2002). A new element in the mechanism of asthma. *New Engl J Med* 346: 857–8.

104 Yazdanbakhsh M, Kermsner P and van Ree R. (2002). Allergy, parasites, and the hygiene hypothesis. *Science* 296: 490–4.

105 Busse W and Lemanske R. (2001). Asthma. *New Engl J Med* 344: 350–362.

106 Black P. (2001). Why is the prevalence of allergy and autoimmunity increasing? *Trends in Immunology* 22: 354–5.

107 Griem P, Wulferink M, Sachs B, Gonzalez J, Gleichmann E. (1998). Allergic and autoimmune reactions to xenobiotics: how do they arise? *Immunology Today* 19: 133–45.

108 James SY, Williams MA, Kelsey SM, Newland AC, Colston KW. (1997). The role of vitamin D derivatives and retinoids in the differentiation of human leukaemic cells. *Biochem Pharmacol* 54: 625–34.

109 James SJ, Williams MA, Kelsey SM, Newland AC, Colston KW. (1997). Interaction of vitamin D derivatives and granulocyte-macrophage colony-stimulating factor in leukaemic cell diferentiation. *Leukemia* 11: 1017–25.

110 James SY, Williams MA, Newland AC, Colston KW. (1999). Leukemia cell differentiation: cellular and molecular interactions of retinoids and vitamin D. *General Pharmacol* 32: 143–54.

111 Hewison M, Freeman L, Hughes SV, et al. (2003). Differential regulation of vitamin D receptor and its ligand in human monocyte-derived dendritic cells. *J Immunol* 170: 5382–90.

112 Adorini L, Penna G, Giarratana N, et al. (2004). Dendritic cells as key targets for immunomodulation by vitamin D receptor ligands. *J Steroid Biochem Mol Biol* 89–90: 437–41.

113 Ben-Zvi I, Aranow C, Mackay M, Stanevsky A, Kamen DL, Marinescu LM, Collins CE, Gilkeson GS, Diamond B, Hardin JA. (2010). The impact of vitamin D on dendritic cell function in patients with systemic lupus erythematosus. *PLoS One* 16;5(2): e9193.

114 Adorini L, Penna G. (2009). Dendritic cell tolerogenicity:a key mechanism in immunomodulation by vitamin D receptor agonists. *Hum Immunol* 70: 345–52.

115 Reichel H, Koeffler HP, Tobler A, Norman AW. (1987). 1 alpha, 25-Dihydroxyvitamin D3 inhibits gamma-interferon synthesis by normal human peripheral blood lymphocytes. *Proc Natl Acad Sci USA* 84: 3385–3389.

116 47. Penna G, Adorini L. (2000). 1 Alpha, 25-dihydroxyvitaminD3 inhibits differentiation, maturation, activation, and survival of dendritic cells leading to impaired alloreactive T cell activation. *J Immunol* 164: 2405–11.

117 Piemonti L, Monti P, Sironi M, et al. (2000). Vitamin D3 affects differentiation, maturation, and function of human monocyte-derived dendritic cells. *J Immunol* 2000; 164: 4443–51.

118 Griffin MD, Lutz WH, Phan VA, Bachman LA, McKean DJ, Kumar R. Potent inhibition of dendritic cell differentiation and maturation by vitamin D analogs. *Biochem Biophys Res Commun* 270: 701–8.

119 Gauzzi MC, Purificato C, Donato K, et al. (2005). Suppressive effect of 1alpha, 25-ihydroxyvitamin D3 on type I IFN-mediated monocyte differentiation into dendritic cells: impairment of functional activities and chemotaxis. *J Immunol* 174: 270–6.

120 Hatch GE, Gardner DE, Menzel DB. (1980). Stimulation of oxidant production in alveolar macrophages by pollutant and latex particles. *Environ Res* 23: 121–36.

121 Hatch GE, Boykin E, Graham JA, Lewtas J, Pott F, Loud K, Mumford JL. (1985). Inhalable particles and pulmonary host defense: in vivo and in vitro effects of ambient air and combustion particles. *Environ Res* 36: 67–80.

122 Norwood J Jr, Ledbetter AD, Doerfler DL, Hatch GE. (2001). Residual oil fly ash inhalation in guinea pigs: influence of absorbate and glutathione depletion. *Toxicol Sci* 61: 144–53.

123 Nel AE, Diaz-Sanchez D, Li N. (2001). The role of particulate pollutants in pulmonary inflammation and asthma: evidence for the involvement of organic chemicals and oxidative stress. *Curr Opin Pulm Med* 7: 20–6

124 Whitekus MJ, Li N, Zhang M, Wang M, Horwitz MA, Nelson SK, Horwitz LD, Brechun N, Diaz-Sanchez D, Nel AE. (2002). Thiol antioxidants inhibit the adjuvant effects of aerosolized diesel exhaust particles in a murine model for ovalbumin sensitization. *J Immunol* 168: 2560–7.

125 Gowdy K, Krantz QT, Daniels M, Linak WP, Jaspers I, Gilmour MI. (2008). Modulation of pulmonary inflammatory responses and antimicrobial defenses in mice exposed to diesel exhaust. Toxicol Appl Pharmacol. 229: 310–19.

126 Sharkhuu T, Doerfler DL, Krantz QT, Luebke RW, Linak WP, Gilmour MI. (2010). Effects of prenatal diesel exhaust inhalation on pulmonary inflammation and development of specific immune responses. *Toxicol Lett* 196: 12–20.
127 Nygaard UC, Alberg T, Bleumink R, Aase A, Dybing E, Pieters R, Løvik M. (2005). Ambient air particles from four European cities increase the primary cellular response to allergen in the draining lymph node. *Toxicology* 207: 241–54.
128 Liu L, Poon R, Chen L, Frescura AM, Montuschi P, Ciabattoni G, Wheeler A, Dales R. (2009). Acute effects of air pollution on pulmonary function, airway inflammation, and oxidative stress in asthmatic children. *Environ Health Perspect* 117: 668–74.
129 Brüske I, Hampel R, Socher MM, Rückerl R, Schneider A, Heinrich J, Oberdörster G, Wichmann HE, Peters A. (2010). Impact of ambient air pollution on the differential white blood cell count in patients with chronic pulmonary disease. *Inhal Toxicol* 22: 245–52.
130 de Hartog JJ, Ayres JG, Karakatsani A, Analitis A, Brink HT, Hameri K, Harrison R, Katsouyanni K, Kotronarou A, Kavouras I, Meddings C, Pekkanen J, Hoek G. (2010). Lung function and indicators of exposure to indoor and outdoor particulate matter among asthma and COPD patients. *Occup Environ Med* 67: 2–10.
131 Gilliland FD. (2009). Outdoor air pollution, genetic susceptibility, and asthma management: opportunities for intervention to reduce the burden of asthma. *Pediatrics 123* Suppl 3: S168–73.
132 Wichmann FA, Müller A, Busi LE, Cianni N, Massolo L, Schlink U, Porta A, Sly PD. (2009). Increased asthma and respiratory symptoms in children exposed to petrochemical pollution. *J Allergy Clin Immunol* 123: 632–8.
133 Tsan MF and Gao B. (2009). Heat shock proteins and immune system. *J Leukoc Biol* 85: 905–10.
134 Blander JM. (2008). Phagocytosis and antigen presentation: a partnership initiated by Toll-like receptors. *Ann Rheum Dis* 67 Suppl 3:iii44–9.
135 Netea MG, van de Veerdonk FL, Kullberg BJ, Van der Meer JW, Joosten LA. (2008). The role of NLRs and TLRs in the activation of the inflammasome. *Expert Opin Biol Ther* 8: 1867–72.
136 Jin MS, Lee JO. (2008). Structures of TLR-ligand complexes. *Curr Opin Immunol* 20: 414–19.
137 Raymond T, Schaller M, Hogaboam CM, Lukacs NW, Rochford R, Kunkel SL. (2007). Toll-like receptors, Notch ligands, and cytokines drive the chronicity of lung inflammation. *Proc Am Thorac Soc* 4: 635–41.
138 Gallucci S, Lolkema M, Matzinger P. (1999). Natural adjuvants: endogenous activators of dendritic cells. *Nat Med* 5: 1249–55.
139 Sauter B, Albert ML, Francisco L, Larsson M, Somersan S, Bhardwaj N. (2000). Consequences of cell death: exposure to necrotic tumor cells, but not primary tissue cells or apoptotic cells, induces the maturation of immunostimulatory dendritic cells. *Exp Med* 191: 423–34.
140 Basu S, Binder RJ, Suto R, Anderson KM, Srivastava PK. (2000). Necrotic but not apoptotic cell death releases heat shock proteins, which deliver a partial maturation signal to dendritic cells and activate the NF-kappa B pathway. *Int Immunol* 12: 1539–46.

141 Somersan S, Larsson M, Fonteneau JF, Basu S, Srivastava P, Bhardwaj N. (2001). Primary tumor tissue lysates are enriched in heat shock proteins and induce the maturation of human dendritic cells. *J Immunol* 167: 4844–52.
142 Moroi Y, Mayhew M, Trcka J, Hoe HM, Takechi Y, Hartl FU, Rothman JE, Houghton AN. (2000). Induction of cellular immunity by immunization with novel hybrid peptides complexed by heat shock protein 70. *Proc Natl Acad Sci USA* 97: 3485–90.
143 Vastava PK, Menoret A, Basu S, Binder RJ, McQuade KL. (1998). Heat shock proteins come of age: primitive functions acquire new roles in an adaptive world. *Immunity* 8: 657–65.
144 Kuppner MC, Gastpar R, Gelwer S, Nössner E, Ochmann O, Scharner A, Issels RD. (2001). The role of heat shock protein (hsp70) in dendritic cell maturation: hsp70 induces the maturation of immature dendritic cells but reduces DC differentiation from monocyte precursors. *Eur J Immunol* 31: 1602–9.
145 Noessner E, Gastpar R, Milani V, Brandl A, Hutzler PJ, Kuppner MC, Roos M, Kremmer E, Asea A, Calderwood SK, Issels RD. (2002). Tumor-derived heat shock protein 70 peptide complexes are cross-presented by human dendritic cells. *J Immunol* 169: 5424–32.
146 Blank F, von Garnier C, Obregon C, Rothen-Rutishauser B, Gehr P, Nicod L. (2008). Role of dendritic cells in the lung: in vitro models, animal models and human studies. *Expert Rev Respir Med* 2: 215–33.
147 Jahnsen FL, Strickland D, Thomas JA, Tobagus IT, Napoli S, Zosky GR, Turner DJ, Sly PD, Stumbles PA, Holt PG. (2006). Accelerated antigen sampling and transport by airway mucosal dendritic cells following inhalation of a bacterial stimulus. *J Immunol* 177: 5861–7.
148 Blank F, Rothen-Rutishauser B, Gehr P. (2007). Dendritic cells and macrophages form a transepithelial network against foreign particulate antigens. *Am J Pathol* 169: 2127–36.
149 Gehr P, Blank F, Rothen-Rutishauser BM. (2006). Fate of inhaled particles after interaction with the lung surface. *Paediatr Respir Rev* 7 Suppl 1: S73–5.
150 Rothen-Rutishauser BM, Kiama SG, Gehr P. (2005). A three-dimensional cellular model of the human respiratory tract to study the interaction with particles. *Am J Respir Cell Mol Biol* 32: 281–9.

2

Asthma: primary immunomodulatory pathways

Timothy D. Bigby and Patricia W. Finn

Abstract: Asthma is a major health problem worldwide that has increased. Much of the prior focus in asthma research has been on adaptive, antigen-dependent immune responses. Recent work suggests that the innate, non-antigen-dependent immune system responses play a critical role in asthma pathogenesis. Here we will focus on key pathways within the innate immune system and their interface with adaptive immunity, highlighting how the innate immune system modulates adaptive allergic immune responses. In particular, we review data on the role of toll-like receptor signaling, including accessory pathways and TRIF-IRF, in modulating allergic pulmonary responses. We will briefly review the role of the growing field of bioinformatics in identifying networks of immune genes involved in allergic responses.

Keywords: asthma, allergy, innate immunity, allergic inflammation, toll-like receptors, hygiene hypothesis, gene-environment interactions, interferon-beta

2.1 Introduction

Asthma is a major health problem worldwide that has increased. Much of the prior focus in asthma research has been on adaptive, antigen-dependent immune responses. Recent work suggests that the innate, non-antigen-dependent immune system responses play a critical role in asthma pathogenesis. One explanation for the asthma increase is termed the "hygiene hypothesis," which suggest that people in the industrialized world are less challenged with infections and more protected from childhood infectious disease.[(1)] Thus, early life events associated with microbial infection, or exposure to molecules unique to microbes, result in deviation of adaptive immune responses from pro-allergic phenotypes. However, simple failure of "immune deviation" does not fully explain the current asthma epidemic, nor does it adequately explain the complex immunobiology of allergic asthma. Moreover, the innate, non-antigen-dependent and adaptive, antigen-dependent immune systems are highly integrated and have substantial cross-talk. Although the cross-talk is bidirectional, innate mechanisms appear to play a major role in regulating the adaptive immune responses in analysis of asthma both in humans and animal models. In this review, we will examine select innate mechanisms that modulate adaptive immune responses, as related to allergic asthma.

2.2 Receptors of the innate immune system and asthma

Lipopolysaccharide (LPS), originally termed endotoxin in 1892 by Pfeiffer, [2] has been the focus of many epidemiological studies of asthma. Children exposed to higher concentrations of LPS early in life have a lower incidence of asthma. [3, 4] Recognition of an association of LPS and asthma has led to a focus on the receptor for LPS, Toll-like receptor 4 (TLR4) and its signaling pathway. LPS contamination of the allergen ovalbumin (OVA) can attenuate allergic inflammation and airway hyperresponsiveness in a murine model. [5] When more directly addressed, both the lipid A component of LPS, signaling via TLR4, and peptidoglycan, signaling via TLR2, can attenuate allergic pulmonary inflammation. [6]

The innate, non-antigen-dependent immune system includes both sensor and effector arms and both of these arms have humoral and cellular elements. The innate system, encoded in the germline DNA, represents not only a first, immediate line of defense against microorganisms, but also helps to inform and direct the adaptive system that is slower and is characterized by the need for gene rearrangement. The innate system immune system is phylogenetically much older than the adaptive immune system and is present in all complex multicellular organisms, whereas the adaptive immune response evolved in vertebrates only. The innate immune system in humans consists not only of at least ten TLRs, but also cytoplasmic as well as extracellular soluble receptors. NOD1 and NOD2 are cytoplasmic receptors characterized by having a nucleotide and oligomerization domain (NOD) but are part of the larger caspase activation and recruitment domain (CARD) family of proteins.[7] Humoral receptors, such as collectins (surfactant protein A and D) [8] and soluble CD14, [9] exist in the extracellular environment. All of these and additional receptors are characterized by recognizing molecules unique to microbes that when engaged trigger a cascade of events contributing to host defense.

2.2.1 Toll-like receptors

TLRs exist as homo- or hetero-dimers and this dimeric structure imparts specificity to their ligand binding via a series of extracellular leucine rich repeats. Although TLRs are membrane bound, their cytoplasmic domain lacks signaling capacity. Instead, TLRs have a cytoplasmic "TLR and interleukin-1 receptor" (TIR) domain that binds to adaptor proteins when a ligand is engaged. These adaptor proteins also have a similar TIR domain and bind to the receptor, in turn, triggering a signaling cascade by binding additional proteins with signaling capacity. The signaling cascade of TLRs is relatively well described, but the mechanisms that impart specificity to the cellular responses are relatively poorly understood. Although there are at least five adaptor proteins, investigative scrutiny has been primarily focused on two: myeloid differentiation factor 88 (MyD88) and TIR domain-containing adaptor inducing IFNβ (TRIF).(10) In the absence of MyD88 and TRIF, no detectable signaling occurs via TLRs.(11, 12)

Signaling via MyD88 is rapid, and primarily responsible for activation of the transcription factor NF-kB. Signaling via TRIF is slower and leads to the activation of IRF3 via TRAF3 and the transcription as well as extracellular release of interferon (IFN).(13) IFNβ induces the expression of co-stimulatory molecules (CD80 and CD86) on the surface of antigen presenting cells(14) Stimulation of TLR4 or TLR3, both TLRs that utilize the TRIF adaptor protein, enhances co-stimulation and in turn, adaptive immune responses. Moreover, TLRs, in general, provide an important adjuvant role in adaptive immune responses.

As noted, early life exposure to LPS is associated with a reduced incidence of asthma in children.(3, 4) This epidemiological finding has been replicated in some murine models, demonstrating LPS treatment reduces the OVA induced pulmonary inflammation.(6) Thus, if LPS is important in modulating the asthma phenotype, a reasonable prediction is that the absence of the receptor for LPS, TLR4, would be associated with an enhanced asthma phenotype. This has been shown to be the case in mice.(15) However, this topic remains complex. Not all clinical studies have found that early life exposure to LPS is associated with reduced risk of asthma and in fact some have found the opposite. For example, one study of a cohort of 499 infants, with one or both parents having asthma or allergy, were studied for LPS levels in their homes during the first three months of life.(16) These investigators noted a modest association with higher concentrations of LPS. Larger studies have suggested an association between levels of household LPS and asthma.(17) These studies underscore that the dose of LPS, as well

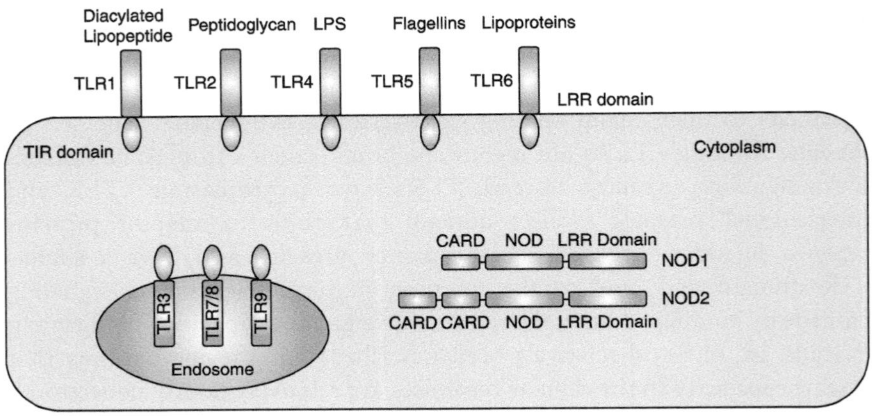

Figure 2.1 Innate immunity receptors.Toll-like receptors (TLRs) are membrane-bound receptors that are present in the plasma membrane (TLR 1,2,4,5,6) or the membrane of endosomes (TLR 3,7/8,9). They consist of a leucine rich repeat (LRR) that is the ligand binding domain and a TLR and interleukin 1 receptor (TIR) domain that is responsible for binding adaptor proteins that then initiate cell signaling. NOD proteins are cytoplasmic receptors that bind ligands through a leucine rich repeat domain and initiate signaling via their nucleotide oligmerization domain (NOD) and a caspase recruitment domain (CARD).

as the timing of exposure, and the environment is important in modulatory allergic adaptive responses.

However, gene–environment interactions are also clinically relevant. Polymorphisms in TLR4 are associated with differences in asthma in groups exposed to LPS. [(18)] A relatively small cohort of Swedish preadolescent schoolchildren were found to have a fourfold higher prevalence of asthma in children having the Asp299Gly polymorphism in TLR4.[(19)] While this data suggest that mutations in TLR4 may make humans more susceptible to the development of asthma, these studies need to be replicated in larger cohorts from different geographic locations and genetic background.

The production of IFNβ might represent one explanation why LPS contamination attenuates the allergic responses in murine models or why TLR4 deficient mice have a heightened allergic response. Consistent with this concept, increased co-stimulatory molecule expression is dependent upon TRIF-mediated IFNγ production. [(14)] Examining the effects of IFN directly, we have found that IFNβ potently attenuates the allergic

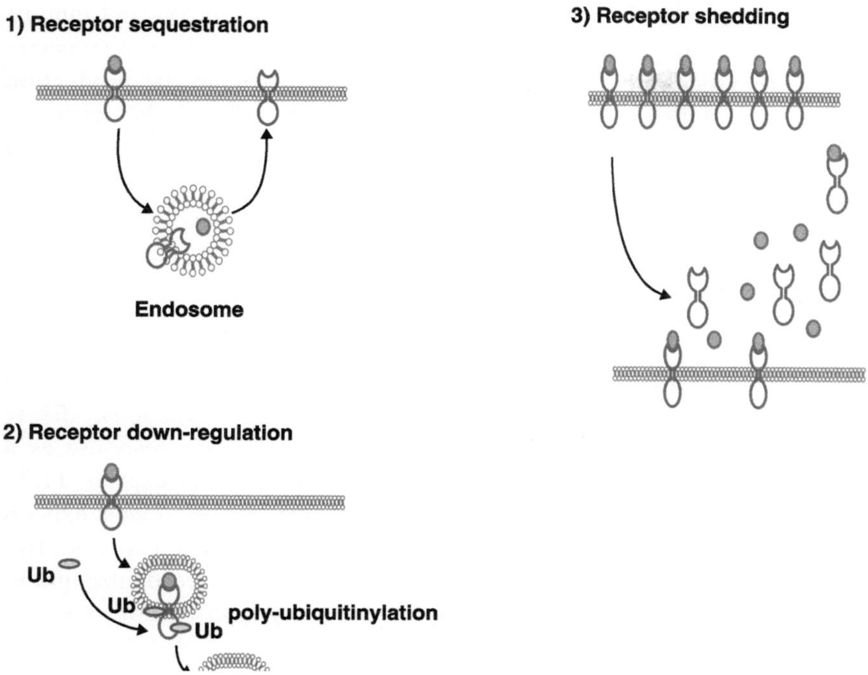

Figure 2.2 TLR4 signaling. Lipopolysaccharide (LPS) binds to TLR4 on the surface of cells in the presence of CD14 and MD2. This induces a conformational change in the cytoplasmic domain of the receptor allowing it to bind the adaptor proteins MyD88, TRIF and Tram. These adaptors production, βinitiate a signaling cascade for NF-kB activation and IFN respectively. NF-kB is activated via IRAK, TRAF6, TAB2, TAK1 and TAB1 leading to the phosphorylation inhibitor of kappa B kinase (IKK) that results in the phosphorylation and degradation of the inhibitor of kappa B (IKB). NF-kB serves as a transcription factor as a heterodimer (p50 and p65) activating a variety of pro-inflammatory genes, many of which are cytokines.

inflammation and airway hyperresponsiveness in a murine model.[20] These data suggest TLR4 signaling via the TRIF adaptor protein attenuates allergic pulmonary inflammation by inducing the production and release of IFNβ.

Similar findings have been shown in a guinea pig allergic model.[21] Examined from a different perspective, human airway epithelial cells from asthmatics have been shown to have deficient IFNβ production when infected with rhinoviruses and, in turn, fail to undergo apoptosis with persistence of the virus.[22] Indeed, exogenous IFNβ applied to these cells restores their ability to undergo virus-induced apoptosis and inhibits viral replication. Airway epithelial cells and mononuclear phagocytes from asthmatics infected with rhinovirus are deficient in the production of Type III interferons, particularly IFNλ, when infected with rhinovirus.[23] Corticosteroids do not restore the ability to undergo viral-induced apoptosis.[22, 23]

2.2.2 Airway epithelial cells

In addition to the ability to generate interferons in response to viral infection as well as many other barrier and transport functions, airway epithelial cells participate in regulating adaptive immune response as a participant in innate host defense. Airway epithelial cells express TLRs including TLR1–6 and TLR9.[24] Notably, airway epithelial cells express low levels of TLR2 and thus recognize and respond to gram-positive organisms poorly. In contrast, airway epithelial cells recognize gram-negative pathogens such as *Pseudomonas aeruginosa* and respiratory syncytial virus (RSV). Interestingly, RSV is a single-stranded RNA virus. Thus, a reasonable postulate would be, in the absence of TLR7 and TLR8, airway epithelial cells would not recognize or respond to RSV. However, within the cell, RSV exists as a double-stranded RNA while replicating, thus stimulating TLR3 and, in turn, IFNγ production.[25] RSV has also been shown to turn off IFNγ production,[26] bi-directed production of the envelope protein G glycoprotein that mediates attachment to the target cell.[27] That protein G diminishes IFNγ production in airway epithelial cells has not yet been established. Regardless, RSV inhibition of IFNβ production is thought to play a significant role in the replication of this virus and may be critical in the response to inhaled antigens in the lung.[28]

Human and non-human bronchial epithelial cells are considered antigen-presenting cells due to their expression of MHC Class II antigens that are essential for external presentation of antigen.[29] In contrast, epithelial cells do have MHC Class I on their surface, but this receptor generates a weak proliferative response of lymphocytes. Human bronchial epithelial cells also express CD40 and ICAM-1 (CD54) in addition to MHC Class II; and these molecules can be upregulated by IFNβ.[30] Bronchial epithelial cells are capable of inducing a proliferative response of mixed lymphocytes in the presence of IFNβ.[30]

2.2.3 NOD receptors

As mentioned, NOD1 and NOD2 are present in the cytoplasm of cells and recognize the natural ligands bacterial diaminopimelic acid or muramyl dipeptide, respectively. Polymorphisms in the NOD2 gene have previously been associated with inflammatory bowel disease,[31, 32] and recent studies have implicated NOD1 in asthma. NOD1 is located on the short arm of chromosome 7 in humans,[33] in a region that has been associated with asthma through linkage analysis of polymorphic markers in human asthmatic populations.[34] An insertion–deletion polymorphism near the beginning of the ninth intron of the NOD1 gene accounts for 7 percent of the variation in IgE in two panels of families.[35] The NOD1 insertion allele was associated with high IgE levels. The same allele was strongly associated with asthma in an independent study of asthmatic children (35). A second report in a German population has shown a correlation with intron 9 of the NOD1 gene with atopy, eczema, asthma and elevated IgE.[36] Again, this study shows a population in Germany raised on farms versus non-farming environments[37] exhibited asthma, hay fever elevated IgE, and in the NOD1 polymorphisms that correlated with the protective effect of being raised on the farm.[37] Together, these data suggest that bacterial products found in the farming environment in humans might protect against the development of asthma and perhaps through NOD1.

2.3 Additional immunoregulatory pathways

2.3.1 Surfactants

The innate immune response has been shown to involve the collectins which include SP-D, a member of the pattern recognition family of collagen containing C- type lectins. The SP-D structure consists of four distinct domains, including an amino terminus, a collagen-like domain, a neck domain, and a lectin or carbohydrate recognition domain (CRD). SP-D exists as a dodecamer which is assembled into a cruciform structure composed of four trimers. SP-D lectin-binding carbohydrate recognition domains at the amino terminus are important in direct binding to infectious agents promoting agglutination, opsonization, and phagocytosis.

Collectins can also promote chemotaxis, respiratory bursts, and immunoglobulin-independent complement activation. Recent studies suggest that SP-D modulate allergic responses.[38–41] Both SP-A and SP-D are associated with decreased allergic responses, suggesting a potential negative regulatory role.[42] Deficiency of SP-D leads to persistent T cell activation.[43] Previous reports have shown that SP-D can inhibit T cell proliferation and interleukin (IL-2) production.[44] Consistent with this observation, we previously showed increased allergic responses in SP-D deficient mice.[41]

2.3.2 CTLA4

CTLA4 is a ligand for the co-stimulatory molecules CD80 and CD86 and, upon T cell activation, transduces a negative feedback signal to decrease immune responses.[45] CTLA4 is also a marker of T regulatory cells (Tregs); T cell suppressor cells that have the potential to decrease allergic responses. CTLA4 deficiency results in systemic autoimmunity, supporting the potent negative regulatory role of CTLA4.[46] The best characterized

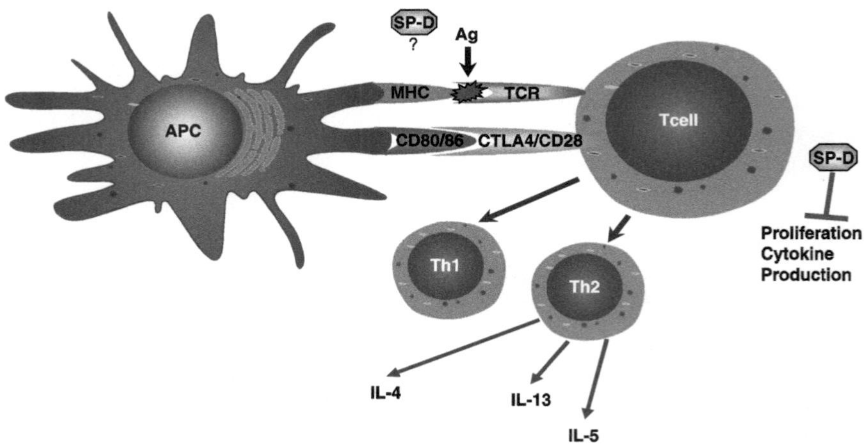

Figure 2.3 Adaptive, antigen-dependent responses that may be mediated by innate surfactant protein D (SP-D). Adaptive immunity is characterized by recognition of antigen (Ag) by an antigen-specific T cell receptor (TCR) in the context of the major histocompatability complex (MHC) on the surface of the antigen presenting cell (APC). The MHC/Ag/TCR interaction results in complete T cell activation with additional co-stimulatory signals (co-stimulation = CD80, CD86 on APC with CD28) on the T cell leading to positive T cell activation. Cytotoxic T cell lymphocyte activator 4 (CTLA4) is an alternative negative receptor present on T cells that binds to CD80 or CD86. SP-D may modify T cell activation, proliferation and T cell subsets including T helper (Th) cells 1 and 2.

negative costimulatory pathways involve the receptors CTLA4 (CD152), described above as a negative regulator and a marker for Tregs, and ICOS on T lymphocytes.[47]

CTLA4 is homologous to the co-stimulatory molecule CD28, and also binds the same co-receptors (CD80 and CD86). However, in contrast to CD28, CTLA4 is a negative signal for T cell activation. Consistent with this function, CTLA4 deficient mice have a lymphoproliferative disorder, and blocking antibodies against CTLA4 can increase allergic responses.[48]

CTLA4, a ligand for CD80 and CD86, is expressed by T cells upon activation, providing a negative feedback signal that limits the immune responses.[45] Systemic administration of CTLA4-Ig during allergen sensitization inhibits the ligation of CD28 with CD80 or CD86, reducing airway inflammation.[49] Inhibition of CD28 with CD80 or CD86 ligation by systemic or intranasal administration of CTLA4 Ig attenuates T helper (Th) 2 cytokine production and airway hyperresponsiveness.[49–52]

2.4 Bioinformatics/systems biology

Allergic immune responses are initiated and maintained by communication between T and other immune cells. Allergic immune responses can be envisioned as multidimensional interaction networks, where interdependency of molecules as a group is elemental. Newer methods of data acquisition (e.g. microarrays) contribute to the expanding knowledge of genomics (information on DNA contained in an organism or a cell, which includes both the chromosomes within the nucleus and the DNA in the mitochondria) and proteomics (protein component of the genome). Multiple powerful data platforms and adaptation of specialized technology have been developed, and are publicly available. These platforms incorporate literature from curated information derived from decades of science across multiple species. Systems biology is a term used for the integration of data from multiple sources. Bioinformatic approaches analyze large numbers of interrelated components of a network comprised of mediators (or "nodes") and interactions (lines in the network connecting the mediators or so-called nodes).

To date, only a few studies have reported network analyses in allergic inflammation.[53] Microarrays have been used to determine differentially expressed genes. Gene expression studies focusing on local airway responses have analyzed bronchial biopsies,[54] smooth muscle cells,[55] airway cells[56] in adults, as well as nasal respiratory epithelium in asthmatic children,[57] and whole lung tissue in animal models including primates.[58] The goal of these approaches is to identify an increased repertoire of novel differentially expressed genes, proteins, and molecules associated with asthma.

2.5 The future

In summary, we have focused on key pathways within the innate immune system and their interface with adaptive immunity, highlighting how the innate immunity modulates the adaptive allergic immune response. In addition, we have described negative regulators such as SP-D, SP-A, or CTLA4, which are promising targets for modulating allergic immune responses, but this remains to be empirically determined. Allergic airway inflammation is not controlled by a single gene or pathway, but is mediated via a network of responses involving numerous genes. Thus, using state-of-the-art approaches, including bioinformatic and network analysis, may be of benefit in elucidating the complex interconnecting allergic immune pathways that define asthma.

Acknowledgments

The authors wish to acknowledge the support of a VA Merit Award (TDB), NIH R01 HL081663 (PWF) and R01 HL077900 (PWF).

References

1 Strachan DP. Hay fever, hygiene, and household size. *BMJ* 1989, 299: 1259–1260.
2 Pfeiffer R. Untersuchungen über das choleragift. *Z Hygeine* 1892, 11: 393–412.
3 Braun-Fahrlander C, Gassner M, Grize L, Neu U, Sennhauser FH, Varonier HS, Vuille JC, Wuthrich B. Prevalence of hay fever and allergic sensitization in farmers' children and their peers living in the same rural community. Scarpol team. Swiss study on childhood allergy and respiratory symptoms with respect to air pollution. *Clin Exp Allergy* 1999, 29: 28–34.
4 Braun-Fahrlander C, Riedler J, Herz U, Eder W, Waser M, Grize L, Maisch S, Carr D, Gerlach F, Bufe A, et al. Environmental exposure to endotoxin and its relation to asthma in school-age children. *N Engl J Med* 2002, 347: 869–877.
5 Watanabe J, Miyazaki Y, Zimmerman GA, Albertine KH, McIntyre TM. Endotoxin contamination of ovalbumin suppresses murine immunologic responses and development of airway hyper-reactivity. *J Biol Chem* 2003, 278: 42361–42368.

6 Velasco G, Campo M, Manrique OJ, Bellou A, He H, Arestides RS, Schaub B, Perkins DL, Finn PW. Toll-like receptor 4 or 2 agonists decrease allergic inflammation. *Am J Respir Cell Mol Biol* 2005, 32: 218–224.
7 Rosenstiel P, Jacobs G, Till A, Schreiber S. NOD-like receptors: Ancient sentinels of the innate immune system. *Cell Mol Life Sci* 2008.
8 Wright JR. Immunoregulatory functions of surfactant proteins. *Nat Rev Immunol* 2005, 5: 58–68.
9 Antal-Szalmas P. Evaluation of cd14 in host defence. *Eur J Clin Invest* 2000, 30: 167–179.
10 Yamamoto M, Sato S, Mori K, Hoshino K, Takeuchi O, Takeda K, Akira S. Cutting edge: A novel toll/il-1 receptor domain-containing adapter that preferentially activates the IFN-beta promoter in the toll-like receptor signaling. *J Immunol* 2002, 169: 6668–6672.
11 Hoebe K, Du X, Georgel P, Janssen E, Tabeta K, Kim SO, Goode J, Lin P, Mann N, Mudd S, et al. Identification of LPS2 as a key transducer of MyD88-independent TIR signalling. *Nature* 2003, 424: 743–748.
12 Yamamoto M, Sato S, Hemmi H, Hoshino K, Kaisho T, Sanjo H, Takeuchi O, Sugiyama M, Okabe M, Takeda K, et al. Role of adaptor trif in the MyD88-independent toll-like receptor signaling pathway. *Science* 2003, 301: 640–643.
13 Hoebe K, Beutler B. Traf3: A new component of the TLR-signaling apparatus. *Trends Mol Med* 2006, 12: 187–189.
14 Hoebe K, Janssen EM, Kim SO, Alexopoulou L, Flavell RA, Han J, Beutler B. Upregulation of costimulatory molecules induced by lipopolysaccharide and double-stranded RNA occurs by TRIF-dependent and TRIF-independent pathways. *Nat Immunol* 2003, 4: 1223–1229.
15 Hollingsworth JW, Whitehead GS, Lin KL, Nakano H, Gunn MD, Schwartz DA, Cook DN. TLR4 signaling attenuates ongoing allergic inflammation. *J Immunol* 2006, 176: 5856–5862.
16 Park JH, Gold DR, Spiegelman DL, Burge HA, Milton DK. House dust endotoxin and wheeze in the first year of life. *Am J Respir Crit Care Med* 2001, 163: 322–328.
17 Thorne PS, Kulhankova K, Yin M, Cohn R, Arbes SJ, Jr., Zeldin DC. Endotoxin exposure is a risk factor for asthma: The national survey of endotoxin in United States housing. *Am J Respir Crit Care Med* 2005, 172: 1371–1377.
18 Werner M, Topp R, Wimmer K, Richter K, Bischof W, Wjst M, Heinrich J. TLR4 gene variants modify endotoxin effects on asthma. *J Allergy Clin Immunol* 2003, 112: 323–330.
19 Fageras Bottcher M, Hmani-Aifa M, Lindstrom A, Jenmalm MC, Mai XM, Nilsson L, Zdolsek HA, Bjorksten B, Soderkvist P, Vaarala O. A TLR4 polymorphism is associated with asthma and reduced lipopolysaccharide-induced interleukin-12(p70) responses in Swedish children. *J Allergy Clin Immunol* 2004, 114: 561–567.
20 Kytasty C, Lin CY, Alvarez LM, Chan A, Ferrada MA, Finn PW, Bigby TD. Interferon β attenuates airway hyperresponsiveness and allergic inflammation in a mouse asthma model. *Am J Respir Crit Care Med* 2007, 175: A504.
21 Satoh Y, Kasama K, Kuwabara M, Yimin, Diao HY, Nakajima H, Kohanawa M, Minagawa T. Suppression of late asthmatic response by low-dose oral

administration of interferon-beta in the guinea pig model of asthma. *J Interferon Cytokine Res* 1999, 19: 887–894.

22 Wark PA, Johnston SL, Bucchieri F, Powell R, Puddicombe S, Laza-Stanca V, Holgate ST, Davies DE. Asthmatic bronchial epithelial cells have a deficient innate immune response to infection with rhinovirus. *J Exp Med* 2005, 201: 937–947.

23 Contoli M, Message SD, Laza-Stanca V, Edwards MR, Wark PA, Bartlett NW, Kebadze T, Mallia P, Stanciu LA, Parker HL, et al. Role of deficient type iii interferon-lambda production in asthma exacerbations. *Nat Med* 2006, 12: 1023–1026.

24 Mayer AK, Muehmer M, Mages J, Gueinzius K, Hess C, Heeg K, Bals R, Lang R, Dalpke AH. Differential recognition of TLR-dependent microbial ligands in human bronchial epithelial cells. *J Immunol* 2007, 178: 3134–3142.

25 Liu P, Jamaluddin M, Li K, Garofalo RP, Casola A, Brasier AR. Retinoic acid-inducible gene I mediates early antiviral response and toll-like receptor 3 expression in respiratory syncytial virus-infected airway epithelial cells. *J Virol* 2007, 81: 1401–1411.

26 Schlender J, Hornung V, Finke S, Gunthner-Biller M, Marozin S, Brzozka K, Moghim S, Endres S, Hartmann G, Conzelmann KK. Inhibition of toll-like receptor 7- and 9-mediated alpha/beta interferon production in human plasmacytoid dendritic cells by respiratory syncytial virus and measles virus. *J Virol* 2005, 79: 5507–5515.

27 Shingai M, Azuma M, Ebihara T, Sasai M, Funami K, Ayata M, Ogura H, Tsutsumi H, Matsumoto M, Seya T. Soluble g protein of respiratory syncytial virus inhibits toll-like receptor 3/4-mediated IFN-beta induction. *Int Immunol* 2008, 20: 1169–1180.

28 Johnston SL. Innate immunity in the pathogenesis of virus-induced asthma exacerbations. *Proc Am Thorac Soc* 2007, 4: 267–270.

29 Vignola AM, Campbell AM, Chanez P, Bousquet J, Paul-Lacoste P, Michel FB, Godard P. HLA-DR and ICAM-1 expression on bronchial epithelial cells in asthma and chronic bronchitis. *Am Rev Respir Dis* 1993, 148: 689–694.

30 Tanaka H, Maeda K, Nakamura Y, Azuma M, Yanagawa H, Sone S. Cd40 and IFN-gamma dependent T cell activation by human bronchial epithelial cells. *J Med Invest* 2001, 48: 109–117.

31 Hugot JP, Chamaillard M, Zouali H, Lesage S, Cezard JP, Belaiche J, Almer S, Tysk C, O'Morain CA, Gassull M, et al. Association of nod2 leucine-rich repeat variants with susceptibility to crohn's disease. *Nature* 2001, 411: 599–603.

32 Ogura Y, Bonen DK, Inohara N, Nicolae DL, Chen FF, Ramos R, Britton H, Moran T, Karaliuskas R, Duerr RH, et al. A frameshift mutation in NOD2 associated with susceptibility to Crohn's disease. *Nature* 2001, 411: 603–606.

33 Inohara N, Koseki T, del Peso L, Hu Y, Yee C, Chen S, Carrio R, Merino J, Liu D, Ni J, et al. Nod1, an APAF-1-like activator of caspase-9 and nuclear factor-kappab. *J Biol Chem* 1999, 274: 14560–14567.

34 Laitinen T, Polvi A, Rydman P, Vendelin J, Pulkkinen V, Salmikangas P, Makela S, Rehn M, Pirskanen A, Rautanen A, et al. Characterization of a common susceptibility locus for asthma-related traits. *Science* 2004, 304: 300–304.

35 Hysi P, Kabesch M, Moffatt MF, Schedel M, Carr D, Zhang Y, Boardman B, von Mutius E, Weiland SK, Leupold W, et al. Nod1 variation, immunoglobulin e and asthma. *Hum Mol Genet* 2005, 14: 935–941.
36 Weidinger S, Klopp N, Rummler L, Wagenpfeil S, Novak N, Baurecht HJ, Groer W, Darsow U, Heinrich J, Gauger A, et al. Association of nod1 polymorphisms with atopic eczema and related phenotypes. *J Allergy Clin Immunol* 2005, 116: 177–184.
37 Eder W, Klimecki W, Yu L, von Mutius E, Riedler J, Braun-Fahrlander C, Nowak D, Holst O, Martinez FD. Association between exposure to farming, allergies and genetic variation in card4/nod1. *Allergy* 2006, 61: 1117–1124.
38 Brandt EB, Mingler MK, Stevenson MD, Wang N, Khurana Hershey GK, Whitsett JA, Rothenberg ME. Surfactant protein d alters allergic lung responses in mice and human subjects. *J Allergy Clin Immunol* 2008, 121: 1140–1147 e1142.
39 Haczku A. Role and regulation of lung collectins in allergic airway sensitization. *Pharmacol Ther* 2006, 110: 14–34.
40 Janssen WJ, McPhillips KA, Dickinson MG, Linderman DJ, Morimoto K, Xiao YQ, Oldham KM, Vandivier RW, Henson PM, Gardai SJ. Surfactant proteins A and D suppress alveolar macrophage phagocytosis via interaction with SIRP alpha. *Am J Respir Crit Care Med* 2008, 178: 158–167.
41 Schaub B, Westlake RM, He H, Arestides R, Haley KJ, Campo M, Velasco G, Bellou A, Hawgood S, Poulain FR, et al. Surfactant protein D deficiency influences allergic immune responses. *Clin Exp Allergy* 2004, 34: 1819–1826.
42 Brinker KG, Garner H, Wright JR. Surfactant protein A modulates the differentiation of murine bone marrow-derived dendritic cells. *Am J Physiol Lung Cell Mol Physiol* 2003, 284: L232–241.
43 Fisher JH, Larson J, Cool C, Dow SW. Lymphocyte activation in the lungs of SP-D null mice. *Am J Respir Cell Mol Biol* 2002, 27: 24–33.
44 Borron PJ, Mostaghel EA, Doyle C, Walsh ES, McHeyzer-Williams MG, Wright JR. Pulmonary surfactant proteins a and d directly suppress CD3+/CD4+ cell function: Evidence for two shared mechanisms. *J Immunol* 2002, 169: 5844–5850.
45 Perez VL, Van Parijs L, Biuckians A, Zheng XX, Strom TB, Abbas AK. Induction of peripheral T cell tolerance in vivo requires CTLA-4 engagement. *Immunity* 1997, 6: 411–417.
46 Tivol EA, Borriello F, Schweitzer AN, Lynch WP, Bluestone JA, Sharpe AH. Loss of CTLA-4 leads to massive lymphoproliferation and fatal multiorgan tissue destruction, revealing a critical negative regulatory role of CTLA-4. *Immunity* 1995, 3: 541–547.
47 Akbari O, Freeman GJ, Meyer EH, Greenfield EA, Chang TT, Sharpe AH, Berry G, DeKruyff RH, Umetsu DT. Antigen-specific regulatory T cells develop via the ICOS-ICOS-ligand pathway and inhibit allergen-induced airway hyperreactivity. *Nat Med* 2002, 8: 1024–1032.
48 Jen KY, Jain VV, Makani S, Finn PW. Immunomodulation of allergic responses by targeting costimulatory molecules. *Curr Opin Allergy Clin Immunol* 2006, 6: 489–494.
49 Krinzman SJ, De Sanctis GT, Cernadas M, Mark D, Wang Y, Listman J, Kobzik L, Donovan C, Nassr K, Katona I, et al. Inhibition of T cell costimulation

abrogates airway hyperresponsiveness in a murine model. *J Clin Invest* 1996, 98: 2693–2699.

50 Umetsu DT, Akbari O, Dekruyff RH. Regulatory T cells control the development of allergic disease and asthma. *J Allergy Clin Immunol* 2003, 112: 480–487; quiz 488.

51 Jenkins MK, Chen CA, Jung G, Mueller DL, Schwartz RH. Inhibition of antigen-specific proliferation of type 1 murine T cell clones after stimulation with immobilized anti-CD3 monoclonal antibody. *J Immunol* 1990, 144: 16–22.

52 Jenkins MK, Mueller D, Schwartz RH, Carding S, Bottomley K, Stadecker MJ, Urdahl KB, Norton SD. Induction and maintenance of anergy in mature T cells. *Adv Exp Med Biol* 1991, 292: 167–176.

53 Lu X, Jain VV, Finn PW, Perkins DL. Hubs in biological interaction networks exhibit low changes in expression in experimental asthma. *Mol Syst Biol* 2007, 3: 98.

54 Laprise C, Sladek R, Ponton A, Bernier MC, Hudson TJ, Laviolette M. Functional classes of bronchial mucosa genes that are differentially expressed in asthma. *BMC Genomics* 2004, 5: 21.

55 Hakonarson H, Halapi E, Whelan R, Gulcher J, Stefansson K, Grunstein MM. Association between IL-1beta/TNF-alpha-induced glucocorticoid-sensitive changes in multiple gene expression and altered responsiveness in airway smooth muscle. *Am J Respir Cell Mol Biol* 2001, 25: 761–771.

56 Lee JH, Kaminski N, Dolganov G, Grunig G, Koth L, Solomon C, Erle DJ, Sheppard D. Interleukin-13 induces dramatically different transcriptional programs in three human airway cell types. *Am J Respir Cell Mol Biol* 2001, 25: 474–485.

57 Guajardo JR, Schleifer KW, Daines MO, Ruddy RM, Aronow BJ, Wills-Karp M, Hershey GK. Altered gene expression profiles in nasal respiratory epithelium reflect stable versus acute childhood asthma. *J Allergy Clin Immunol* 2005, 115: 243–251.

58 Zou J, Young S, Zhu F, Gheyas F, Skeans S, Wan Y, Wang L, Ding W, Billah M, McClanahan T, et al. Microarray profile of differentially expressed genes in a monkey model of allergic asthma. *Genome Biol* 2002, 3: research0020.

3

Environmental lung injury and pattern recognition receptors

Zhuowei Li, Stavros Garantziotis, Paul W. Noble, and John W. Hollingsworth

Abstract. The lung is continuously exposed to a variety of inhaled toxicants. Host factors play an important role in recognition and clearance of inhaled foreign material. Tight regulation of the inflammatory response promotes effective clearance of toxicants, while limiting the severity of associated lung injury. Immediate and precise host recognition of environmental toxicants and associated lung injury is required for effective maintenance of normal lung function. Recent advances support the central role of pattern recognition receptors in host innate immune recognition during both inhaled foreign material and lung injury. Pattern recognition receptors (PRR) facilitate recognition of pathogen associated molecular patterns (PAMP) and endogenous damage-associated molecular patterns (DAMP). Coincidently, these receptors contribute to the biological response to pathogens, air pollutants, and oxidant stress. Signal transduction of pattern recognition receptors can directly impact a number of human lung diseases. In this chapter, we review the complex interaction between commonly encountered environmental toxicants and pulmonary innate immunity.

Keywords: pulmonary biology, experimental lung injury, immunotoxicology, pattern-recognition receptors, pathogen associated molecular patterns (PAMP), endogenous damage-associated molecular patterns (DAMP), allergic asthma, innate immunity, adaptive immunity, ozone, viral infection

3.1 Introduction

Unlike other organs in the body, the lung is continuously exposed to many airborne environmental factors. The lung structure results in a high exposure area with abundant blood supply, which facilitates direct contact between the host and the ambient environment. The lung is exposed to both gaseous toxins and aerosolized solid matter. Commonly encountered environmental gaseous hazards include ozone, carbon monoxide, sulphur dioxide and nitrogen monoxide/dioxide, which enter the lung via inhalation and impair lung function or cause lung injury depending on their chemical features such as the solubility, concentration and oxidative/reductive capabilities. In addition, various solid environmental hazards come into direct contact with the lung, including particulate matter, house dust, and microbes. It is now recognized that bacteria, fungi, virus and their toxic components can either be aerosolized and directly inhaled or bound to house dust and particulate matter. Co-exposure to inhaled toxicants is common. The host factors that regulate the immediate biological response to these common exposures are an area of considerable clinical interest. Recent advances in this field provide evidence supporting the theory that innate immunity is central to host response to both gaseous and solid inhaled environmental toxicants.

An accurate and tightly regulated immune system has evolved to maintain pulmonary homeostasis despite continuous environmental challenges. This system includes an immediate response (innate immune system) and an acquired response (adaptive immune system). Innate immunity requires immediate recognition and clearance of invading pathogens or non-biological toxicants. In contrast, adaptive immunity is delayed and gains memory for subsequent antigen-specific response. The innate immune system broadly consists of structural barriers, microbial phagocytosis, and specific microbial pattern recognition. Immediate and precise host recognition facilitates clearance of foreign material. Regulated control of the innate response prevents excessive tissue injury in response to external stimuli. An important advance in this field was the discovery of pattern recognition receptors (PRR).

The first pattern recognition receptors identified were the scavenger receptors.[1, 2] The role of pattern recognition receptors on immunologic response was advanced through the pioneering vision of Charles Janeway. He proposed that the host immune system differentiates infectious non-self from non-infectious self through receptors or ligands recognizing various exogenous and endogenous molecular patterns.[3] A seminal contribution to this field was completely unrelated to immunology. Drosophila Toll was originally identified to regulate early embryogenesis (4). Subsequently, drosophila Toll was identified to regulate host defense to fungal aspergillus infection.[5] The mammalian homologue of drosophila Toll, toll-like receptor 4 (TLR4), was cloned and discovered to regulate adaptive immune response.[6] This gene, TLR4, was then identified as the elusive receptor for gram-negative bacterial lipopolysaccharide (LPS) in mice.[7, 8] The functional implication of human TLR4 was initially identified in a model of environmental airways disease.[9] We now recognize that the TLR family of pattern recognition receptors (PRR) represent a large group of highly conserved molecules expressed on many cell-types of immune system and play a central role in host immune function. PRR recognize specific molecular patterns from microorganisms, which are now known as pathogen-associated molecular patterns (PAMP). Previously described pathogen sources of PRR-ligands include bacteria, fungi, and viruses. Recently, PRR have also been implicated in recognition signals from endogenous cellular stress, which are termed danger-associated molecular patterns (DAMP). These observations suggest that pattern recognition receptors can regulate immunologic response through recognition of both exogenous and endogenous ligands. The number of both ligands and PRRs continues to grow with thirteen mammalian toll-like receptors currently identified. Inhaled environmental exposures of the lung include microbiotic pathogen-associated molecular patterns (PAMPs), but even sterile lung injury results in the release of DAMPs. Therefore, the role of innate immunity in many forms of environmental lung disease could result from either exogenous or endogenous ligands of PRRs.

In this chapter, we focus on the prototypic pattern recognition receptor, toll-like receptor 4 (TLR4), in the biological response to various commonly inhaled environmental exposures. We will discuss the complex interaction between common inhaled toxicants and the innate immune response. It is now clear that TLR4 contributes to the pathogenesis of many common pulmonary diseases. Recent advances support divergent roles of TLR4 in the pathogenesis of various forms of lung disease dependent on the context, intensity, and duration of environmental exposure.

3.2 Toll-like receptor 4 signaling

Cellular surface recognition of bacterial lipopolysaccharide (LPS) involves an intricate mechanism of membrane receptors, soluble co-receptors and intracellular adaptor molecules. In addition to TLR4, recognition of LPS is facilitated by an extracellular complex of LPS binding protein (LBP) and CD14. LBP is an extracellular soluble protein, which directly binds to LPS and conveys LPS to cell surface receptor CD14. CD14 is a glycosylphosphatidylinositol (GPI)-anchored protein located on the surface of mononuclear cells. CD14 does not trigger an intracellular signal, but functions to concentrate cell surface LPS and present LPS to another receptor complex TLR4/MD-2. In addition, LBP and soluble CD14 also facilitate the clearance of LPS by accelerating the movement of LPS to lipoprotein particles by which LPS undergoes neutralization and becomes biologically inactive.[10, 11] However, the presence of CD14 is not necessary for LPS-induced TNF-a and IL-1β production, given the fact that cellular responses persist with exposure to high concentration of LPS in the absence of CD14. In contrast, both MD-2 and TLR4 are essential to trigger cell response to LPS.[12, 13] MD-2/TLR4 binding is intracellular with cytosolic MD-2 regulating TLR4 trafficking from Golgi to cell surface membrane[14] possibly through the N-linked glycosylation of MD-2.[15] Therefore, the formation of MD-2/TLR4 complex appears essential for transmembrane signaling in response to LPS stimulation.

Upon surface binding of LPS to MD-2/TLR4 complex, TLR4 mediated signal transduction is initiated. LPS-induced TLR4 signal transduction activates MyD88-dependent and TRIF-dependent pathways leading to NFκB activation and the induction of type 1 interferon (IFN-β). Classically, in response to LPS stimulation, the cytosolic TIR domain of TLR4 recruits TIR domain-containing adaptor protein TIRAP to the membrane on the cytosolic side. TIRAP is important for the link between TLR4 and MyD88. A series of downstream molecules are also recruited by the activation of MyD88, including IL-1 receptor-associated kinases (IRAKs) and TNF receptor-associated factor 6 (TRAF6). TRAF6 then leads to the activation of NFκB in mitogen-activated protein kinases (MAPKs)-dependent or independent manner. MyD88 pathway is conserved among most of TLRs. However, LPS-stimulated macrophages and dendritic-cells deficient in MyD88 can be activated by a MyD88-independent pathway leading to the induction of IFN-γ inducible protein (IP10) and the type 1 interferon (IFN-β).[16, 17] In TLR4/MD-2 expressing HEK293 cells, which naturally lack MyD88, LPS increased production of RANTES and IP10 entirely independently of MyD88.[18] Both TIR domain containing adaptor molecules TRIF and TRAM appear to be required for LPS-TLR4 signaling to activate the MyD88-independent pathway in response to LPS.

Collectively, TLR4 plays an important role in innate immune surface recognition of bacterial endotoxin and intracellular signaling. LPS-TLR4 binding-initiated signal cascade not only leads to an inflammatory response, but also participates in the directed migration of inflammatory cells. Growing evidence supports a fundamental role of toll-like receptors in environmental lung injury. While we focus our discussion on TLR4, the

TLR family of pattern recognition receptors are now recognized as a major component of host immunity, including antibacterial host defense, innate-adaptive crosstalk, and many other pro-inflammatory conditions. Toll-like receptor signaling in the lung can modify each of these components of pulmonary immunity. Consistently, TLR-signaling appears to have profound impact on the pathogenesis of many common lung diseases. We are only beginning to understand the complex interactions between TLR-dependent signaling and common environmental exposures in both the development and progression of human lung disease.

3.3 Bacterial endotoxin contributes to environmental airways disease

3.3.1 Inhaled LPS contributes to occupational lung disease

Ligands of TLRs are ubiquitous in the environment and are therefore frequently inhaled. The health effects of exposure to bacterial endotoxin have primarily been studied during occupational exposures. While the methods to measure environmental levels of endotoxin have not been standardized, elevated levels of endotoxin have been documented with sampling of airborne dust in many settings, including biofuel plants,[19, 20] composting facilities,[21] cattle ranches,[22] pig farms,[23] cotton mills,[24–26] and grain silos.[27–29] Additionally, bacterial endotoxin is commonly found in dust collected from domestic[30] and occupational environments[31] and can contribute to the biological response to bioaerosols.[32] Acute exposure to high levels of aerosolized bacterial endotoxin, as encountered in many occupational settings, can lead to both respiratory and systemic symptoms, including chest pain, shortness of breath, decrements in lung function, chills, and fever.[33] Repeated occupational exposure to endotoxin-contaminated bioaerosols can result in chronic loss of lung function.[34] In fact, in subjects with exposure to cotton dust, the severity of airflow obstruction is more closely associated with levels of endotoxin exposure than levels of cotton dust exposure.[25]

These findings support that inhaled endotoxin can contribute to the development of both acute and chronic human lung disease. It remains plausible that other microbial products are as ubiquitous as endotoxin. However, these microbial products have not been as widely examined as the assays used to measure their concentrations are generally less sensitive. The environmental levels at which individual microbial products can impact human lung disease remain unknown.

3.3.2 Murine studies with toll-like receptors in environmental airways disease

Using a variety of animal models, TLR4 has been recognized as a critical component in the pathogenesis of LPS-induced lung inflammation which may contribute to acute lung injury, respiratory distress syndrome, and airways disease. It has long been recognized that the C3H/HeJ mouse is unresponsive to LPS. This phenotype was associated with functional mutations in TLR4.[7, 8] The genetically engineered TLR4-deficient mouse confirmed the essential role of TLR4 in the response to LPS.[35] Inhaled aerosols of endotoxin have many features common in occupational lung disease, including neutrophil infiltration, cytokine production, airway hyperreactivity, vascular endothelial and alveolar epithelial injury caused protein leakage. The role of TLR4 in acute response to aerosolized endotoxin has been confirmed in both the C3H/HeJ[36] and TLR4-deficient[37] mouse. Repeated exposure to endotoxin can results in persistent changes to the airway that include sub-epithelial remodeling.[29, 38] These findings support that TLR4 plays a central role in the biological response to clinically relevant levels of endotoxin in bioaerosols.

Recent evidence supports that the level of TLR4 expression is directly related to the functional response to a given level of endotoxin. A gene dosage response relationship between LPS exposure and lung inflammation was established using TLR4-transgenic mice expressing variable copy numbers of TLR4.[39] Higher copy numbers of TLR4 were associated with enhanced response to LPS. These observations support that TLR4 is a key regulator of LPS-induced lung disease. Furthermore, both the dose of endotoxin and level of TLR4 expression can regulate the intensity of the innate immune response mounted by the host. Additionally, genes other than TLR4 modify the response to LPS. For example, mice with normal genomic TLR4 have variable responses to LPS.[40] These findings support a complex relationship between host genetics and environmental challenges. Furthermore, this relationship suggests that the level of environmental exposure should be considered when determining the role of genes of innate immunity in pulmonary diseases.

3.3.3 Human studies of inhaled LPS and toll-like receptors

Human exposure to inhaled endotoxin has been most extensively studied in the context of occupational lung disease, where repeated exposures can lead to chronic bronchitis, emphysema, and occupational asthma. Experimental findings with humans are consistent with these epidemiological observations, and further demonstrate that the clinical and biological consequences of endotoxin inhalation depend on the length of the exposure.[41, 42] A single exposure to inhaled endotoxin, which activates signaling through TLR4, results in symptoms including fever, cough, and dyspnea,[27, 36, 43, 44] neutrophilic inflammation, production of pro-inflammatory cytokines, and the development of airway hyperresponsiveness that commences within minutes of challenge and can persist for up to 48 hours.[45] However, it has been widely observed that the individual response to inhaled LPS is highly variable.[45] This phenomenon strongly suggests a role of genetic background on the regulation of host susceptibility. This observation led to the initial discovery of functional polymorphisms of TLR4 (Asp299Gly) in humans which is associated with diminished airway response to short-term exposure to aerosolized endotoxin.[9, 46] While this observation in the lung has been replicated in several cohorts, the functional implications of these common polymorphisms in PBMC remain unclear.[47] However, recent advances support the observation that both minor alleles of TLR4 (Asp299Gly and Thr399lle) lead to changes of protein structure that affect the translocation of TLR4 receptor from cytoplasm to cell surface membrane.[48] Therefore, minor alleles of TLR4 (Asp299Gly and Thr399lle) could influence binding with ligands or co-receptors through altering the structure of the binding site. Accordingly, we speculate that the effects of these common polymorphisms will have cell-type specific and tissue specific responses to ligands. Future studies are warranted to clarify the functional implications of common and uncommon variants of TLR4 in human disease. However, current evidence supports that TLR4s play a central role in pulmonary response to inhaled endotoxin.

3.4 Microbial contamination of aerosolized biomass

Inhalation of bacterial or microbial products is common in both outdoor and indoor air pollutants. For example, endotoxin is ubiquitous in the environment. Detectable levels of endotoxin have been detected in dust from the home environment, tobacco smoke, indoor ventilation systems, particulate matter in air pollution, and in a wide variety of workplace environments.[27, 43, 49–54] There is currently no evidence supporting the suggestion that toll-like receptors can directly bind aerosolized biomass. However, aerosolized solid matter frequently contains biologically significant amounts of endotoxin,[53, 55] suggesting that part of the inflammatory response to this environmental pollutant might be due to this organic content. *In vitro*, low levels of microbial products within particulate matter contribute to the inflammatory response, which appears to be TLR-dependent.[50, 56] Thus, the primary mechanism of TLR-dependent signaling following exposure to inhaled particulate air pollutants is likely related to contamination with biologic material.

Particulate matter (PM) is a heterogeneous mixture of small airborne particles commonly found in urban environments. The health effect of particulate matter is widely divergent and appears to be dependent on the chemical content. Exposure to particulate matter leads to pulmonary inflammation[57, 58] and increased all-cause mortality.[59] It is clear that transition metal contents or an insoluble core of PM contributes to inflammatory reactions in epithelial and macrophage cells by inducing intracellular oxidative stress. However, recent evidence suggests that microbial products bound to the surface of PM can also contribute to the inflammatory response. These conclusions are based on *in vitro* studies, in which LBP and polymixin B were used to demonstrate reduced inflammation due to the blocking of LPS effects. Rodent studies further support that the level of endotoxin, but not soluble metals, can contribute to the pulmonary inflammatory response.[60] In fact, pure particle fractions such as silica, volcanic ash and residual oil fly ash, do not stimulate human alveolar macrophages to produce pro-inflammatory cytokines, whereas when mixed with environmental relevant numbers of dead bacteria they induced significant cytokine production which is TLR4 mediated.[50, 61] Although it is difficult to directly compare PM studies due to variable metal compositions, there is good evidence to suggest that bacterial contamination can contribute to the biologic activity of these common outdoor air pollutants.

Dust is a common source of indoor air pollution and can also be contaminated with immunostimulatory microbial products. Air sampling of homes and offices reveals gram-positive bacteria, gram-negative bacteria, and fungal products.[62] Generally, the number and level of airborne gram-negative bacteria and endotoxin is much lower in homes than the workplace. However, home exposure to endotoxin can contribute to the severity of airways disease.[30] The role of TLR4 with house dust appears to extend beyond bacterial endotoxin exposure. This is supported by studies where cultured bone marrow-derived dendritic cells were stimulated with house dust extract. House dust extract induced pro-inflammatory cytokines and expression of co-stimulatory molecules. Interestingly, immunostimmulatory properties of dust extract were dependent on TLR4/MyD88 and independent from endotoxin content.[63] This finding suggests that environmental factors, in addition to endotoxin, may contribute to the biological effects of house dust. Clearer understandings of the environmental factors which can interact with pattern recognition receptors are required and are not limited to bacterial endotoxin.

3.5 The role of toll-like receptors in sterile lung injury

There is a growing body of literature supporting the role of toll-like receptors in sterile lung injury. Pattern recognition receptors were initially identified to recognize pathogen-associated molecular patterns. However, the role of pattern recognition receptors now extends beyond recognition of microbial products. There is now evidence that pattern recognition receptors can contribute to the pulmonary response after exposure to ozone, hyperoxia, and bleomycin. These findings are consistent with a growing body of literature suggesting that pattern recognition receptors can contribute to the host response to non-infectious tissue injury.

3.5.1 Ozone and pattern recognition receptors

Ozone is a commonly encountered urban air pollutant that significantly contributes to increased morbidity in human populations.[64–67] This gaseous air pollutant has an extremely short half-life with rapid conversion to a number of reactive oxygen species that react with cellular proteins and lipids. It has been estimated that each year strict adherence to the established eight-hour ozone standard would result in reductions of 800 premature deaths, 4,500 hospital admissions, 900,000 school absences, and more than 1 million restricted activity days with an estimated $5 billion annual economic burden.[68] Recent estimates support that for each 10-ppb increase in one-hour daily maximum of ozone there is an increase in mortality between 0.39 and 0.87 percent.[65, 66, 69, 70] Experimental exposures to ambient ozone are clinically relevant and occur in the absence of contamination of any microbial product.

The discovery that the pattern recognition receptor, TLR4, plays a role in airway injury in response to ozone was made through fine mapping of a QTL and characterization of the C3H/HeJ mouse.[71, 72] Subsequently, O_3-induced airway hyperresponsiveness was identified to be dependent on both TLR4[37] and MyD88.[73] Furthermore, previous work suggests that the biologic response to ozone is, in part, dependent on the downstream signal and the transcription regulator, NF-kB p50.[74, 75] Based on these observations, it is plausible that TLR4-dependent signaling can lead to

MyD88-dependent activation of NF-kB and transcription of downstream pro-inflammatory factors leading to the response to ambient ozone. However, the TLR4-ligand, which contributes to the biological response to ozone, remains unknown. It is known that ozonolysis products (eicosanoid release and generation of peroxyl radicals) of epithelial membrane fatty acids can function as early transducers of ozone reactions at the epithelial surface.[76] Lipid ozonation products (hydrogen peroxide and aldehydes) have been suggested to act as signal transduction molecules in both the lung and extrapulmonary tissues.[77, 78] These observations suggest that ozone could modify lipid products and modify subsequent systemic innate immune response. However, the mechanisms, which link the biologic response to ozone and innate immunity, remain poorly understood.

In addition to the pattern recognition receptor TLR4, recent work supports the role of a macrophage scavenger receptor in response to ambient ozone. *Marco* (macrophage receptor with collagenous structure) was highly upregulated in lungs of C3H/HeJ (TLR4-mutant mice) after exposure to ozone and found to be functionally important. This scavenger receptor contributes to clearance of pro-inflammatory oxidized lipids.[79] These findings suggest TLR4-deficiency is associated with enhanced scavenger receptor-dependent clearance of oxidized lipids. Together, these observations support an important role of toll-like receptors and scavenger receptors in the response to ambient ozone. Cumulatively, these data strongly support that the complete response to ozone is dependent on many components of the innate immune system.

3.5.2 Hyperoxia and toll-like receptor 4

Exposure to high levels of oxygen (hyperoxia) is common in critically ill patients and can be associated with the development of acute lung injury (ALI). Prolonged exposure to hyperoxia results in the local generation of reactive oxygen species, which can lead to damage of viable tissue. Consistent with the hypothesis that pattern recognition receptors can recognize non-infectious tissue injury and modify oxidant stress, previous work supports a role for toll-like receptor 4 in response to hyperoxia-induced lung injury. The severity of hyperoxia-induced lung injury is dependent on the intensity of exposure and genetic background. Previous work supports that the C3H/HeJ (TLR4-mutant) strain of mice is relatively *resistant* to the effects of hyperoxia when compared to other congenic strains of mice.[80, 81] However, studies using the BXH recombinant inbred strain (C3H/HeJ x C57BL/6) of mice demonstrate that part of the protective effects observed in the C3H/HeJ mouse are resultant from differences in the transcription factor *Nrf2* (nuclear factor related factor 2),[82] which play an essential role in antioxidant stress.[83, 84] Studies directly comparing C3H/HeJ (TLR4-mutant) and C3H/HeN (TLR4-wild type) suggest that TLR4-defınciency can be protective when mice are exposed to 80 percent oxygen.[85] However, it remains conceivable that other strain-dependent genetic differences could exist between these two congenic mouse strains accounting for the observed differences. Studies using genetically modified animals (TLR4-/-) exposed to hyperoxia (100% oxygen) are remarkably consistent. Interestingly, these studies suggest that TLR4 confers *protection* against hyperoxic lung injury. Specifically, TLR4-deficient animals increased lung injury, apoptosis, and mortality.[86] Similarly, transgenic mice with inducible expression of TLR4 are protected against lung injury, apoptosis, and mortality.[87] Each of these effects appears dependent on TLR4-dependent activation of heme oxygenase-1 and Bcl-2. However, the role of TLR4 signaling remains less clear with lower levels of oxidant stress.[88] These observations suggest that toll-like receptor signaling can provide host anti-oxidant protection under certain environmental conditions.

3.5.3 Bleomycin lung injury and toll-like receptors

The role of pattern recognition receptors in sterile lung injury has been observed with bleomycin lung injury. While bleomycin is not an environmental toxicant, the mechanism of bleomycin-induced lung injury has similarities with other environmental exposures. Bleomycin injures cells through DNA damage and cellular injury through the formation of reactive oxygen species and lipid peroxidation. Recent work demonstrates a role of TLR2 and TLR4 in bleomycin-induced lung injury.[89] In this study, findings suggest that the gylcosaminoglycan, hyaluronan, can function as an endogenous ligand to these toll-like receptors. Specifically, bleomycin injury leads to the formation of immuno-stimulatory short fragments of hyaluronan. These fragments appear to interact with toll-like receptors on alveolar macrophages contributing to chemokine production and possibly neutrophil recruitment into the airspace.[89] In this model, TLR2 and TLR4 are also protective to the severity of lung injury, interstitial inflammation, and cellular apoptosis. This apparent paradox in compartmentalized TLR-dependent response remains an area of considerable interest. However, the role of ROS-dependent fragmentation of hyaluronan and inflammatory cell recruitment into the airspace is also supported in a model of asbestos-induced lung injury.[90] It remains unclear whether these pattern recognition receptors play a role in tissue repair and fibrosis of the lung after oxidative lung injury as a result of inhaled toxicants. However, recent evidence from a murine model of scleroderma utilizing subcutaneous injection of bleomycin supports that hyaluronan can stimulate B-cells to produce pro-fibrogenic cytokines, mainly through TLR4, which the authors speculate could contribute to the development of fibrosis in both the skin and lung.[91] These data further support a role of toll-like receptors in oxidative lung injury and suggest a possible role in pulmonary fibrosis. However, the precise mechanisms which confer TLR-dependent protection during oxidative stress remain unclear.

3.5.4 Lung injury and endogenous ligands of toll-like receptors

There is a growing evidence to support the role of endogenous ligands of toll-like receptors. This specific response of the innate immune system to tissue injury is believed to be a conserved mechanism to limit tissue injury. The successful repair of tissue injury requires a precise and well-coordinated response by the host. The endogenous danger signal can, in part, be attributed to "danger-associated molecular patterns" or "DAMPs". These factors are released during tissue injury and believed to be recognized by pattern recognition receptors. While the study of endogenous ligands of toll-like receptors is challenging resultant from the ubiquitous nature of microbial contamination of reagents,[92] many lines of evidence support the role of toll-like receptors in non-infectious tissue injury and suggest an important role of endogenous ligands in this context. Collectively, these data suggest that the innate immune system has evolved to recognize "danger signals" generated by the host during tissue injury.[93]

Putative endogenous ligands of toll-like receptors are generally derived from damaged cells or the cellular response to stress. Endogenous pro-inflammatory factors, which have been implicated in TLR-dependent signaling include mRNA,[94] fibrinogen,[95] and surfactant protein A,[96] several heat shock proteins (hsp60, hsp70, gp96),[97-99] β-defensin 2,[100] high-mobility group box 1 protein (HMGB1),[101] myeloid-related protein-8 and 14,[102] hyaluronan,[103, 104] heparan sulfate,[105] and fibronectin extra domain A.[106] However, many previous studies did not directly measure the level of endotoxin contamination and did not consider the possibility of contamination by other microbial products. For example, in the case of heat shock proteins, subsequent studies using LPS-free preparations suggest that previous reports may be the result of bacterial contamination.[107–110] Despite the controversy surrounding initial reports of endogenous ligands of pattern recognition receptors, several models of non-infectious tissue injury, as outlined, support the role of endogenous danger-associated molecular patterns in host-innate immune response to tissue injury and repair. Future studies of non-infectious tissue injury are warranted to better understand the role of putative endogenous ligands and pattern recognition receptors in host response to common environmental insults.

3.6 Toll-like receptor 4 and other human lung diseases

3.6.1 Emphysema and toll-like receptors

Emphysema is a component of chronic obstructive pulmonary disease (COPD), which is characterized by enlarged airspaces, destruction of alveolar walls and capillaries surrounding the alveoli, and inflammatory cell infiltration in airway and parenchyma. The mechanisms of pathogenesis of emphysema include genetic factors, inflammatory injury, and oxidative stress. A recent human study suggests that TLR4 could be an important host factor contributing to the development of emphysema. In humans, the TLR4 (Asp299Gly) minor allele was associated with protection from COPD.[111] Particularly interesting in that study was that among the 24 non-smoking COPD patients, the TLR4 (Asp299Gly) minor allele was not detected. This observation suggests that TLR4-signaling could contribute to the development of COPD, and might be related to environmental factors other than tobacco smoke. This association was not observed in an earlier cohort of subjects with COPD.[112] However, the TLR4 (Asp299Gly) minor allele is associated with diminished response to LPS in the lung (9). Given the increased prevalence of bacterial infection in the lungs of patients with COPD, the authors suggest that TLR4-mediated inflammatory response to bacterial colonization might contribute to the pathogenesis of COPD. This speculation is supported by recent animal studies. Chronic exposure to inhaled LPS contributes to airspace enlargement in a murine model, which appears dependent on neutrophilic inflammation.[113] Interestingly, cigarette smoking also induces neutrophilic inflammation in the lung dependent on the TLR4/MyD88 signaling pathway but independent of LPS.[114] Cigarette-smoke condensate has also been shown to induce TLR4-dependent pro-inflammatory response in both murine macrophages and human monocytes.[115] These data suggest that both exogenous and endogenous ligands of toll-like receptors can contribute to the pathogenesis of emphysema.

Seemingly in contrast, spontaneous emphysema has recently been reported in TLR4-deficient mice at three months of age.[116] TLR4-deficient mice exhibit both increased oxidant burden and decreased antioxidant capacity. Through upregulating NOX3 expression, TLR4-deficiency results in increased production of reactive oxygen species and elastolytic activity in the lung and endothelial cells. This observation suggested that TLR4 plays a key role for lung homeostasis by maintaining oxidant/antioxidant balance under normal conditions. Nonetheless, it is not always the case that increased ROS generation leads to emphysema change. For example, $p47^{phox}$ and $gp91^{phox}$ deficient mice with reduced ROS production are more susceptible to cigarette smoke-induced lung inflammation and emphysema.[117] In those mice, cigarette smoke exposure significantly increased TLR4 mRNA expression and augmented TLR4-mediated signal transduction, which was ROS independent. Therefore, depending on both host factors and environmental conditions, the role of TLR4 in the development of airspace enlargement may prove divergent. It remains plausible that a low level TLR4-dependent signal is protective while a high level of TLR4-signal is harmful to the lung parenchyma.

In addition, it has been observed that lung infection during a vulnerable period of neonatal lung development could contribute to airspace enlargement. It has been appreciated that the C3H/HeJ (TLR4-mutant) strain of mouse is predisposed to airspace enlargement.[118] TLR4-deficiency is also associated with predisposition to gram-negative bacterial infections. Consistently, C3H/HeJ mice were found carrying higher bacterial colonization at seven days old and enlarged alveolar spaces developed 14 days later.[119] This observation suggests that TLR4-deficiency may predispose to neonatal opportunistic microbial infections leading to enhanced TLR4-independent inflammation in the lung and associated airspace enlargement later in life. It remains unclear whether the antioxidant properties of TLR4-signaling are a direct effect on lung parenchyma or a secondary effect resultant from more effective neonatal bacterial clearance during a vulnerable period of lung development.

These observations again suggest that the role of toll-like receptors in the pathogenesis of lung disease must be considered in context of environmental exposures. The detrimental role of toll-like receptor signaling is suggested in an association study of subjects with COPD and an animal model of occupational lung disease related to high levels of endotoxin exposure. However, it appears that in the absence of toxicant exposure the presence of toll-like receptor-signaling can be protective. Clear understanding of the role of pattern recognition receptors in the pathogenesis of emphysema will require careful analysis of both host genetics and relevant environmental conditions.

3.7 Allergic airways disease and toll-like receptors

The role of endotoxin and toll-like receptors in allergic airways disease initially appears highly contradictory. It is increasingly evident that the role of innate immunity in allergic asthma must be carefully considered in the context of environmental exposures. For example, endotoxin has been reported to both exacerbate allergic asthma and diminish its incidence. Consideration of both the timing and level of exposure to endotoxin can provide some insight into this apparent paradox. To better understand the role of innate immunity in allergic airways disease, we divide current studies by the context of exposure. Current evidence supports that pattern recognition receptors do indeed play a fundamental role in development and progression of allergic airways disease. While it is likely that many microbial products and pattern recognition receptors contribute to asthma, we focus this discussion on the evidence supporting a potential role of endotoxin and TLR4 on this complex disease.

Multiple epidemiologic studies support that exposure to TLR ligands can be protective against development of allergic asthma. This general observation is commonly referred to as the "*hygiene hypothesis*". This hypothesis is supported by several epidemiological observations: individuals living on farms have a reduced risk of developing hay fever or asthma;[(120–122)] episodes of fever early in life affect the natural history of asthma by preventing the development of atopy;[(123)] the risk of developing asthma is decreased with increased numbers of siblings;[(124)] and levels of endotoxin in the bedding of school-aged children are inversely proportional to the incidence of hay fever and atopic asthma.[(125)] Consistent with this hypothesis, some studies support that asthmatic individuals bearing the Asp299Gly minor allele of TLR4, associated with *reduced* function, have an *increased* severity of atopy[(126)] and an *increased* incidence of atopic asthma.[(127)] Consistent with these observations, rodent models of prolonged antigen challenge demonstrate that low doses of endotoxin can suppress allergic inflammation in both mice[(128–131)] and rats.[(132–135)] Similar suppression of allergic inflammation in murine models has been observed with ligands of TLR2,[(136, 137)] TLR9,[(138)] and ligands of TLR4 other than endotoxin.[(139)] The suppression of experimental allergic airways disease by chronic low doses of TLR ligands is consistent with the hygiene hypothesis. While the mechanisms of TLR4-dependent suppression of allergic inflammation remain unknown, recent evidence supports TLR2-ligands can both enhance proliferation of T-regulatory cells and suppress the function of T-regulatory cells during tonic stimulation.[140] Each of these findings suggests that very low-level exposure to TLR-ligands can be protective in the development of allergic asthma.

Seemingly in contrast, endotoxin has been reported to enhance allergic asthma through either adjuvant activity during antigen sensitization or exacerbating pre-existing airways disease. Murine studies support the theory that endotoxin-free antigen alone cannot sensitize mice. However, when mixed with small amounts of endotoxin, antigen acquires immunogenic properties dependent on the presence of TLR4.[141] Interestingly, if higher concentrations of LPS are added to antigen in this method of sensitization, increased numbers of neutrophils are seen in the inflammatory infiltrate following antigen challenge.[141] It is known that severe asthmatics can present with relatively high numbers of neutrophils in the airways,[142] which could be the result of inhalation of environmental toxins. In some subjects with documented dust mite allergy, the level of endotoxin in the home environment was more closely related to exacerbations of asthma and wheeze than the levels of specific antigen.[143–145] These findings suggest that higher levels of endotoxin could contribute to exacerbations of pre-existing disease. Indeed, animal models of exposure to moderate levels of TLR-ligands increase the severity allergic response when the period of challenge is relatively short.[141, 146–148] While the mechanism of this response remains unclear, recruitment of Th2 cells into the lung associated with endotoxin exposure can occur independent of a specific allergic antigen.[148] Consistent with these observations, a study of asthma specifically associated with endotoxin in house dust showed that people with the TLR4 (Asp299Gly) minor allele had a decreased risk of airway hyperreactivity.[149] Human studies with moderate levels of endotoxin have revealed that endotoxin, and its receptor, TLR4, can be associated with exacerbations of allergic asthma.[144, 150–152]

Given the opposing effects of endotoxin, it is perhaps not unexpected that some studies have not revealed an effect of the common TLR4 (Asp299Gly) minor allele on the overall incidence of asthma.[149, 153, 154] Recent work supports the need to consider level of environmental exposure when evaluating genes of innate immunity. For example, polymorphisms of the accessory molecule CD14 are associated with increased levels of soluble CD14 and an enhanced biological response to endotoxin. Polymorphisms of CD14 have been associated with both a decrease in total serum IgE in asthmatic children with low-level exposure[155] and a decrease in lung function among endotoxin exposed farmers with high-level exposure.[156] The observation among children is consistent with the hygiene hypothesis with attenuation of allergic symptoms with enhanced response to LPS. The enhanced biologic response among farmers with exposure to high levels of occupational LPS would be expected to demonstrate decreased lung function, as was observed. When the level of LPS exposure in the home is considered, the effect of CD14 is remarkably consistent.[157, 158] In subjects exposed to low concentrations of LPS, the T allele for CD14/-159 (associated with increased soluble CD14) was protective. However, at high concentrations of LPS exposure the opposite was observed. These studies highlight the importance of gene–environment interactions when evaluating a complex disease such as allergic asthma.

The association between airway disease and activation of the innate immune system is not limited to TLR4/CD14. Signaling through TLR9 can suppress the development of atopic airway disease and can reverse established eosinophilic inflammation.[159] TLR9-agonists consistently attenuate multiple components of the allergic phenotype including eosinophilic airway inflammation, serum IgE, T_H2 cytokines, airway hyperresponsiveness, sub-epithelial fibrosis, and goblet cell metaplasia.[138, 160–166] Given the central role of innate immunity in the development and progression of allergic airways disease, modification of TLR-signaling could have important future therapeutic implications for human allergic disease.[167]

3.8 Transplantation and pattern recognition receptors

Historically, adaptive immunity has been the main focus of transplantation immunology and the primary therapeutic target of post-transplant immunosuppression, while innate immunity was simply considered a first line of defense against invasive pathogens. However, this paradigm of adaptive immunity as the driving force in allograft rejection has been modified in recent years by the recognition of innate-adaptive immune cross-talk.[168] Recent observations suggest that innate immune activation informs adaptive immune responses by influencing antigen presenting cell maturation,[6] regulatory T-cell activation, and effector cell function.[169] Furthermore, the spectrum of innate immune ligands is now recognized to include endogenous "danger-associated" molecular patterns,[93] which can be released in non-infectious tissue damage. These observations provide us with new insight into potential mechanisms associated with the pathogenesis of allograft rejection.

Dysregulation of innate immunity is evident early in many organ transplants and could contribute to acute allograft rejection. Cadaveric solid organ transplants require significant cold ischemic time for the allograft, and for more than 15 percent of lung allografts cold ischemic time lasts for more than six hours.[170] Ischemia-reperfusion (I/R) injury induces the release of endogenous innate immune ligands such as hyaluronan, HMGB1, and biglycan.[171–173] I/R also leads to upregulation of innate immune receptors such as TLR4.[173] Thus, increased TLR4 reactivity is found after ischemic injury in many examined organs such as lung, liver and spleen.[174] In human lung allografts, TLR4 expression correlates positively with levels of inflammatory cytokines both before and after reperfusion.[174] In animal models, TLR4 signaling is required for both "warm" I/R injury in liver[175] and kidney,[173] but also in "cold" I/R in a murine liver transplantation model.[176] Finally, early inflammation after solid organ transplantation presents with cellular infiltration, cytokine release and chemokine receptor expression that are independent of adaptive immunity.[177] Interestingly, pre-treatment of heart, kidney or liver with moderate doses of endogenous or exogenous innate immune ligands confers protection from I/R injury,[178–180] although it is unclear what the mechanism of this action is, and whether this "preconditioning" translates into protection from later rejection as well. Collectively these data suggest that innate immunity is both activated by and necessary for the development of I/R injury, which is a major cause of early graft dysfunction in lung transplantation.

Several recent studies have addressed the role of innate immunity in chronic tissue allograft rejection. Goldstein et al. investigated the effect of deficiency in TLR2, TLR4, or their adaptor molecule MyD88 in minor-antigen mismatched skin transplantation. These investigators found that MyD88, but not TLR2 or TLR4 alone, is necessary for the rejection of minor antigen-incompatible grafts in a murine model of skin rejection. MyD88 deficient mice had impaired accumulation of dendritic cells in draining lymph nodes, diminished graft-reactive CD8+ T cells in the spleen and generally reduced Th1 immunity (assessed by IFN-γ gene expression), but intact Th2 immunity (assessed by IL-4 gene expression) MyD88 presence in either donor or recipient was sufficient to reproduce the rejection phenotype.[181] MyD88 seems to contribute to a lesser extent in the alloimmune response to major antigen-mismatched cardiac and skin grafts.[182] The ligand which ultimately requires MyD88 signaling is unknown, but hyaluronan may be a strong candidate molecule. Indeed, hyaluronan was recently shown to be released in tissue injury, and it requires MyD88 and both TLR2 and TLR4 to unfold its cell-protective effect.[89] Hyaluronan was also found to be elevated in skin allografts in a murine transplant model, as well as in the lavage fluid of patients with obliterative bronchiolitis after lung transplantation.[183] Furthermore, stimulation of dendritic cells with low molecular weight hyaluronan fragments leads to dendritic cell maturation, MyD88-dependent production of TNF-alpha, and MyD88-independent but TIRAP-dependent upregulation of co-stimulatory molecules like CD40, CD86, and CCR7.[183] Collectively, these data suggest that endogenous innate immune ligands, like hyaluronan, may be an important trigger of alloimmune tissue injury in transplantation.

Human research data also support the role of innate immunity in the pathogenesis of transplant rejection. Functional genetic polymorphisms in pattern recognition receptors may underlie individual susceptibility to lung transplant rejection. For example, lung transplant recipients bearing the TLR4 Asp299Gly or the Thr399Ile minor alleles, which render patients hypo-responsive to TLR4 activation,[9] had significantly reduced severity, frequency, and onset of both acute and chronic rejection compared with transplant recipients bearing the major allele.[184, 185] On the contrary, patients with a common promoter polymorphism of CD14 (CD14-159 TT), which is associated with enhanced innate immune response, demonstrate earlier onset of acute and chronic rejection and decreased graft survival.[186] The mechanism underlying these associations has been investigated in a murine model of alloimmune lung injury, where inhaled endotoxin induced adaptive immune activation and lymphocytic bronchiolitis, without evidence of systemic alloimmunity.[187] Furthermore, in a rat model of primary graft dysfunction induced by autoimmune activation against collagen (V), CD14+ cells were necessary for the induction of hypersensitivity to ColV that leads to primary graft dysfunction.[188] Cumulatively, these findings suggest an important role of both TLR4/CD14 in pulmonary allograft rejection.

A less well-studied family of innate immune receptors are the defensins, which bind and permeabilize lipid bilayers of bacterial walls, and mannose-binding lectin, which is part of the lectin complement pathway. Human α-defensins are also known as human neutrophil peptides (HNP). In an analysis of lavage fluid from 101 lung transplant recipients, higher levels of HNP were reported in lung transplant recipients compared to normal controls. Furthermore, high levels of HNP beyond the initial post-transplant period predicted early development of chronic rejection.[189] Human β defensins can activate the adaptive immune system through chemokine CCR6 and act as a ligand for TLR4 receptors.[100, 190] Human β defensin type 2 was found to be elevated in patients with chronic lung allograft rejection.[191] Mannose-binding lectin is involved in complement activation and complement-dependent inflammation in kidney and heart I/R injury.[192] Furthermore, high mannose-binding lectin plasma levels are associated with decreased graft survival in kidney transplant recipients.[193] Complement deposition in endothelial walls is observed in humoral lung rejection[194] and deposition in bronchial walls was seen in patients with chronic rejection.[195] These observations suggest that many pattern recognition receptors contribute to the pathogenesis of allograft rejection.

In conclusion, innate immunity is increasingly recognized as an important contributor in the host response to solid organ allograft. The role of innate immunity in lung transplantation is complex and involves bi-directional adaptive-innate immune cross-talk. Pattern recognition receptors appear to contribute to ischemia/reperfusion injury, acute rejection, and chronic rejection. Clear understanding of the innate immune mechanisms that contribute to allograft rejection could lead to novel therapeutic approaches and improve patient survival.

3.9 Environmental co-exposures and pattern recognition receptors

The lung is continuously exposed to a variety of environmental toxicants. While the role of pattern recognition receptors in response to specific toxicants can be effectively studied in experimental models, it is also important to understand that co-exposure to environmental factors can have a profound impact on host immunologic response. The effect of each toxicant in modifying subsequent host innate immunity can be not only dependent on the specific toxicant, but also appears dependent on the timing, dose, and duration of each exposure. Additionally, specific toxicants can have divergent effects on each cell type in the lung. Each of these factors needs to be considered when determining the clinical implications of environmental co-exposures. Effective antibacterial host defense requires sufficient activation of pulmonary innate immune response without uncontrolled inflammation and associated tissue injury. Previous epidemiologic and experimental studies demonstrate that exposure to particulate matter, diesel particles, or ozone can impair antibacterial host defense.[64, 196, 197] Considerable evidence suggests that many forms of environmental stress can either enhance or suppress host innate immune response depending on the specific toxicant and context of exposure.

Common inhaled toxicants can modify innate immune response through either altered transcription of pattern recognition receptors or modification of cellular distribution of these receptors. Results from many of these studies have seemingly contradictory results, which are likely the result of experimental conditions or microbial contamination of reagents. For example, exposure to diesel exhaust particles can either down-regulate TLR4 expression [198] and suppress response to LPS [199–201] or up-regulate TLR4 expression and enhance response to LPS. [202] Similar discordant results exist for particulate matter. For example, both combustion source particulate matter and nanoparticles can enhance TLR4 protein in the lung [203] and functional response to bacterial endotoxin. [204, 205] Seemingly in contrast, both coarse and fine ambient air particulate matter can decrease the expression of TLR4 on macrophages and the functional response to LPS. [61] These observed differences could certainly be related to the biochemical content of toxicants used in each experimental model. Becker et al. suggest that low levels of microbial contamination could contribute to the divergent biological effects of toll-like receptor ligands observed after pre-exposure to airborne particulate matter. [50, 61] To further complicate the situation, recent evidence now suggests that TLR4 contribute to the response to diesel exhaust particles [206] and TLR2 may contribute to the response to particulate matter. [61] Cumulatively, these observations suggest that the biological response to complex airborne particulate matter may be, in part, dependent on pattern recognition receptors and that exposure to particulate matter can modify the subsequent functional response to toll-like receptor ligands.

The effects of ambient ozone on pulmonary innate immune response are also seemingly contradictory. Experimental studies using ozone demonstrate that ozone can either enhance [207] or suppress [208] response to LPS. When evaluating the effects of ozone immediately after exposure, the response to LPS was suppressed [208] despite an elevated TLR4 mRNA message. [209] However, this observation is consistent with the known immediate cytotoxic effects of ozone on airway epithelia in the context of the central role of airway epithelia in response to LPS. [210] By 24 hours after ozone exposure, the response to LPS was enhanced but without detectible differences in mRNA expression of TLR4. However, ozone altered the distribution of TLR4 on macrophages, which was associated with an enhanced functional response to LPS. [207] Similar effects on trafficking of toll-like receptors have been observed in macrophages after hemorrhagic shock. [211] Recent human data suggest that ozone exposure can also enhance surface expression of the TLR4 co-receptor CD14 on airway macrophages and monocytes,[212] which would be expected to modify the functional response to LPS.

The lung is continuously exposed to a variety of inhaled toxicants. To better understand the clinically relevant effects of common environmental exposures, careful consideration of the effects of co-exposure is required. The effects of inhaled environmental toxicants are dependent on the dose and duration of exposure, as well as the timing after exposure. Studies of environmental co-exposures provide important insight into the pathogenesis of human disease and the role of pattern recognition receptors in response to common inhaled toxicants.

3.10 Conclusion

TLR-dependent signaling in the lung appears to be a double-edged sword. Precise regulation of the TLR-dependent signal is required to optimize normal inflammatory response, antibacterial host defense, and resolution of injury. While effective innate immune response is critical for effective clearance of microbial pathogens, an exaggerated response can be associated with increased tissue injury and disease progression. Tight regulation of the inflammatory response to infection or tissue injury is required to maintain tissue homeostasis. Low-level activation of toll-like receptor signaling is required to protect against infection and possibly resolution of tissue injury. High-level activation of toll-like receptors can result in uncontrolled tissue injury or cellular death. Dysregulation of host innate immunity in either direction appears to contribute to the pathogenesis of many common pulmonary diseases. The host response after some inhaled toxicant exposures is dependent on toll-like receptors and growing evidence supports the theory that common environmental exposures can also modify host innate immunity. If we are to gain a better understanding of the pathogenesis of common inflammatory lung diseases, we need a more detailed understanding of the complex interaction between common environmental exposures and fundamental homeostatic mechanisms which regulate host innate immunity.

Acknowledgements

JWH gratefully receives support from the National Heart Lung and Blood Institute (HL91335) and the National Institute of Environmental Health Sciences (ES011961, ES016126). SG is supported through the

Intramural Research Program, National Institute of Environmental Health Sciences.

References

1 Goldstein, J.L., Ho, Y.K., Basu, S.K., and Brown, M.S. 1979. Binding site on macrophages that mediates uptake and degradation of acetylated low density lipoprotein, producing massive cholesterol deposition. *Proc Natl Acad Sci USA* 76: 333–337.

2 Kodama, T., Freeman, M., Rohrer, L., Zabrecky, J., Matsudaira, P., and Krieger, M. 1990. Type I macrophage scavenger receptor contains alpha-helical and collagen-like coiled coils. *Nature* 343: 531–535.

3 Janeway, C.A., Jr. 1992. The immune system evolved to discriminate infectious nonself from noninfectious self. *Immunol Today* 13: 11–16.

4 Anderson, K.V., Jurgens, G., and Nusslein-Volhard, C. 1985. Establishment of dorsal-ventral polarity in the Drosophila embryo: genetic studies on the role of the Toll gene product. *Cell* 42: 779–789.

5 Lemaitre, B., Nicolas, E., Michaut, L., Reichhart, J.M., and Hoffmann, J.A. 1996. The dorsoventral regulatory gene cassette *spatzle/Toll/cactus* controls the potent antifungal response in Drosophila adults. *Cell* 86: 973–983.

6 Medzhitov, R., Preston-Hurlburt, P., and Janeway, C.A. 1997. A human homologue of the *Drosophila* Toll protein signals activation of adaptive immunity. *Nature* 388: 394–397.

7 Poltorak, A., He, X., Smirnova, I., Liu, M.-Y., Van Huffel, C., Du, X., Birdwell, D., Alejos, E., Silva, M., Galanos, C., et al. 1998. Defective LPS signaling in C3H/Hej and C57BL/10ScCr mice: mutations in Tlr4 gene. *Science* 282: 2085–2088.

8 Poltorak, A., Smirnova, I., He, X., Liu, M.Y., Van Huffel, C., Birdwell, D., Alejos, E., Silva, M., Du, X., Thompson, P., et al. 1998. Genetic and physical mapping of the *Lps* locus: Identification of the Toll-4 receptor as a candidate gene in the critical region. *Blood Cells, Molecules, and Diseases* 24: 340–355.

9 Arbour, N.C., Lorenz, E., Schutte, B., Zabner, J., Kline, J., Jones, M., Frees, K., Watt, J.L., and Schwartz, D.A. 2000. TLR4 mutations are associated with endotoxin hyporesponsiveness in humans. *Nat Genet* 25: 187–191.

10 Wurfel, M.M., Kunitake, S.T., Lichenstein, H., Kane, J.P., and Wright, S.D. 1994. Lipopolysaccharide (LPS)-binding protein is carried on lipoproteins and acts as a cofactor in the neutralization of LPS. *J Exp Med* 180: 1025–1035.

11 Kitchens, R.L., Thompson, P.A., Viriyakosol, S., O'Keefe, G.E., and Munford, R.S. 2001. Plasma CD14 decreases monocyte responses to LPS by transferring cell-bound LPS to plasma lipoproteins. *J Clin Invest* 108: 485–493.

12 Shimazu, R., Akashi, S., Ogata, H., Nagai, Y., Fukudome, K., Miyake, K., and Kimoto, M. 1999. MD-2, a molecule that confers lipopolysaccharide responsiveness on Toll-like receptor 4. *J Exp Med* 189: 1777–1782.

13 Perera, P.Y., Vogel, S.N., Detore, G.R., Haziot, A., and Goyert, S.M. 1997. CD14-dependent and CD14-independent signaling pathways in murine macrophages from normal and CD14 knockout mice stimulated with lipopolysaccharide or taxol. *J Immunol* 158: 4422–4429.

14 Nagai, Y., Akashi, S., Nagafuku, M., Ogata, M., Iwakura, Y., Akira, S., Kitamura, T., Kosugi, A., Kimoto, M., and Miyake, K. 2002. Essential role of MD-2 in LPS responsiveness and TLR4 distribution. *Nat Immunol* 3: 667–672.
15 Ohnishi, T., Muroi, M., and Tanamoto, K. 2001. N-linked glycosylations at Asn(26) and Asn(114) of human MD-2 are required for toll-like receptor 4mediated activation of NF-kappaB by lipopolysaccharide. *J Immunol* 167: 3354–3359.
16 Kawai, T., Takeuchi, O., Fujita, T., Inoue, J., Muhlradt, P.F., Sato, S., Hoshino, K., and Akira, S. 2001. Lipopolysaccharide stimulates the MyD88-independent pathway and results in activation of IFN-regulatory factor 3 and the expression of a subset of lipopolysaccharide-inducible genes. *J Immunol* 167: 5887–5894.
17 De Trez, C., Pajak, B., Brait, M., Glaichenhaus, N., Urbain, J., Moser, M., Lauvau, G., and Muraille, E. 2005. TLR4 and Toll-IL-1 receptor domain-containing adapter-inducing IFN-beta, but not MyD88, regulate Escherichia coli-induced dendritic cell maturation and apoptosis in vivo. *J Immunol* 175: 839–846.
18 Fitzgerald, K.A., Rowe, D.C., Barnes, B.J., Caffrey, D.R., Visintin, A., Latz, E., Monks, B., Pitha, P.M., and Golenbock, D.T. 2003. LPS-TLR4 signaling to IRF-3/7 and NF-kappaB involves the toll adapters TRAM and TRIF. *J Exp Med* 198: 1043–1055.
19 Madsen, A.M. 2006. Airborne endotoxin in different background environments and seasons. *Ann Agric Environ Med* 13: 81–86.
20 Madsen, A.M. 2006. Exposure to airborne microbial components in autumn and spring during work at Danish biofuel plants. *Ann Occup Hyg* 50: 821–831.
21 Bunger, J., Schappler-Scheele, B., Hilgers, R., and Hallier, E. 2007. A 5-year follow-up study on respiratory disorders and lung function in workers exposed to organic dust from composting plants. *Int Arch Occup Environ Health* 80: 306–312.
22 Schierl, R., Heise, A., Egger, U., Schneider, F., Eichelser, R., Neser, S., and Nowak, D. 2007. Endotoxin concentration in modern animal houses in southern Bavaria. *Ann Agric Environ Med* 14: 129–136.
23 Portengen, L., Preller, L., Tielen, M., Doekes, G., and Heederik, D. 2005. Endotoxin exposure and atopic sensitization in adult pig farmers. *J Allergy Clin Immunol* 115: 797–802.
24 Castellan, R.M., Olenchock, S.A., Hankinson, J.L., Millner, P.D., Cocke, J.B., Bragg, C.K., Perkins, H.H., Jr., and Jacobs, R.R. 1984. Acute bronchoconstriction induced by cotton dust: dose-related responses to endotoxin and other dust factors. *Ann Intern Med* 101: 157–163.
25 Castellan, R.M., Olenchock, S.A., Kinsley, K.B., and Hankinson, J.L. 1987. Inhaled endotoxin and decreased spirometric values. An exposure-response relation for cotton dust. *N Engl J Med* 317: 605–610.
26 Christiani, D.C., Wang, X.R., Pan, L.D., Zhang, H.X., Sun, B.X., Dai, H., Eisen, E.A., Wegman, D.H., and Olenchock, S.A. 2001. Longitudinal changes in pulmonary function and respiratory symptoms in cotton textile workers. A 15-year follow-up study. *Am J Respir Crit Care Med* 163: 847–853.

27 Schwartz, D.A., Thorne, P.S., Yagla, S.J., Burmeister, L.F., Olenchock, S.A., Watt, J.L., and Quinn, T.J. 1995. The role of endotoxin in grain dust-induced lung disease. *Am J Respir Crit Care Med* 152: 603–608.
28 Clapp, W.D., Thorne, P.S., Frees, K.L., Zhang, X., Lux, C.R., and Schwartz, D.A. 1993. The effects of inhalation of grain dust extract and endotoxin on upper and lower airways. *Chest* 104: 825–830.
29 George, C.L., Jin, H., Wohlford-Lenane, C.L., O'Neill, M.E., Phipps, J.C., O'Shaughnessy, P., Kline, J.N., Thorne, P.S., and Schwartz, D.A. 2001. Endotoxin responsiveness and subchronic grain dust-induced airway disease. *Am J Physiol Lung Cell Mol Physiol* 280: L203–213.
30 Thorne, P.S., Kulhankova, K., Yin, M., Cohn, R., Arbes, S.J., Jr., and Zeldin, D.C. 2005. Endotoxin exposure is a risk factor for asthma: the national survey of endotoxin in United States housing. *Am J Respir Crit Care Med* 172: 1371–1377. Epub 2005 Sep 1371.
31 1998. Respiratory health hazards in agriculture. *Am J Respir Crit Care Med* 158: S1–S76.
32 Jagielo, P., Thorne, P., Kern, J., Quinn, T., and Schwartz, D. 1996. Role of endotoxin in grain dust-induced lung inflammation in mice. *Am J Physiol (Lung Cell Mol Physiol)* 270: L1052–L1059.
33 Michel, O., Nagy, A.M., Schroeven, M., Duchateau, J., Neve, J., Fondu, P., and Sergysels, R. 1997. Dose–response relationship to inhaled endotoxin in normal subjects. *Am J Respir Crit Care Med* 156: 1157–1164.
34 Wang, X.R., Zhang, H.X., Sun, B.X., Dai, H.L., Hang, J.Q., Eisen, E.A., Wegman, D.H., Olenchock, S.A., and Christiani, D.C. 2005. A 20-year follow-up study on chronic respiratory effects of exposure to cotton dust. *Eur Respir J* 26: 881–886.
35 Hoshino, K., Takeuchi, O., Kawai, T., Sanjo, H., Ogawa, T., Takeda, Y., Takeda, K., and Akira, S. 1999. Cutting edge: toll-like receptor 4 (TLR4)-deficient mice are hyporesponsive to lipopolysaccharide: evidence for TLR4 as the *Lps* gene product. *J Immunol* 162: 3749–3752.
36 Schwartz, D., Thorne, P., Jagielo, P., White, G., Bleuer, S., and Frees, K. 1994. Endotoxin responsiveness and grain dust-induced inflammation in the lower respiratory tract. *Am J Physiol (Lung Cell Mol Physiol)* 267: L609–L617.
37 Hollingsworth, J.W., Cook, D.N., Brass, D.M., Walker, J.K., Morgan, D.L., Foster, W.M., and Schwartz, D.A. 2004. The role of Toll-like receptor 4 in environmental airway injury in mice. *Am J Respir Crit Care Med* 170: 126–132.
38 Brass, D.M., Savov, J.D., Gavett, S.H., Haykal-Coates, N., and Schwartz, D.A. 2003. Subchronic endotoxin inhalation causes persistent airway disease. *Am J Physiol Lung Cell Mol Physiol* 285: L755–761.
39 Togbe, D., Schnyder-Candrian, S., Schnyder, B., Couillin, I., Maillet, I., Bihl, F., Malo, D., Ryffel, B., and Quesniaux, V.F. 2006. TLR4 gene dosage contributes to endotoxin-induced acute respiratory inflammation. *J Leukoc Biol* 80: 451–457.
40 Lorenz, E., Jones, M., Wohlford-Lenane, C., Meyer, N., Frees, K.L., Arbour, N.C., and Schwartz, D.A. 2001. Genes other than TLR4 are involved in the response to inhaled LPS. *Am J Physiol Lung Cell Mol Physiol* 281: L1106–1114.

41 Jagielo, P.J., Thorne, P.S., Watt, J.L., Frees, K.L., Quinn, T.J., and Schwartz, D.A. 1996. Grain dust and endotoxin inhalation challenges produce similar inflammatory responses in normal subjects. *Chest* 110: 263–270.
42 O'Grady, N.P., Preas, H.L., Pugin, J., Fiuza, C., Tropea, M., Reda, D., Banks, S.M., and Suffredini, A.F. 2001. Local inflammatory responses following bronchial endotoxin instillation in humans. *Am J Respir Crit Care Med* 163: 1591–1598.
43 Schwartz, D.A. 1996. Grain dust, endotoxin, and airflow obstruction. *Chest* 109: 57S–63S.
44 Simpson, J.C., Niven, R.M., Pickering, C.A., Fletcher, A.M., Oldham, L.A., and Francis, H.M. 1998. Prevalence and predictors of work related respiratory symptoms in workers exposed to organic dusts. *Occup Environ Med* 55: 668–672.
45 Kline, J., Cowden, J., Hunninghake, G., Schutte, B., Watt, J., Wohlford-Lenane, C., Powers, L., Jones, M., and Schwartz, D. 1999. Variable airway responsiveness to inhaled lipopolysaccharide. *Am J Respir Crit Care Med* 160: 297–303.
46 Michel, O., LeVan, T.D., Stern, D., Dentener, M., Thorn, J., Gnat, D., Beijer, M.L., Cochaux, P., Holt, P.G., Martinez, F.D., et al. 2003. Systemic responsiveness to lipopolysaccharide and polymorphisms in the Toll-like receptor 4 gene in human beings. *J Allergy Clin Immunol* 112: 923–929.
47 Erridge, C., Stewart, J., and Poxton, I.R. 2003. Monocytes heterozygous for the Asp299Gly and Thr399Ile mutations in the Toll-like receptor 4 gene show no deficit in lipopolysaccharide signalling. *J Exp Med* 197: 1787–1791. Epub 2003 Jun 1789.
48 Rallabhandi, P., Bell, J., Boukhvalova, M.S., Medvedev, A., Lorenz, E., Arditi, M., Hemming, V.G., Blanco, J.C., Segal, D.M., and Vogel, S.N. 2006. Analysis of TLR4 polymorphic variants: new insights into TLR4/MD-2/CD14 stoichiometry, structure, and signaling. *J Immunol* 177: 322–332.
49 Hasday, J.D., Bascom, R., Costa, J.J., Fitzgerald, T., and Dubin, W. 1999. Bacterial endotoxin is an active component of cigarette smoke. *Chest* 115: 829–835.
50 Becker, S., Fenton, M.J., and Soukup, J.M. 2002. Involvement of microbial components and tToll-like receptors 2 and 4 in cytokine responses to air pollution particles. *Am J Respir Cell Mol Biol* 27: 611–618.
51 Mueller-Anneling, L., Avol, E., Peters, J.M., and Thorne, P.S. 2004. Ambient endotoxin concentrations in PM10 from Southern California. *Environ Health Perspect* 112: 583–588.
52 Carty, C.L., Gehring, U., Cyrys, J., Bischof, W., and Heinrich, J. 2003. Seasonal variability of endotoxin in ambient fine particulate matter. *J Environ Monit* 5: 953–958.
53 Soukup, J.M., and Becker, S. 2001. Human alveolar macrophage responses to air pollution particulates are associated with insoluble components of coarse material, including particulate endotoxin. *Toxicol Appl Pharmacol* 171: 20–26.
54 Ozesmi, M., Aslan, H., Hillerdal, G., Rylander, R., Ozesmi, C., and Baris, Y.I. 1987. Byssinosis in carpet weavers exposed to wool contaminated with endotoxin. *Br J Ind Med* 44: 479–483.

55 Dong, W., Lewtas, J., and Luster, M.I. 1996. Role of endotoxin in tumor necrosis factor alpha expression from alveolar macrophages treated with urban air particles. *Exp Lung Res* 22: 577–592.
56 Arimoto, T., Kadiiska, M.B., Sato, K., Corbett, J., and Mason, R.P. 2005. Synergistic production of lung free radicals by diesel exhaust particles and endotoxin. *Am J Respir Crit Care Med* 171: 379–387. Epub 2004 Oct 2011.
57 Becker, S., Soukup, J.M., Gilmour, M.I., and Devlin, R.B. 1996. Stimulation of human and rat alveolar macrophages by urban air particulates: effects on oxidant radical generation and cytokine production. *Toxicol Appl Pharmacol* 141: 637–648.
58 Carter, J.D., Ghio, A.J., Samet, J.M., and Devlin, R.B. 1997. Cytokine production by human airway epithelial cells after exposure to an air pollution particle is metal-dependent. *Toxicol Appl Pharmacol* 146: 180–188.
59 Pope, C.A., 3rd, Thun, M.J., Namboodiri, M.M., Dockery, D.W., Evans, J.S., Speizer, F.E., and Heath, C.W., Jr. 1995. Particulate air pollution as a predictor of mortality in a prospective study of U.S. adults. *Am J Respir Crit Care Med* 151: 669–674.
60 Schins, R.P., Lightbody, J.H., Borm, P.J., Shi, T., Donaldson, K., and Stone, V. 2004. Inflammatory effects of coarse and fine particulate matter in relation to chemical and biological constituents. *Toxicol Appl Pharmacol* 195: 1–11.
61 Becker, S., Mundandhara, S., Devlin, R.B., and Madden, M. 2005. Regulation of cytokine production in human alveolar macrophages and airway epithelial cells in response to ambient air pollution particles: Further mechanistic studies. *Toxicol Appl Pharmacol* 207: 269–275.
62 Huttunen, K., Rintala, H., Hirvonen, M.R., Vepsalainen, A., Hyvarinen, A., Meklin, T., Toivola, M., and Nevalainen, A. 2008. Indoor air particles and bioaerosols before and after renovation of moisture-damaged buildings: the effect on biological activity and microbial flora. *Environ Res* 107: 291–298.
63 Batzer, G., Lam, D.P., Paulus, P., Boasen, J., Ng, N., and Horner, A.A. 2007. Using house dust extracts to understand the immunostimulatory activities of living environments. *Immunobiology* 212: 491–498.
64 Dockery, D.W., Pope, C.A., Xu, X., Spengler, J.D., Ware, J.H., Fay, M.E., Ferris, B.G., and Speizer, F.E. 1993. An association between air pollution and mortality in six U.S. cities. *N Engl J Med* 329: 1754–1759.
65 Bell, M., McDermott, A., Zeger, S., Samet, J., and Dominici, F. 2004. Ozone and short-term mortality in 95 US urban communities, 1987–2000. *JAMA* 292: 2372–2378.
66 Gryparis, A., Forsberg, B., Katsouyanni, K., Analitis, A., Touloumi, G., Schwartz, J., Samoli, E., Medina, S., Anderson, H.R., Niciu, E.M., et al. 2004. Acute Effects of Ozone on Mortality from the "Air Pollution and Health: A European Approach" Project. *Am J Respir Crit Care Med* 28: 28.
67 Katsouyanni, K., Zmirou, D., Spix, C., Sunyer, J., Schouten, J.P., Ponka, A., Anderson, H.R., Le Moullec, Y., Wojtyniak, B., Vigotti, M.A., et al. 1995. Short-term effects of air pollution on health: a European approach using epidemiological time-series data. The APHEA project: background, objectives, design. *Eur Respir J* 8: 1030–1038.
68 Hubbell, B.J., Hallberg, A., McCubbin, D.R., and Post, E. 2005. Health-related benefits of attaining the 8-hr ozone standard. *Environ Health Perspect* 113: 73–82.

69 Ito, K., De Leon, S.F., and Lippmann, M. 2005. Associations between ozone and daily mortality: analysis and meta-analysis. *Epidemiology* 16: 446–457.
70 Levy, J.I., Chemerynski, S.M., and Sarnat, J.A. 2005. Ozone exposure and mortality: an empiric bayes metaregression analysis. *Epidemiology* 16: 458–468.
71 Kleeberger, S.R., Reddy, S., Zhang, L.Y., and Jedlicka, A.E. 2000. Genetic susceptibility to ozone-induced lung hyperpermeability: role of Toll-like receptor 4. *Am J Respir Cell Mol Biol* 22: 620–627.
72 Kleeberger, S.R., Reddy, S.P., Zhang, L.Y., Cho, H.Y., and Jedlicka, A.E. 2001. Toll-like receptor 4 mediates ozone-induced murine lung hyperpermeability via inducible nitric oxide synthase. *Am J Physiol Lung Cell Mol Physiol* 280: L326–333.
73 Williams, A.S., Leung, S.Y., Nath, P., Khorasani, N.M., Bhavsar, P., Issa, R., Mitchell, J.A., Adcock, I.M., and Chung, K.F. 2007. Role of TLR2, TLR4 and MyD88 in ozone-induced airway hyperresponsiveness and neutrophilia. *J Appl Physiol.*
74 Fakhrzadeh, L., Laskin, J.D., and Laskin, D.L. 2004. Ozone-induced production of nitric oxide and TNF-alpha and tissue injury are dependent on NF-kappaB p50. *Am J Physiol Lung Cell Mol Physiol* 287: L279–285.
75 Cho, H.Y., Morgan, D.L., Bauer, A.K., and Kleeberger, S.R. 2007. Signal transduction pathways of tumor necrosis factor-mediated lung injury induced by ozone in mice. *Am J Respir Crit Care Med* 175: 829–839.
76 Leikauf, G.D., Zhao, Q., Zhou, S., and Santrock, J. 1995. Activation of eicosanoid metabolism in human airway epithelial cells by ozonolysis products of membrane fatty acids. *Res Rep Health Eff Inst*:1–15; discussion 19–26.
77 Pryor, W.A., Das, B., and Church, D.F. 1991. The ozonation of unsaturated fatty acids: aldehydes and hydrogen peroxide as products and possible mediators of ozone toxicity. *Chem Res Toxicol* 4: 341–348.
78 Pryor, W.A., Squadrito, G.L., and Friedman, M. 1995. The cascade mechanism to explain ozone toxicity: the role of lipid ozonation products. *Free Radic Biol Med* 19: 935–941.
79 Dahl, M., Bauer, A., Arredouani, M., Soininen, R., Tryggvason, K., Kleeberger, S., and Kobzik, L. 2007. Protection against inhaled oxidants through scavenging of oxidized lipids by macrophage receptors MARCO and SR-AI/II. *J Clin Invest* 117: 757–764.
80 Hudak, B.B., Zhang, L.Y., and Kleeberger, S.R. 1993. Inter-strain variation in susceptibility to hyperoxic injury of murine airways. *Pharmacogenetics* 3: 135–143.
81 Whitehead, G.S., Burch, L.H., Berman, K.G., Piantadosi, C.A., and Schwartz, D.A. 2006. Genetic basis of murine responses to hyperoxia-induced lung injury. *Immunogenetics* 58: 793–804.
82 Cho, H.Y., Jedlicka, A.E., Reddy, S.P., Kensler, T.W., Yamamoto, M., Zhang, L.Y., and Kleeberger, S.R. 2002. Role of NRF2 in protection against hyperoxic lung injury in mice. *Am J Respir Cell Mol Biol* 26: 175–182.
83 Cho, H.Y., Jedlicka, A.E., Reddy, S.P., Zhang, L.Y., Kensler, T.W., and Kleeberger, S.R. 2002. Linkage analysis of susceptibility to hyperoxia. Nrf2 is a candidate gene. *Am J Respir Cell Mol Biol* 26: 42–51.
84 Cho, H.Y., Reddy, S.P., and Kleeberger, S.R. 2006. Nrf2 defends the lung from oxidative stress. *Antioxid Redox Signal* 8: 76–87.

85 Ogawa, Y., Tasaka, S., Yamada, W., Saito, F., Hasegawa, N., Miyasho, T., and Ishizaka, A. 2007. Role of Toll-like receptor 4 in hyperoxia-induced lung inflammation in mice. *Inflamm Res* 56: 334–338.
86 Zhang, X., Shan, P., Qureshi, S., Homer, R., Medzhitov, R., Noble, P.W., and Lee, P.J. 2005. Cutting edge: TLR4 deficiency confers susceptibility to lethal oxidant lung injury. *J Immunol* 175: 4834–4838.
87 Qureshi, S.T., Zhang, X., Aberg, E., Bousette, N., Giaid, A., Shan, P., Medzhitov, R.M., and Lee, P.J. 2006. Inducible activation of TLR4 confers resistance to hyperoxia-induced pulmonary apoptosis. *J Immunol* 176: 4950–4958.
88 Kubo, H., and Ishizawa, K. 2006. Comment on "Cutting edge: TLR4 deficiency confers susceptibility to lethal oxidant lung injury". *J Immunol* 176: 3856–3857; author reply 3857.
89 Jiang, D., Liang, J., Fan, J., Yu, S., Chen, S., Luo, Y., Prestwich, G.D., Mascarenhas, M.M., Garg, H.G., Quinn, D.A., et al. 2005. Regulation of lung injury and repair by Toll-like receptors and hyaluronan. *Nat Med* 11: 1173–1179. Epub 2005 Oct 1123.
90 Gao, F., Koenitzer, J.R., Tobolewski, J.M., Jiang, D., Liang, J., Noble, P.W., and Oury, T.D. 2008. Extracellular superoxide dismutase inhibits inflammation by preventing oxidative fragmentation of hyaluronan. *J Biol Chem* 283: 6058–6066.
91 Yoshizaki, A., Iwata, Y., Komura, K., Ogawa, F., Hara, T., Muroi, E., Takenaka, M., Shimizu, K., Hasegawa, M., Fujimoto, M., et al. 2008. CD19 regulates skin and lung fibrosis via Toll-like receptor signaling in a model of bleomycin-induced scleroderma. *Am J Pathol* 172: 1650–1663.
92 Tsan, M.F., and Gao, B. 2004. Endogenous ligands of Toll-like receptors. *J Leukoc Biol* 76: 514–519.
93 Matzinger, P. 2002. The danger model: a renewed sense of self. *Science* 296: 301–305.
94 Kariko, K., Ni, H., Capodici, J., Lamphier, M., and Weissman, D. 2004. mRNA is an endogenous ligand for Toll-like receptor 3. *J Biol Chem* 279: 12542–12550.
95 Smiley, S.T., King, J.A., and Hancock, W.W. 2001. Fibrinogen stimulates macrophage chemokine secretion through Toll-like receptor 4. *J Immunol* 167: 2887–2894.
96 Guillot, L., Balloy, V., McCormack, F.X., Golenbock, D.T., Chignard, M., and Si-Tahar, M. 2002. Cutting edge: the immunostimulatory activity of the lung surfactant protein-A involves Toll-like receptor 4. *J Immunol* 168: 5989–5992.
97 Ohashi, K., Burkart, V., Flohe, S., and Kolb, H. 2000. Cutting edge: heat shock protein 60 is a putative endogenous ligand of the Toll-like receptor-4 complex. *J Immunol* 164: 558–561.
98 Asea, A., Rehli, M., Kabingu, E., Boch, J.A., Bare, O., Auron, P.E., Stevenson, M.A., and Calderwood, S.K. 2002. Novel signal transduction pathway utilized by extracellular HSP70: role of Toll-like receptor (TLR) 2 and TLR4. *J Biol Chem* 277: 15028–15034.
99 Vabulas, R.M., Braedel, S., Hilf, N., Singh-Jasuja, H., Herter, S., Ahmad-Nejad, P., Kirschning, C.J., Da Costa, C., Rammensee, H.G., Wagner, H., et al. 2002. The endoplasmic reticulum-resident heat shock protein Gp96 activates dendritic cells via the Toll-like receptor 2/4 pathway. *J Biol Chem* 277: 20847–20853.

100 Biragyn, A., Ruffini, P.A., Leifer, C.A., Klyushnenkova, E., Shakhov, A., Chertov, O., Shirakawa, A.K., Farber, J.M., Segal, D.M., Oppenheim, J.J., et al. 2002. Toll-like receptor 4-dependent activation of dendritic cells by beta-defensin 2. *Science* 298: 1025–1029.
101 Park, J.S., Svetkauskaite, D., He, Q., Kim, J.Y., Strassheim, D., Ishizaka, A., and Abraham, E. 2004. Involvement of Toll-like receptors 2 and 4 in cellular activation by high mobility group box 1 protein. *J Biol Chem* 279: 7370–7377.
102 Vogl, T., Tenbrock, K., Ludwig, S., Leukert, N., Ehrhardt, C., van Zoelen, M.A., Nacken, W., Foell, D., van der Poll, T., Sorg, C., et al. 2007. Mrp8 and Mrp14 are endogenous activators of Toll-like receptor 4, promoting lethal, endotoxin-induced shock. *Nat Med* 13: 1042–1049.
103 Taylor, K.R., Trowbridge, J.M., Rudisill, J.A., Termeer, C.C., Simon, J.C., and Gallo, R.L. 2004. Hyaluronan fragments stimulate endothelial recognition of injury through TLR4. *J Biol Chem* 279: 17079–17084. Epub 12004 Feb 17075.
104 Termeer, C., Benedix, F., Sleeman, J., Fieber, C., Voith, U., Ahrens, T., Miyake, K., Freudenberg, M., Galanos, C., and Simon, J.C. 2002. Oligosaccharides of Hyaluronan activate dendritic cells via Toll-like receptor 4. *J Exp Med* 195: 99–111.
105 Johnson, G.B., Brunn, G.J., Kodaira, Y., and Platt, J.L. 2002. Receptor-mediated monitoring of tissue well-being via detection of soluble heparan sulfate by Toll-like receptor 4. *J Immunol* 168: 5233–5239.
106 Okamura, Y., Watari, M., Jerud, E.S., Young, D.W., Ishizaka, S.T., Rose, J., Chow, J.C., and Strauss, J.F., 3rd. 2001. The extra domain A of fibronectin activates Toll-like receptor 4. *J Biol Chem* 276: 10229–10233.
107 Bausinger, H., Lipsker, D., Ziylan, U., Manie, S., Briand, J.P., Cazenave, J.P., Muller, S., Haeuw, J.F., Ravanat, C., de la Salle, H., et al. 2002. Endotoxin-free heat-shock protein 70 fails to induce APC activation. *Eur J Immunol* 32: 3708–3713.
108 Gao, B., and Tsan, M.F. 2003. Recombinant human heat shock protein 60 does not induce the release of tumor necrosis factor alpha from murine macrophages. *J Biol Chem* 278: 22523–22529.
109 Gao, B., and Tsan, M.F. 2003. Endotoxin contamination in recombinant human heat shock protein 70 (Hsp70) preparation is responsible for the induction of tumor necrosis factor alpha release by murine macrophages. *J Biol Chem* 278: 174–179.
110 Reed, R.C., Berwin, B., Baker, J.P., and Nicchitta, C.V. 2003. GRP94/gp96 elicits ERK activation in murine macrophages. A role for endotoxin contamination in NF-kappa B activation and nitric oxide production. *J Biol Chem* 278: 31853–31860.
111 Rohde, G., Klein, W., Arinir, U., Hagedorn, M., Duerig, N., T, T.B., Gillissen, A., Schultze-Werninghaus, G., and J, T.E. 2006. Association of the ASP299GLY TLR4 polymorphism with COPD. *Respir Med* 100: 892–896.
112 Sabroe, I., Whyte, M.K., Wilson, A.G., Dower, S.K., Hubbard, R., and Hall, I. 2004. Toll-like receptor (TLR) 4 polymorphisms and COPD. *Thorax* 59: 81.
113 Brass, D.M., Hollingsworth, J.W., Cinque, M., Li, Z., Potts, E., Toloza, E., Foster, W.M., and Schwartz, D.A. 2008. Chronic LPS inhalation causes

emphysema-like changes in mouse lung that is associated with apoptosis. *Am J Respir Cell Mol Biol.*
114 Doz, E., Noulin, N., Boichot, E., Guenon, I., Fick, L., Le Bert, M., Lagente, V., Ryffel, B., Schnyder, B., Quesniaux, V.F., et al. 2008. Cigarette smoke-induced pulmonary inflammation is TLR4/MyD88 and IL-1R1/MyD88 signaling dependent. *J Immunol* 180: 1169–1178.
115 Karimi, K., Sarir, H., Mortaz, E., Smit, J.J., Hosseini, H., De Kimpe, S.J., Nijkamp, F.P., and Folkerts, G. 2006. Toll-like receptor-4 mediates cigarette smoke-induced cytokine production by human macrophages. *Respir Res* 7: 66.
116 Zhang, X., Shan, P., Jiang, G., Cohn, L., and Lee, P.J. 2006. Toll-like receptor 4 deficiency causes pulmonary emphysema. *J Clin Invest* 116: 3050–3059.
117 Yao, H., Edirisinghe, I., Yang, S.R., Rajendrasozhan, S., Kode, A., Caito, S., Adenuga, D., and Rahman, I. 2008. Genetic ablation of NADPH oxidase enhances susceptibility to cigarette smoke-induced lung inflammation and emphysema in mice. *Am J Pathol* 172: 1222–1237.
118 Soutiere, S.E., Tankersley, C.G., and Mitzner, W. 2004. Differences in alveolar size in inbred mouse strains. *Respir Physiol Neurobiol* 140: 283–291.
119 Sampath, V., Davis, K., Senft, A.P., Richardson, T.R., Kitzmiller, J.A., Berclaz, P.Y., and Korfhagen, T.R. 2006. Altered postnatal lung development in C3H/HeJ mice. *Pediatr Res* 60: 663–668.
120 Adler, A., Tager, I., and Quintero, D.R. 2005. Decreased prevalence of asthma among farm-reared children compared with those who are rural but not farm-reared. *J Allergy Clin Immunol* 115: 67–73.
121 Leynaert, B., Neukirch, C., Jarvis, D., Chinn, S., Burney, P., and Neukirch, F. 2001. Does living on a farm during childhood protect against asthma, allergic rhinitis, and atopy in adulthood? *Am J Respir Crit Care Med* 164: 1829–1834.
122 Braun-Fahrlander, C., Gassner, M., Grize, L., Neu, U., Sennhauser, F.H., Varonier, H.S., Vuille, J.C., and Wuthrich, B. 1999. Prevalence of hay fever and allergic sensitization in farmer's children and their peers living in the same rural community. SCARPOL team. Swiss Study on Childhood Allergy and Respiratory Symptoms with Respect to Air Pollution. *Clin Exp Allergy* 29: 28–34.
123 Calvani, M., Jr., Alessandri, C., and Bonci, E. 2002. Fever episodes in early life and the development of atopy in children with asthma. *Eur Respir J* 20: 391–396.
124 Salam, M.T., Li, Y.F., Langholz, B., and Gilliland, F.D. 2004. Early-life environmental risk factors for asthma: findings from the Children's Health Study. *Environ Health Perspect* 112: 760–765.
125 Braun-Fahrlander, C., Riedler, J., Herz, U., Eder, W., Waser, M., Grize, L., Maisch, S., Carr, D., Gerlach, F., Bufe, A., et al. 2002. Environmental exposure to endotoxin and its relation to asthma in school-age children. *N Engl J Med* 347: 869–877.
126 Yang, I.A., Barton, S.J., Rorke, S., Cakebread, J.A., Keith, T.P., Clough, J.B., Holgate, S.T., and Holloway, J.W. 2004. Toll-like receptor 4 polymorphism and severity of atopy in asthmatics. *Genes Immun* 5: 41–45.
127 Fageras Bottcher, M., Hmani-Aifa, M., Lindstrom, A., Jenmalm, M.C., Mai, X.M., Nilsson, L., Zdolsek, H.A., Bjorksten, B., Soderkvist, P., and Vaarala, O.

2004. A TLR4 polymorphism is associated with asthma and reduced lipopolysaccharide-induced interleukin-12(p70) responses in Swedish children. *J Allergy Clin Immunol* 114: 561–567.
128 Watanabe, J., Miyazaki, Y., Zimmerman, G.A., Albertine, K.H., and McIntyre, T.M. 2003. Endotoxin contamination of ovalbumin suppresses murine immunologic responses and development of airway hyper-reactivity. *J Biol Chem* 278: 42361–42368. Epub 42003 Aug 42308.
129 Rodriguez, D., Keller, A.C., Faquim-Mauro, E.L., de Macedo, M.S., Cunha, F.Q., Lefort, J., Vargaftig, B.B., and Russo, M. 2003. Bacterial lipopolysaccharide signaling through Toll-like receptor 4 suppresses asthma-like responses via nitric oxide synthase 2 activity. *J Immunol* 171: 1001–1008.
130 Velasco, G., Campo, M., Manrique, O.J., Bellou, A., He, H., Arestides, R.S., Schaub, B., Perkins, D.L., and Finn, P.W. 2005. Toll--ike receptor 4 or 2 agonists decrease allergic inflammation. *Am J Respir Cell Mol Biol* 32: 218–224. Epub 2004 Dec 2002.
131 Hollingsworth, J., Whitehead, G., Lin, K., Nakano, H., Gunn, M., Schwartz, D., and Cook, D. 2006. TLR4 signaling attenuates ongoing allergic inflammation. *J Immunol* 176: 5856–5862.
132 Tulic, M.K., Wale, J.L., Holt, P.G., and Sly, P.D. 2000. Modification of the inflammatory response to allergen challenge after exposure to bacterial lipopolysaccharide. *Am J Respir Cell Mol Biol* 22: 604–612.
133 Tulic, M.K., Knight, D.A., Holt, P.G., and Sly, P.D. 2001. Lipopolysaccharide inhibits the late-phase response to allergen by altering nitric oxide synthase activity and interleukin-10. *Am J Respir Cell Mol Biol* 24: 640–646.
134 Tulic, M.K., Holt, P.G., and Sly, P.D. 2002. Modification of acute and late-phase allergic responses to ovalbumin with lipopolysaccharide. *Int Arch Allergy Immunol* 129: 119–128.
135 Tulic, M.K., Fiset, P.O., Manoukian, J.J., Frenkiel, S., Lavigne, F., Eidelman, D.H., and Hamid, Q. 2004. Role of Toll-like receptor 4 in protection by bacterial lipopolysaccharide in the nasal mucosa of atopic children but not adults. *Lancet* 363: 1689–1697.
136 Akdis, C.A., Kussebi, F., Pulendran, B., Akdis, M., Lauener, R.P., Schmidt-Weber, C.B., Klunker, S., Isitmangil, G., Hansjee, N., Wynn, T.A., et al. 2003. Inhibition of T helper 2-type responses, IgE production and eosinophilia by synthetic lipopeptides. *Eur J Immunol* 33: 2717–2726.
137 Campo M., V.G., Manrique O.J., Bellou A., He H., Arestides R.S., Schaub B., Mueller T.F., Ting L., Perkins D.L., Finn P.W. 2004. TLR2 stimulation decreases allergen induced eosinophilia. *AJRCCM* 169: A202.
138 Kline, J.N., Waldschmidt, T.J., Businga, T.R., Lemish, J.E., Weinstock, J.V., Thorne, P.S., and Krieg, A.M. 1998. Modulation of airway inflammation by CpG oligodeoxynucleotides in a murine model of asthma. *J Immunol* 160: 2555–2559.
139 Tsuji, R.F., Hoshino, K., Noro, Y., Tsuji, N.M., Kurokawa, T., Masuda, T., Akira, S., and Nowak, B. 2003. Suppression of allergic reaction by lambda-carrageenan: toll-like receptor 4/MyD88-dependent and -independent modulation of immunity. *Clin Exp Allergy* 33: 249–258.
140 Sutmuller, R.P., den Brok, M.H., Kramer, M., Bennink, E.J., Toonen, L.W., Kullberg, B.J., Joosten, L.A., Akira, S., Netea, M.G., and Adema, G.J. 2006.

Toll-like receptor 2 controls expansion and function of regulatory T cells. *J Clin Invest* 116: 485–494.
141 Eisenbarth, S.C., Piggott, D.A., Huleatt, J.W., Visintin, I., Herrick, C.A., and Bottomly, K. 2002. Lipopolysaccharide-enhanced, toll-like receptor 4-dependent T helper cell type 2 responses to inhaled antigen. *J Exp Med* 196: 1645–1651.
142 Wenzel, S.E., Szefler, S.J., Leung, D.Y., Sloan, S.I., Rex, M.D., and Martin, R.J. 1997. Bronchoscopic evaluation of severe asthma. Persistent inflammation associated with high dose glucocorticoids. *Am J Respir Crit Care Med* 156: 737–743.
143 Park, J.H., Gold, D.R., Spiegelman, D.L., Burge, H.A., and Milton, D.K. 2001. House dust endotoxin and wheeze in the first year of life. *Am J Respir Crit Care Med* 163: 322–328.
144 Michel, O., Kips, J., Duchateua, J., Vertongen, F., Robert, L., Collet, H., Pauwels, R., and Sergysels, R. 1996. Severity of asthma is related to endotoxin in house dust. *Am J Respir Crit Care Med* 154: 1641–1646.
145 Rizzo, M.C., Naspitz, C.K., Fernandez-Caldas, E., Lockey, R.F., Mimica, I., and Sole, D. 1997. Endotoxin exposure and symptoms in asthmatic children. *Pediatr Allergy Immunol* 8: 121–126.
146 Delayre-Orthez, C., de Blay, F., Frossard, N., and Pons, F. 2004. Dose-dependent effects of endotoxins on allergen sensitization and challenge in the mouse. *Clin Exp Allergy* 34: 1789–1795.
147 Wan, G.H., Li, C.S., and Lin, R.H. 2000. Airborne endotoxin exposure and the development of airway antigen-specific allergic responses. *Clin Exp Allergy* 30: 426–432.
148 Stephens, R., and Chaplin, D.D. 2002. IgE cross-linking or lipopolysaccharide treatment induces recruitment of Th2 cells to the lung in the absence of specific antigen. *J Immunol* 169: 5468–5476.
149 Werner, M., Topp, R., Wimmer, K., Richter, K., Bischof, W., Wjst, M., and Heinrich, J. 2003. TLR4 gene variants modify endotoxin effects on asthma. *J Allergy Clin Immunol* 112: 323–330.
150 Michel, O., Ginanni, R., Le Bon, B., Content, J., Duchateau, J., and Sergysels, R. 1992. Inflammatory response to acute inhalation of endotoxin in asthmatic patients. *Am Rev Respir Dis* 146: 352–357.
151 Michel, O., Ginanni, R., Duchateau, J., Vertongen, F., Le Bon, B., and Sergysels, R. 1991. Domestic endotoxin exposure and clinical severity of asthma. *Clin Exp Allergy* 21: 441–448.
152 Michel, O., Duchateau, J., and Sergysels, R. 1989. Effect of inhaled endotoxin on bronchial reactivity in asthmatic and normal subjects. *J Appl Physiol* 66: 1059–1064.
153 Raby, B.A., Klimecki, W.T., Laprise, C., Renaud, Y., Faith, J., Lemire, M., Greenwood, C., Weiland, K.M., Lange, C., Palmer, L.J., et al. 2002. Polymorphisms in Toll-like receptor 4 are not associated with asthma or atopy-related phenotypes. *Am J Respir Crit Care Med* 166: 1449–1456. Epub 2002 Sep 1425.
154 Noguchi, E., Nishimura, F., Fukai, H., Kim, J., Ichikawa, K., Shibasaki, M., and Arinami, T. 2004. An association study of asthma and total serum immunoglobin E levels for Toll-like receptor polymorphisms in a Japanese population. *Clin Exp Allergy* 34: 177–183.

155 Baldini, M., Lohman, I.C., Halonen, M., Erickson, R.P., Holt, P.G., and Martinez, F.D. 1999. A Polymorphism* in the 5' flanking region of the CD14 gene is associated with circulating soluble CD14 levels and with total serum immunoglobulin E. *Am J Respir Cell Mol Biol* 20: 976–983.
156 Levan, T.D., Von Essen, S., Romberger, D.J., Lambert, G.P., Martinez, F.D., Vasquez, M.M., and Merchant, J.A. 2004. Polymorphisms in the CD14 Gene are Associated with Pulmonary Function in Farmers. *Am J Respir Crit Care Med* 10: 10.
157 Eder, W., Klimecki, W., Yu, L., von Mutius, E., Riedler, J., Braun-Fahrlander, C., Nowak, D., and Martinez, F.D. 2005. Opposite effects of CD 14/-260 on serum IgE levels in children raised in different environments. *J Allergy Clin Immunol* 116: 601–607.
158 Simpson, A., John, S.L., Jury, F., Niven, R., Woodcock, A., Ollier, W.E., and Custovic, A. 2006. Endotoxin exposure, CD14, and allergic disease: an interaction between genes and the environment. *Am J Respir Crit Care Med* 174: 386–392.
159 Jain, V.V., Kitagaki, K., and Kline, J.N. 2003. CpG DNA and immunotherapy of allergic airway diseases. *Clin Exp Allergy* 33: 1330–1335.
160 Ikeda, R.K., Nayar, J., Cho, J.Y., Miller, M., Rodriguez, M., Raz, E., and Broide, D.H. 2003. Resolution of airway inflammation following ovalbumin inhalation: comparison of ISS DNA and corticosteroids. *Am J Respir Cell Mol Biol* 28: 655–663.
161 Youn, C.J., Miller, M., Baek, K.J., Han, J.W., Nayar, J., Lee, S.Y., McElwain, K., McElwain, S., Raz, E., and Broide, D.H. 2004. Immunostimulatory DNA reverses established allergen-induced airway remodeling. *J Immunol* 173: 7556–7564.
162 Cho, J.Y., Miller, M., Baek, K.J., Han, J.W., Nayar, J., Rodriguez, M., Lee, S.Y., McElwain, K., McElwain, S., Raz, E., et al. 2004. Immunostimulatory DNA inhibits transforming growth factor-beta expression and airway remodeling. *Am J Respir Cell Mol Biol* 30: 651–661. Epub 2003 Nov 2014.
163 Broide, D.H., Stachnick, G., Castaneda, D., Nayar, J., Miller, M., Cho, J.Y., Roman, M., Zubeldia, J., Hayashi, T., and Raz, E. 2001. Systemic administration of immunostimulatory DNA sequences mediates reversible inhibition of Th2 responses in a mouse model of asthma. *J Clin Immunol* 21: 175–182.
164 Sur, S., Wild, J.S., Choudhury, B.K., Sur, N., Alam, R., and Klinman, D.M. 1999. Long term prevention of allergic lung inflammation in a mouse model of asthma by CpG oligodeoxynucleotides. *J Immunol* 162: 6284–6293.
165 Broide, D., Schwarze, J., Tighe, H., Gifford, T., Nguyen, M.D., Malek, S., Van Uden, J., Martin-Orozco, E., Gelfand, E.W., and Raz, E. 1998. Immunostimulatory DNA sequences inhibit IL-5, eosinophilic inflammation, and airway hyperresponsiveness in mice. *J Immunol* 161: 7054–7062.
166 Banerjee, B., Kelly, K.J., Fink, J.N., Henderson, J.D., Jr., Bansal, N.K., and Kurup, V.P. 2004. Modulation of airway inflammation by immunostimulatory CpG oligodeoxynucleotides in a murine model of allergic aspergillosis. *Infect Immun* 72: 6087–6094.
167 Ulevitch, R.J. 2004. Therapeutics targeting the innate immune system. *Nat Rev Immunol* 4: 512–520.

168 Pasare, C., and Medzhitov, R. 2005. Toll-like receptors: linking innate and adaptive immunity. *Adv Exp Med Biol* 560: 11–18.
169 Schnare, M., Barton, G.M., Holt, A.C., Takeda, K., Akira, S., and Medzhitov, R. 2001. Toll-like receptors control activation of adaptive immune responses. *Nat Immunol* 2: 947–950.
170 Novick, R.J., Bennett, L.E., Meyer, D.M., and Hosenpud, J.D. 1999. Influence of graft ischemic time and donor age on survival after lung transplantation. *J Heart Lung Transplant* 18: 425–431.
171 Andrade, C.F., Kaneda, H., Der, S., Tsang, M., Lodyga, M., Chimisso Dos Santos, C., Keshavjee, S., and Liu, M. 2006. Toll-like receptor and cytokine gene expression in the early phase of human lung transplantation. *J Heart Lung Transplant* 25: 1317–1323.
172 Tsung, A., Sahai, R., Tanaka, H., Nakao, A., Fink, M.P., Lotze, M.T., Yang, H., Li, J., Tracey, K.J., Geller, D.A., et al. 2005. The nuclear factor HMGB1 mediates hepatic injury after murine liver ischemia-reperfusion. *J Exp Med* 201: 1135–1143.
173 Wu, H., Chen, G., Wyburn, K.R., Yin, J., Bertolino, P., Eris, J.M., Alexander, S.I., Sharland, A.F., and Chadban, S.J. 2007. TLR4 activation mediates kidney ischemia/reperfusion injury. *J Clin Invest* 117: 2847–2859.
174 Paterson, H.M., Murphy, T.J., Purcell, E.J., Shelley, O., Kriynovich, S.J., Lien, E., Mannick, J.A., and Lederer, J.A. 2003. Injury primes the innate immune system for enhanced Toll-like receptor reactivity. *J Immunol* 171: 1473–1483.
175 Tsung, A., Hoffman, R.A., Izuishi, K., Critchlow, N.D., Nakao, A., Chan, M.H., Lotze, M.T., Geller, D.A., and Billiar, T.R. 2005. Hepatic ischemia/reperfusion injury involves functional TLR4 signaling in nonparenchymal cells. *J Immunol* 175: 7661–7668.
176 Shen, X.D., Ke, B., Zhai, Y., Gao, F., Tsuchihashi, S., Lassman, C.R., Busuttil, R.W., and Kupiec-Weglinski, J.W. 2007. Absence of Toll-like receptor 4 (TLR4) signaling in the donor organ reduces ischemia and reperfusion injury in a murine liver transplantation model. *Liver Transpl* 13: 1435–1443.
177 He, H., Stone, J.R., and Perkins, D.L. 2003. Analysis of differential immune responses induced by innate and adaptive immunity following transplantation. *Immunology* 109: 185–196.
178 Chatterjee, P.K., Zacharowski, K., Cuzzocrea, S., Brown, P.A., Stewart, K.N., Mota-Filipe, H., and Thiemermann, C. 2002. Lipoteichoic acid from Staphylococcus aureus reduces renal ischemia/reperfusion injury. *Kidney Int* 62: 1249–1263.
179 Eising, G.P., Mao, L., Schmid-Schonbein, G.W., Engler, R.L., and Ross, J. 1996. Effects of induced tolerance to bacterial lipopolysaccharide on myocardial infarct size in rats. *Cardiovasc Res* 31: 73–81.
180 Izuishi, K., Tsung, A., Jeyabalan, G., Critchlow, N.D., Li, J., Tracey, K.J., Demarco, R.A., Lotze, M.T., Fink, M.P., Geller, D.A., et al. 2006. Cutting edge: high-mobility group box 1 preconditioning protects against liver ischemia-reperfusion injury. *J Immunol* 176: 7154–7158.
181 Goldstein, D.R., Tesar, B.M., Akira, S., and Lakkis, F.G. 2003. Critical role of the Toll-like receptor signal adaptor protein MyD88 in acute allograft rejection. *J Clin Invest* 111: 1571–1578.

182 Tesar, B.M., Zhang, J., Li, Q., and Goldstein, D.R. 2004. TH1 immune responses to fully MHC mismatched allografts are diminished in the absence of MyD88, a Toll–like receptor signal adaptor protein. *Am J Transplant* 4: 1429–1439.
183 Tesar, B.M., Jiang, D., Liang, J., Palmer, S.M., Noble, P.W., and Goldstein, D.R. 2006. The role of hyaluronan degradation products as innate alloimmune agonists. *Am J Transplant* 6: 2622–2635.
184 Palmer, S.M., Burch, L.H., Davis, R.D., Herczyk, W.F., Howell, D.N., Reinsmoen, N.L., and Schwartz, D.A. 2003. The role of innate immunity in acute allograft rejection after lung transplantation. *Am J Respir Crit Care Med* 168: 628–632. Epub 2003 May 2028.
185 Palmer, S.M., Burch, L.H., Trindade, A.J., Davis, R.D., Herczyk, W.F., Reinsmoen, N.L., and Schwartz, D.A. 2005. Innate immunity influences long-term outcomes after human lung transplant. *Am J Respir Crit Care Med* 171: 780–785.
186 Palmer, S.M., Klimecki, W., Yu, L., Reinsmoen, N.L., Snyder, L.D., Ganous, T.M., Burch, L., and Schwartz, D.A. 2007. Genetic regulation of rejection and survival following human lung transplantation by the innate immune receptor CD14. *Am J Transplant* 7: 693–699.
187 Garantziotis, S., Palmer, S.M., Snyder, L.D., Ganous, T., Chen, B.J., Wang, T., Cook, D.N., and Schwartz, D.A. 2007. Alloimmune lung injury induced by local innate immune activation through inhaled lipopolysaccharide. *Transplantation* 84: 1012–1019.
188 Bobadilla, J.L., Love, R.B., Jankowska-Gan, E., Xu, Q., Haynes, L.D., Braun, R.K., Hayney, M.S., Munoz del Rio, A., Meyer, K., Greenspan, D.S., et al. 2008. Th-17, monokines, collagen type V, and primary graft dysfunction in lung transplantation. *Am J Respir Crit Care Med* 177: 660–668.
189 Nelsestuen, G.L., Martinez, M.B., Hertz, M.I., Savik, K., and Wendt, C.H. 2005. Proteomic identification of human neutrophil alpha-defensins in chronic lung allograft rejection. *Proteomics* 5: 1705–1713.
190 Yang, D., Chertov, O., Bykovskaia, S.N., Chen, Q., Buffo, M.J., Shogan, J., Anderson, M., Schroder, J.M., Wang, J.M., Howard, O.M., et al. 1999. Beta-defensins: linking innate and adaptive immunity through dendritic and T cell CCR6. *Science* 286: 525–528.
191 Ross, D.J., Cole, A.M., Yoshioka, D., Park, A.K., Belperio, J.A., Laks, H., Strieter, R.M., Lynch, J.P., 3rd, Kubak, B., Ardehali, A., et al. 2004. Increased bronchoalveolar lavage human beta-defensin type 2 in bronchiolitis obliterans syndrome after lung transplantation. *Transplantation* 78: 1222–1224.
192 Jordan, J.E., Montalto, M.C., and Stahl, G.L. 2001. Inhibition of mannose-binding lectin reduces postischemic myocardial reperfusion injury. *Circulation* 104: 1413–1418.
193 Berger, S.P., Roos, A., Mallat, M.J., Fujita, T., de Fijter, J.W., and Daha, M.R. 2005. Association between mannose-binding lectin levels and graft survival in kidney transplantation. *Am J Transplant* 5: 1361–1366.
194 Magro, C.M., Deng, A., Pope-Harman, A., Waldman, W.J., Bernard Collins, A., Adams, P.W., Kelsey, M., and Ross, P. 2002. Humorally mediated

posttransplantation septal capillary injury syndrome as a common form of pulmonary allograft rejection: a hypothesis. *Transplantation* 74: 1273–1280.
195 Magro, C.M., Ross, P., Jr., Kelsey, M., Waldman, W.J., and Pope-Harman, A. 2003. Association of humoral immunity and bronchiolitis obliterans syndrome. *Am J Transplant* 3: 1155–1166.
196 Gilmour, M., Park, P., Doerfler, D., and Selgrade, M. 1993. Factors that influence the suppression of pulmonary antibacterial defenses in mice exposed to ozone. *Exp Lung Res* 19: 299–314.
197 Goldstein, E., Tyler, W., Hoeprich, P., and Eagle, C. 1971. Ozone and the antibacterial defense mechanisms of the murine lung. *Arch Intern Med* 127: 1099–1102.
198 Porter, M., Karp, M., Killedar, S., Bauer, S.M., Guo, J., Williams, D., Breysse, P., Georas, S.N., and Williams, M.A. 2007. Diesel-enriched particulate matter functionally activates human dendritic cells. *Am J Respir Cell Mol Biol* 37: 706–719.
199 Amakawa, K., Terashima, T., Matsuzaki, T., Matsumaru, A., Sagai, M., and Yamaguchi, K. 2003. Suppressive effects of diesel exhaust particles on cytokine release from human and murine alveolar macrophages. *Exp Lung Res* 29: 149–164.
200 Inoue, K., Takano, H., Yanagisawa, R., Sakurai, M., Ueki, N., and Yoshikawa, T. 2006. Effects of diesel exhaust on lung inflammation related to bacterial endotoxin in mice. *Basic Clin Pharmacol Toxicol* 99: 346–352.
201 Inoue, K., Takano, H., Yanagisawa, R., Sakurai, M., Ueki, N., and Yoshikawa, T. 2007. Effects of diesel exhaust particles on cytokine production by splenocytes stimulated with lipopolysaccharide. *J Appl Toxicol* 27: 95–100.
202 Takano, H., Yanagisawa, R., Ichinose, T., Sadakane, K., Yoshino, S., Yoshikawa, T., and Morita, M. 2002. Diesel exhaust particles enhance lung injury related to bacterial endotoxin through expression of proinflammatory cytokines, chemokines, and intercellular adhesion molecule-1. *Am J Respir Crit Care Med* 165: 1329–1335.
203 Gilmour, P.S., Schladweiler, M.C., Richards, J.H., Ledbetter, A.D., and Kodavanti, U.P. 2004. Hypertensive rats are susceptible to TLR4-mediated signaling following exposure to combustion source particulate matter. *Inhal Toxicol* 16 Suppl 1: 5–18.
204 Inoue, K., Takano, H., Yanagisawa, R., Hirano, S., Kobayashi, T., Fujitani, Y., Shimada, A., and Yoshikawa, T. 2007. Effects of inhaled nanoparticles on acute lung injury induced by lipopolysaccharide in mice. *Toxicology* 238: 99–110.
205 Inoue, K., Takano, H., Yanagisawa, R., Hirano, S., Sakurai, M., Shimada, A., and Yoshikawa, T. 2006. Effects of airway exposure to nanoparticles on lung inflammation induced by bacterial endotoxin in mice. *Environ Health Perspect* 114: 1325–1330.
206 Inoue, K., Takano, H., Yanagisawa, R., Hirano, S., Ichinose, T., Shimada, A., and Yoshikawa, T. 2006. The role of Toll-like receptor 4 in airway inflammation induced by diesel exhaust particles. *Arch Toxicol* 80: 275–279.
207 Hollingsworth, J.W., Maruoka, S., Li, Z., Potts, E.N., Brass, D.M., Garantziotis, S., Fong, A., Foster, W.M., and Schwartz, D.A. 2007. Ambient ozone primes pulmonary innate immunity in mice. *J Immunol* 179: 4367–4375.

208 Johnston, C.J., Holm, B.A., and Finkelstein, J.N. 2005. Sequential exposures to ozone and lipopolysaccharide in postnatal lung enhance or inhibit cytokine responses. *Exp Lung Res* 31: 431–447.
209 Johnston, C.J., Holm, B.A., Gelein, R., and Finkelstein, J.N. 2006. Postnatal lung development: immediate-early gene responses post ozone and LPS exposure. *Inhal Toxicol* 18: 875–883.
210 Skerrett, S.J., Liggitt, H.D., Hajjar, A.M., Ernst, R.K., Miller, S.I., and Wilson, C.B. 2004. Respiratory epithelial cells regulate lung inflammation in response to inhaled endotoxin. *Am J Physiol Lung Cell Mol Physiol* 287: L143–152. Epub 2004 Mar 2026.
211 Powers, K., Szaszi, K., Khadaroo, R., Tawadros, P., Marshall, J., Kapus, A., and Rotstein, O. 2006. Oxidative stress generated by hemorrhagic shock recruits Toll-like receptor 4 to the plasma membrane in macrophages. *J Exp Med* 203: 1951–1961. Epub 2006 Jul 1917.
212 Alexis, N.E., Becker, S., Bromberg, P.A., Devlin, R., and Peden, D.B. 2004. Circulating CD11b expression correlates with the neutrophil response and airway mCD14 expression is enhanced following ozone exposure in humans. *Clin Immunol* 111: 126–131.

4

Asthma exacerbations: a paradigm of synergy between allergens, pollutants and viruses

Antoine Magnan, Karine Botturi, Anaïs Pipet, Arnaud Cavaillès, Damien Reboulleau, Marie Langelot and Yannick Lacoeuille, assisted by Emilie Berthoux and Bérangère Neveu

Abstract. Exacerbations represent a major clinical issue in asthma management, leading to hospitalizations, acute respiratory failure and sometimes death. They induce the main costs of asthma management in terms of care recourse and loss of working days. Their mechanisms must be carefully elucidated to design new drugs able to prevent them. Exacerbations are mainly caused by viral infection, and also allergen and pollutant exposure. These triggers induce exacerbations in asthmatic subjects already displaying a chronic bronchial inflammation caused itself by allergy, pollutants and/or perhaps infection. Exacerbations therefore result from two additive immunological signals. Both signals involve innate immunity via the activation of epithelial and dendritic cells. The first signal induces chronic epithelium damage and activation. By stimulating cytokine production and coreceptors expression by dendritic cells, it determines the type of inflammatory response leading to T cell activation and polymorphonuclear cells homing and activation. The second signal acutely enhances the chronic inflammation and eventually adds a distinct type of inflammation to the first chronic response. These mechanisms will be discussed in the context of the various triggers involved, both from an epidemiologic and immunologic point of view.

Keywords: allergic asthma, inflammation, allergens, house-dust mite antigen, virus, pollutants, atopy, IgE response, innate immunity, T cells, regulatory T cells (Tregs), interferon-gamma, bronchial epithelium, pattern-recognition receptors, disease exacerbations, dendritic cells

4.1 Introduction

Asthma is a chronic respiratory disease whose prevalence is growing worldwide, reaching more than 10 per cent of people in childhood and young adulthood in some industrialized countries.[1] Efficient drugs have been developed and brought on to the market during the last twenty years, which control the disease by limiting inflammation (inhaled steroids) and relaxing bronchial smooth muscle (long-acting and short-acting beta-2 agonists). These controllers, however, do not modify the natural history of the disease, do not definitely prevent the occurrence of severe exacerbations, and remain insufficient to control the most severe cases of refractory asthma. This is why a considerable effort is being made in research and development to design drugs targeting specifically relevant molecules involved in asthmatic inflammation, or to cure the disease through immunotherapies aiming to reverse the course of the disease itself. These strategies are driven from the extensive knowledge accumulated during the last two decades about the immunopathology of asthma. However, if some drugs such as anti-IgE monoclonal antibodies proved to be efficient in some patients,[2] most tested molecules to date, including anti-IL-5[3] and anti-TNF,[4] remained unsuccessful in most patients. These disappointments could be due to the incomplete picture of asthma mechanisms obtained through studies of stable patients versus healthy controls, rather than exacerbating asthmatics versus stable counterparts or versus themselves in a quiet period. Indeed, the inflammatory reaction occurring during exacerbations cannot be entirely comparable to the inflammatory reaction leading to the disease itself, otherwise patients would not be controlled at any time. Factors triggering exacerbations are many, and drive various inflammatory events that lead to symptoms in asthmatics only and not in healthy subjects. This shows that an immune synergy is necessary between mechanisms involved in the inception of asthma and those triggered by causative agents of exacerbations to induce symptoms. It is this immune synergy, allying innate and adaptive immunity, that we propose to discuss in this chapter.

4.2 Immunopathology of controlled asthma

4.2.1 Definition and natural history of asthma

Asthma is defined by the GINA consortium as "a chronic inflammatory disorder of the airways in which many cells and cellular elements play a role. The chronic inflammation is associated with airway hyperresponsiveness that leads to recurrent episodes of wheezing, breathlessness, chest tightness, and coughing". [1] This definition clearly affirms inflammation as the primary mechanism of asthma. Asthma is a non-predicable chronic disease, usually starting in infancy or childhood, and lasting throughout the whole life. More or less durable periods of remission can occur, than can last for years without treatment. In most patients, however, control (i.e. minimal level of symptoms compatible with a normal life and activity) is achieved only when triggering factors are identified and avoided, or under controller therapy. Therefore, after entering into the disease by an inaugural attack, periods of controlled asthma alternate with periods of exacerbating asthma all through life. Exacerbations are defined by a progressive increase of symptoms over a short period of time, inducing an emergency visit for asthma and/or a treatment with systemic steroids. Severe exacerbations can lead to hospitalization and sometimes death.

The decline of pulmonary function is more rapid and accentuated in asthmatics compared to the general population. This progressive limitation results from the development of a bronchial remodeling, due to structural modifications of the bronchial wall associated with collagen deposition, smooth muscle and goblet cell hyperplasia. From a clinical point of view, remodelling results in a persistent respiratory limitation sometimes leading to heavy handicap.

This view of the natural history of asthma clearly indicates that research for improving asthma treatments must focus on preventive strategies targeting exacerbations and bronchial remodelling (Fig. 4.1).

4.2.2 Role of atopy

Atopy can be defined as an individual's predisposition of developing an IgE and eosinophillic-mediated disease such as allergic asthma, atopic dermatitis and chronic allergic rhino-conjunctivitis, which are often concurrently associated within the same individual or as successive episodes. This background is detected by the presence of IgEs specific for environmental allergens such as house dust mites (HDM), pollens or moistures, revealed by skin prick tests. Atopy is found among 70 per cent of asthmatics, which does not mean that allergens are responsible, either for the disease or for exacerbations of the disease. Indeed, the role of allergens in the inception of asthma is unclear, and most exacerbations are not allergen-driven. However, the role of IgEs in this kind of asthma is proved by the modest but real efficacy of anti-IgE monoclonal antibodies in preventing exacerbations in severe atopic asthma. [2]

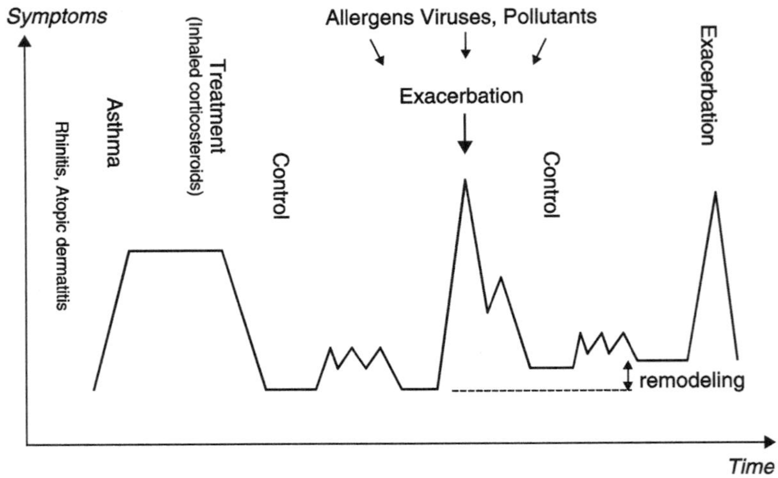

Figure 4.1 Natural history of asthma. After a variable period of allergic rhinitis and/or atopic dermatitis, the first asthma attack occurs, leading to administration of a controller treatment, and the course of the disease then consists in the succession of periods of control, interrupted by exacerbations. In the long term, the return to baseline can be incomplete, due to bronchial remodeling.

Thirty per cent of asthmatics are not atopic. Non-atopic asthma usually occurs later, during the fourth decade of life, is more severe and is unrelated to allergy.[5] It can be associated to nasal polyposis more than chronic rhinosinusitis, and to intolerance to non steroid anti-inflammatory drugs or sulfites. In non-atopic asthma, more similarities than differences are found regarding cells and mediators involved, notably with eosinophilic bronchitis being the main hallmark of both kinds of asthma.[6]

4.2.3 Gene/environment interactions

It is in the field of atopy and especially atopic asthma that the relationships between genes and environment have been best studied and are clearest. Asthma and atopy are largely hereditary, and many genetic studies have found various genes segregating with atopy and/or asthma, depending on the population studied. Some of these genes are regularly found, and particularly in the 5q region, containing loci coding for a series of mediators involved in atopy and asthma such as IL-5 or IL-4.[7]

Gene transmission is not sufficient for the expression of atopy or asthma. The role of environmental factors has been extensively demonstrated by epidemiological studies. Many studies performed in the early 2000s in the US and the north of Europe demonstrated an inverse relationship between the risk of being atopic and early exposure to microorganisms.[8] This finding was the origin of the hygiene hypothesis, which could explain at least in part the rising prevalence of atopy and related diseases in developed countries during the last few decades.

4.3 Adaptive immunity, from atopy to asthma

As atopy and asthma are clearly related to the presence of IgEs, a class of immunoglobulins under the control of interleukin (IL)-4 and IL-13, the importance of the T helper (Th) 2 cell population in the inception of these conditions was suspected as soon as the discovery of this T cell subset was made.[9] Indeed, Th2 cells represent a population of CD4+ T cells producing IL4 and IL13. They also produce IL5, a cytokine involved in eosinophil maturation, migration and proliferation. Th2 cells are defined by opposition to the Th1 subset, characterized by the production of IL-2 and IFN-γ, a cytokine responsible for the activation of CD8+ cytotoxic T cells notably, and involved in the anti-tumour and anti-viral immunity. Th1 and Th2 cells are known to antagonize each other, so that inflammatory responses are polarized as Th1 or Th2 responses.

Th2 cells were found to be elevated in blood from atopic children as early as birth,[10] and to increase as allergic sensitization develops. In addition, Th2 cells are predominant in the nasal mucosa of patients displaying allergic rhinitis[11] and in skin from patients with atopic dermatitis.[12] In asthma, a Th2 cell predominance was found in bronchoalveolar lavages (BAL) and in bronchial biopsies.[13] This Th2 activation in asthma was found whatever the atopic status.[6]

It appears therefore that atopy, as a result of the combined action of both genetic and environmental factors, reflects a predisposition to develop a Th2 response to allergens reaching the nose, the skin and/or the lung. The hygiene hypothesis can at that stage be interpreted as a deficient Th1 activation against microbes because of a too low exposure, opening the possibility for Th2 cells to emerge and proliferate.[14]

However, how can we explain why most atopic subjects will not develop asthma when their exposure to allergens is equivalent to that of asthmatics? The first part of the answer could be that the T cell activation in asthma is not limited to Th2 activation.[14] Indeed, several studies have found a Th1 activation to be associated to asthma. T cell IFN-γ production was demonstrated to be present in asthma, independently of atopy.[15]

IFN-$\tilde{\gamma}$ producing T cells are also found in situ, both in BAL and induced sputum, in higher proportions than in controls.[15, 16, 17] Circulating Th1 cells are strongly correlated to bronchial hyperresponsiveness, a hallmark of asthma whatever the atopic status.[15] Although in the context of atopy Th1 cells specific of allergens could have regulatory properties by counteracting the Th2 activation, in the context of asthma they appear as amplifiers of inflammation and tissue damage.

The second part of the answer could come from the implication of a third subset of T cells, recently identified and called T regulatory cells (Treg). The Treg population represents several small subsets differing in their tissue localization and their membrane antigens expression but all being anti-inflammatory through their production of IL-10 and/or TGF-beta, two cytokines able to deactivate immune cells. The T cell-induced regulation intervenes primarily by inducing tolerance to non-dangerous antigens, or secondarily to stop an inflammatory reaction and induce the phase of tissue repair. Natural Treg cells emerge directly from the thymus. They express the α chain of the IL-2 receptor (CD25) at a high level and CD127 at an intermediate level, which renders easy their detection by flow cytometry, even though they represent less than 1 per cent of circulating T cells. These Treg cells also express the Fox p 3 transcription factor, which seems directly related to their immunosuppressive properties.[18]

Treg cells have been shown to display a deficient activation in the context of atopy, more precisely of allergic rhinitis.[19, 20] Indeed in symptomatic allergic subjects, they failed to inhibit the ex vivo proliferation of peripheral T cells induced by the allergen. In asthma, we have demonstrated a decreased proportion of Treg cells in blood.[21, 22] Their importance in allergy was further demonstrated indirectly by immunotherapy. Allergen specific immunotherapy consists in inducing tolerance by administrating increasing doses of allergens via the subcutaneous or the sublingual route. This treatment induces a Th2 to Th1 shift of the specific T cell activation and an increase in activated Treg cells.[23]

Recently, we investigated in more details the relationships between T cell activation, asthma and allergy in an ex-vivo model of allergen stimulation.[22] Unexpectedly, we demonstrated that in asthma, the decreased proportion of Treg cells was constitutive and independent of any allergen stimulation. Constitutive also was the higher proportion of Th1 cells in blood. These intrinsic properties were found both in atopic and non-atopic asthma. After allergen stimulation, a Th2 profile was induced and the Treg cell decrease was amplified in allergic subjects only. It seems therefore that inflammation in asthma consists in a mixed Th1 and Th2 activation, the former being constitutive and antigen-independent, and the

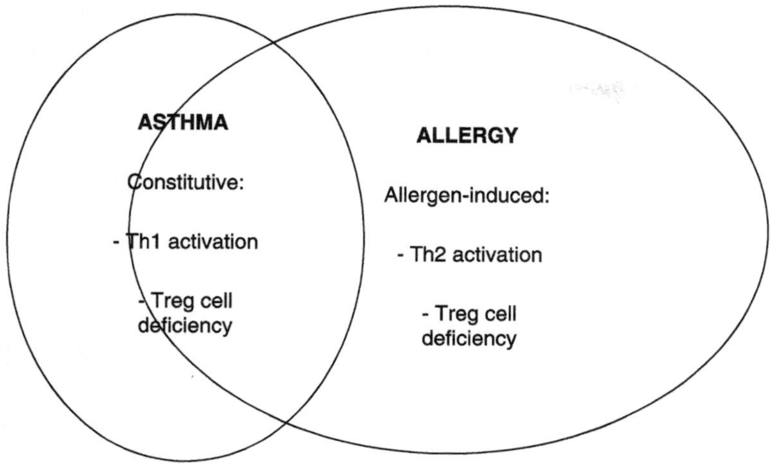

Figure 4.2 Immunopathology of allergy and asthma.

Although allergy is characterized by a Th2 inflammation with a Treg deficiency inducible upon allergen stimulation, in asthma a constitutive defect in the Treg activation is accompanied by a basal Th1 deviation. In atopic asthma, both inflammatory characteristics are mixed together.

latter being induced by allergen in atopic subjects. In non-atopic asthmatics the Th2 part of inflammation would be triggered by unknown antigens (Figure 4.2). These data introduce the concept of two signals being necessary to induce asthma symptoms: the first signal would induce the disease itself and the second would trigger the symptoms

Because the Th2 activation seen in asthma results from stimulation by specific antigens (purified Der p1 in our experiments), it is usually considered that activated T cells are specific to the allergen used. From *in vivo* experiments, it is also widely considered that T cells infiltrating tissues after allergen challenge are specific to the allergen used. However, it is likely that most T cells seen in these situations are bystander T cells with other specificities.[24] Indeed, the proportion of activated T cells after allergen stimulation is much higher than expected if these cells were all recognizing specifically the cognate allergen. The importance of bystander T cells is probably best illustrated by the prevention of further sensitization in children "specifically" desensitized to an allergen.[25] The mechanisms leading to the activation of T cells independently of the allergen stimulation include necessarily the implication of other antigens, for example viral antigens found during exacerbations of asthma, and also immune cells involved in innate rather than adaptive immunity. Thus we will now describe the implication of innate cells involved in asthma and then go into the pathophysiology of asthma exacerbations which best illustrates the implication of innate cells and bystander T cells during this chronic inflammatory disease.

4.4 Innate immunity from atopy to asthma

4.4.1 Epithelial cell

As a mucosal organ open to the environment, the respiratory system has to organize very tightly its protection against not only microbial agents but also pollutants and various irritants including tobacco smoke. The bronchial epithelium is encountered at first by antigens reaching the airways, and constitutes an efficient, intelligent barrier. Bronchial epithelial cells (BEC) are indeed very powerful in inducing and maintaining tolerance towards non-pathogenic environmental agents and in organizing the defence against viruses and bacteria. These functions are based both on the mechanical action of BEC and on their immune properties. BEC constitute a pseudo stratified, cubic epithelium. They are polarized, ciliated at their apical pole. The muco-ciliar escalator is efficient in scavenging continuously from the distal airways to the glottis any inhaled particle. BEC are strongly joined to one another through regions of adherence called tight junctions, offering an efficient barrier preventing any particle from getting through the epithelium and invading the submucosa.[(26)] Tight junctions are constituted of membrane proteins of the occludin and claudin family, and are associated to zonula occludens proteins. Some enzymes with protease activity have the ability to break down the tight junctions and facilitate the penetration of exogenous substances and micro-organisms. Some of these proteases are in addition capable of inducing a specific inflammatory response, which can be an allergic response in predisposed individuals. Indeed, many allergens exert such protease activity and therefore promote access of inhaled antigens, including themselves to the submucosa.[(27)]

In addition to these physical properties, BEC are able to express pattern recognition receptors (PRR), adhesion molecules, class II MHC proteins, and to produce a wide range of pro-inflammatory and anti-inflammatory cytokines. BEC are therefore able to reinforce tolerance towards particles and antigens that will be eliminated without any inflammation, and to trigger an inflammatory response when judged necessary. Especially relevant to their permanent function of tolerance induction, BEC constitutively and normally produce TGF-β, an immunosuppressive cytokine that can be detected at their apical pole in normal conditions.[28] In inflammatory conditions such as asthma, the BEC TGF-β immunostaining intensity decreases.[29]

In inflammatory conditions, BEC can be activated through PRR such as Toll-like receptors (TLR) but also protease-associated receptors (PAR) and Nod-like receptors. Relevant to asthma, some allergens such as HDM allergens, as proteases, are able to activate PAR2 and induce BEC to produce chemokine and pro-inflammatory cytokines such as TNF, IL-6 and GMCSF, all cytokines involved in inflammation and immune cell activation.

4.4.2 Dendritic cells

Dendritic cells (DCs) are professional antigen presenting cells, which make the decision of inducing or not an adaptive antigen-specific response. In addition they decide on the type of response induced, which can be tolerant or inflammatory, of one type or of another, namely Th1, Th2 or Th17. In bronchi, DCs constitute a large network covering the whole bronchial surface. They lie beneath BEC, in the submucosa, and exert a permanent sentinel periscope function through dendrites emitted into tight junctions and bound to BEC via adhesion molecules and molecules belonging to the claudin family.[30, 31] In this position, DCs are able to detect at any time the existence of any unwanted particle that gets through the mucosal blanket and would be susceptible to induce a bronchial injury. As sensors, DCs use their innate receptors, the PRR, including TLR and PAR. These receptors recognize molecular motifs associated to inhaled substances including microbes and allergens, called pathogen-associated molecular patterns (PAMPS). PAMPS include polysaccharides such as lipopolysacharides associated to gram negative bacteria, oligonucleotides such as CpGs, which are abundant in prokaryotic genomes, single-strand RNA which is the molecular signature of some viruses. These PAMPS are recognized by TLR 4, TLR9, TLR 7 and TLR8 respectively. According to the PRR involved, but also to the type of dendritic cell, this very early step of recognition induces the expression of coreceptors by DCs, which will in turn determine the type of T cell that will be associated to the subsequent adaptive response. This step also triggers the DC production of a pattern of cytokines that will help differentiate T cells into regulatory or proinflammatory Th1, Th2 or Th17 cells. According to the current literature it is not possible to clearly consider that one coreceptor will be associated to one T cell response, and if it is fairly clear that the expression of CD86, the CTLA4 ligand is involved in tolerance, ICOS ligand, CD80 and PD1 can be involved in diverse inflammatory responses according to the relative balance between these receptors and the amount of molecules expressed. For example the ICOS–ICOSL interaction can induce a Th1, Th2 or Treg response according to the density of coreceptors engaged.[32, 33] Among cytokines involved in the T cell differentiation, again the balance between them is crucial. IL-10 and TGF-β induce tolerance and Treg cell maturation, albeit IL-12 and IL-18 are major mediators involved in Th1 differentiation. Regarding IL-17, the mechanisms of differentiation are still unclear, but the production of TGF-β together with IL-6 seems to be the main cytokine combination required.[34]

These mechanisms of early differentiation of T cells also depend on genetics, and to go back to the hygiene hypothesis, some polymorphisms of TLR 4, one of the LPS receptors, were found to be associated with atopy (35). The altered recognition of LPS could impair the normal Th1 differentiation and therefore favour the Th2 deviation induced by allergens.

4.4.3 NK T cells

An abundant literature has considered relationships between natural killer T cells (NKT) and allergy in the recent years. This small subset of T cells (0.5 to 1 per cent of circulating T cells) belongs to the innate rather than the adaptive immunity in that they bear an invariant TCR, Vα24Vβ12 in humans, recognizing endogenous lipid antigens presented by the MHC class I related CD1d molecule. Their capacity to produce rapidly a high amount of cytokines makes them a crucial population in the induction of inflammatory responses. According to the context of inflammation, NKT cells are able to produce IL-4 and thus favour a Th2 response or IFN-γ and therefore drive a Th1 reaction. In mice, a subset of NKT cells express CD4, the other being CD4-CD8, although in humans there is also a subset of CD8αα positive cells. We have shown in the past that circulating CD4+ NKT cells were elevated in atopic subjects, and correlated with serum IgE levels.[36] This was in keeping with results obtained in mice that showed NKT cells to be mandatory to induce an IgE-mediated allergic response.[37] More recently, contradictory results were obtained, with α-galacosylceramide, the natural ligand of CD1d recognized by NK T cells, being capable of inducing or inhibiting an allergic reaction in mice.[38, 39]

In asthma, we did not find NKT cells to be differently regulated in blood compared to healthy subjects.[36] In BAL, it was first showed in a paediatric survey that NKT cells were very scarce in lungs,[40] with no variation in asthma compared to controls although they were significantly elevated during infection. In adults, a first study found high proportions of

NK T cells in BAL from asthmatics.[41] These NKT cells were producing IL-4 and IL-13 but no IFN-γ, suggesting their role in the Th2 deviation seen in asthma. As controls, BAL from patients with a Th1-mediated autoimmune disease, sarcoidosis, contained a normal amount of NKT cells. However, these results were largely contradicted in another study, which showed NK T cells to be equally represented in asthmatics, patients with COPD, a tobacco-related inflammatory panbronchitis, and controls.[42] At that stage, if it is shown that NKT cell are important in the inception of allergy, their role in asthma remains unclear.

4.5 Immunopathology of exacerbations

The rationale for studying the immunopathological events occurring during asthma exacerbations comes from the natural history of the disease and from the importance of developing drugs or treatment strategies targeting exacerbations specifically. Indeed, exacerbations represent a major clinical issue in asthma care, leading to hospitalizations, acute respiratory failure and sometimes death. They induce the main costs of asthma management in terms of care recourse and loss of working days. However, the large majority of works in the field of asthma immunopathology have compared stable patients to healthy controls. This has provided very important data on the mechanisms of asthma itself but not so much on those leading to symptoms and exacerbations; this pitfall could explain the relative failure of drugs targeting very specifically the Th2 inflammation.[3] Studies investigating the same patients in stable conditions and during exacerbations are few, mainly due to the difficulty of obtaining *in situ* samples more than once, especially during uncomfortable symptomatic periods.

Nevertheless, some data are available and will be discussed below. These data come from human surveys, but also experimental *in vitro* or animal studies. Results obtained in humans during exacerbations, whatever the cause, will be discussed first, and then we will consider the specificities provided by triggering factors of exacerbations and discuss the pivotal importance of the synergy between these triggers.

4.5.1 Immunopathological findings during exacerbations

Many results were obtained during the last decade through the generalization of induced sputum (IS) usage to explore the cellular events occurring during exacerbations. Indeed IS represents a non-invasive method of recovering bronchial cells, which can be repeated in the same patients in stable conditions or during exacerbation without any serious adverse event.[43]

In studies experimentally inducing exacerbations by interruption of anti-inflammatory treatment, a bronchial eosinophilia occurs, predicting the imminence of symptoms.[44] This predictive property of IS eosinophilia has been used successfully in preventive strategies in moderate to severe asthmatics, by adapting asthma treatment according to IS eosinophilia.[45,46] Such a strategy, however, seems limited in most severe cases of refractory asthma, probably because exacerbations are often related in these patients to neutrophil rather than eosinophil-mediated inflammation.[47] Indeed, in severe refractory asthmatics, the IS profile is heterogeneous, with some patients with an increase in IS eosinophila, other patients with an increase in IS neutrophilia and other with a stable IS profile.[47,48] It is noteworthy that in the latter patients, stable IS is abnormal with a high percentage of IS neutrophils at a basal stage.[47,49] It is clear therefore that IS cellularity, although easy to study, does not provide a complete picture of exacerbation immunopathology, and that mediators related to cell activation must be considered as well.

Norzila et al.[50] sampled IS in 38 children admitted to an emergency room, followed up two weeks later with another IS. They showed an influx in IS neutrophils and eosinophils, associated to a significant increase of myeloperoxydase and eosinophil cationic protein, and of IL-8 and IL-5. All of these parameters decreased in the post-exacerbation samples. This work is a clear illustration of the mixed neutrophil-related and eosinophil-related inflammation in asthma exacerbations. In adults, studies of asthma exacerbations are few. Qiu et al.[51] have obtained bronchial biopsies in 15 patients with exacerbations and compared them to 15 biopsies from stable asthmatic controls and 15 non-asthmatics. In addition to an increase in eosinophils and neutrophils, they found an increase of CXC chemokines and chemokine receptors in the exacerbating group compared to others, notably in BEC, but mainly in the sub-epithelial area.

We prospectively studied the T cell activation in blood and induced sputum from severe refractory asthmatics.[21] Patients were sampled every month over 18 months and were selected as having displayed at least two exacerbations within the last 12 months before inclusion. This gave us the opportunity to get samples at a distance from any exacerbations, and before, during and after exacerbations. T cell activation was studied by flow cytometry. We showed at baseline an increase in blood Th2 cell and a decrease in Treg cell proportions in asthmatics compared to controls. During exacerbations, there was an increase in both Th1 and Th2 cells, and a decrease of Treg cells. This profile was found both in the whole T cell population and at the level of CD8+ T cells. It was found both in blood and IS. More recently, using the same approach, we observed an increase of T cells expressing ICOS and a decrease of T cells expressing CTLA-4 before exacerbations.

This variation in coreceptor expression suggests a determinant role for innate immunity in the process of exacerbations, which must be investigated further. We did not document causes of exacerbations in this survey, but the cytokine profile found was roughly homogeneous from one exacerbation to another, thus suggesting that the mixed Th1/Th2 activation was a hallmark of exacerbations, whatever their cause. The Th17 pathway, recently identified, is probably relevant as well as far as the neutrophil-driven inflammation is concerned, but has not been explored yet in the context of asthma exacerbations.[(52)]

4.6 Immunopathology according to triggering factors

4.6.1 Viruses

Viral infections are considered as the main cause of asthma exacerbations, both in children and adults.[(53)] The viruses implicated are essentially rhinovirus (RV), influenza and respiratory syncitial virus (RSV). As other environmental pathogens, viruses first encounter and infect BEC, leading to extensive necrosis (influenza) or a patchy destruction (RV) of the epithelium.[(54)] In any case, the viral infection of BEC activates these cells, which switch their phenotype from tolerant to pro-inflammatory. The effect of RV on BEC has been extensively studied on cell lines, and in mouse models. Some data were also obtained in humans after experimental RV infection: briefly, after PAMP recognition by BEC TLR, adherence molecule (ICAM-1, VCAM), coreceptors (CD80, CD86), cytokine, and chemokine genes are expressed, allowing BEC to attract and activate immune cells including effector T cells.

Viruses are also recognized by TLR bared by DCs, activated as well as BEC. In response to viruses recognized notably through TLR3, TLR7 and TLR9, DCs overexpress CD80 and CD86 and produce IL-12, inducing a strong Th1 and Tc1 response. Although it is still uncertain if and to what extent asthmatic subjects are more susceptible than normal to infection, it is clear that asthma and atopy modify the anti-viral response, and that could be relevant to exacerbations. Viral bronchial infection induces a bronchial hyperreactivity detected by an increased response to an acetyl-choline analogue, metacholine. This increased response lasts a few weeks in non-atopic subjects but is delayed to a few months in atopics.[55]

Primary cultures of BEC have been widely studied and compared in asthma versus controls. BEC from asthmatics are resistant to early apoptosis.[56] In addition there is a clear defect, both in vitro and in vivo in their IFN-β and IFN-λ production,[56, 57] both mediators involved in the anti-viral response. These abnormalities could be relevant to the increased viral replication and the delayed viral clearance from asthmatic epithelium.

Apart from these anomalies, it must be discussed that although asthma is dominated by a Th2 inflammation, viral infections mainly drive a Th1 response. Indeed, one would expect viral infection to attenuate rather than exacerbate the asthmatic phenotype and to prevent rather than trigger the asthmatic symptoms in patients. It appears in fact that although viruses still induce a Th1 activation in asthmatic bronchi they also exacerbate the Th2 pre-existing activation in these patients, thus increasing the asthmatic-related inflammation. Indeed, it was demonstrated that BEC from asthmatics not only produce IL-8 and GMCSF, but also the pro-eosinophilic eotaxin. In addition, exposure of PBMCs to RV leads to an impaired production of IFN-γ in asthmatics, but also to an increased production of IL-4. The virus-driven Th1 inflammation can also enhance the allergic disease by inducing a mature phenotype of DCs.[58, 59]

Nevertheless, it is likely that the virus-induced Th1 activation is also deleterious for the asthmatic phenotype itself. Indeed, as developed above, there is an intrinsic Th1 activation in asthma that can be exacerbated during infection (Figure 4.2).[22] In addition it was showed that IP-10, a chemokine involved in Th1 cell homing, is increased in BEC culture supernatants obtained from asthmatics displaying a viral infection compared to non-asthmatics. This chemokine was even proposed as a novel biomarker of RV-induced exacerbations.[60] Furthermore, cytotoxic T cells, which are strongly solicited during viral infection and are related to a Th1 inflammation, seem to be highly relevant to asthma exacerbations. Indeed, it was demonstrated that the bronchial infiltration of CD8+ T cells was associated to asthma exacerbations and asthma death.[61]

It appears therefore that in asthmatics, response to viruses is different than in healthy subjects. The question that arises is whether these differences are related to the asthmatic or atopic status itself or whether other environmental stimulation such as allergen exposure also intervenes in these differences.

Recently, Bartlett et al.[62] developed a model of infection in mice that provided new insights into the relationships between asthma and viral infection. In this model, mice are sensitized to ovalbumin, a protein largely used in mouse models of asthma, and challenged intra-nasally. This classically induces a specific IgE response and a pulmonary infiltrate of eosinophils with airways reactivity detected by response to methacholine. In this model, mice are additionally infected by RV and the inflammation resulting from both allergen and viral stimulation is studied at successive time points by BAL analysis and measurement of metacholine-induced airways resistances. Results elegantly demonstrate (i) that allergic challenge is necessary to induce a Th2 activation (BAL IL-4 and IL-13 detection) that is amplified by virus infection, (ii) that conversely viral infection induces a Th1 response (BAL IFN-γ production, neutrophil influx) which is amplified by allergen challenge, and (iii) that airways hyperresponsiveness dramatically increases when mice are both challenged and infected compared to mice receiving one stimulation only. In addition, this model provides kinetics of inflammation showing that lung lymphocyte infiltration is maximal at seven days after infection. These results clearly demonstrate a synergy between the allergic and the viral inflammation, leading to a dramatic Th1 + Th2 response. Such synergy was previously reported in experimental conditions, leading to an even more drastic phenotype but probably less relevant to real life: Coyle et al.[(63)] used mice transgenic for a TCR specific of LCMV, a virus with a pulmonary tropism in mice. In these mice 80 per cent of T cells bear the cognate TCR, and they develop a strong Th1 lung response to the virus infection. After sensitization and challenge with ovalbumin, the cognate response becomes a huge Th2 response, indicating that the allergen primes T cells to respond in a Th2 manner to virus.

Several results from these important papers are reminiscent of observations realized in human asthma in experimental conditions. Indeed an increase of bronchial hyperreactivity after RV infection was reported in allergic patients challenged with a relevant allergen before infection.[(64)] Interestingly however, in already infected patients, allergen challenge had no effect on BHR, but it appears that the timing of both stimulations, one related to the other, is pivotal in modifying the synergy between both kinds of inflammation.[(65)] More importantly results reported by Bartlett et al. seem concordant with results obtained in real-life conditions in humans during exacerbations: in severe refractory asthma we observed a mixed Th1/Th2 response;[(21)] virus-induced bronchial hyperresponsiveness is increased and delayed in asthmatics;[(66)] the combined exposure to viruses and allergens in sensitized children increases the risk of hospital admission for asthma exacerbation.[(67)] Nevertheless, it remains unclear if the atopic/asthmatic status itself is sufficient to modify the response to viruses or if the concomitant exposure to allergen/other environmental factor is necessary.

To go back to considerations related to innate immunity, the results discussed above, by proving interactions between two types of antigen stimulation, clearly indicate that non-specific (innate) mechanisms involved in both types of responses orchestrate this synergy. Cells and mediators involved are unknown, but it can be speculated that BEC and DCs, by inducing signals of homing to neutrophils, eosinophils and lymphocytes, play a determinant role in this process. It appears therefore that lymphocytes infiltrating the bronchi or recovered during exacerbations in IS display various specificities, including specificity to the cognate viruses or allergens, but also to other allergens the patient would be sensitized to. This presence of bystander T cells during exacerbations, relevant to allergen-virus interaction but also to allergen–other allergen and allergen–pollutants interactions is probably of great importance in asthma and needs to be explored further. BEC and DCs are also pivotal in orientating the response to the Th1 or Th2 pathway, and they could be responsible for the mixed response seen, educating bystander T cells to produce both kinds of cytokines.[21]

4.6.2 Pollutants

Inhaled pollutants are composed of various organic and non-organic particles and gas, and their effect on the immune system is very difficult to study and most unclear. However, it appears that a number of inhaled pollutants act as amplifiers of adaptive responses, probably through their action on BEC or on other cells belonging to the innate immune system. Pollutants considered as relevant in asthma exacerbations are ozone, sulphur dioxide (SO_2), nitrate dioxide (NO_2), diesel exhaust particles (DEP) and tobacco smoke. Several epidemiological studies have now established that if exposure to inhaled pollutants is not related to an increased prevalence of asthma, it decreases the threshold of symptom triggering in already asthmatic subjects. Recently, it was elegantly demonstrated that for an equal amount of physical exercise, exposure to urban pollution (Oxford Street in London) decreases the functional parameters in asthmatics compared to the same subjects in a nearby park (Hyde Park).[68] Exposure to pollutants thus increases both frequency and severity of respiratory symptoms in asthmatics but not in healthy subjects. This is a paradigm illustration of a gene–environment interaction.

Experimental exposure to ozone in healthy volunteers induces an alteration of the pulmonary function.[69] Exposure to ozone at a concentration of 0.1 to 0.4 ppm during one hour induces a neutrophil-mediated inflammation that persists during 24 hours. In asthmatics, experimental exposure to ozone coupled to exposure to an allergen induces an aggravation of the bronchial response with an increase in the IS eosinophilia.[70]

SO_2 also decreases the threshold for asthma symptom triggering, with an effect found in asthmatics at a concentration of 0.25 ppm, which is ineffective in healthy volunteers.[71] NO_2 probably triggers bronchial inflammation as a precursor of ozone. Again, this pollutant amplifies the effect of allergens.[72] It also seems to increase the effect of viruses on asthma exacerbation.

DEP have been shown to facilitate the IgE specific response in several studies conducted by the Diaz-Sanchez group.[73] Indeed these authors showed that pre-exposure of the nasal mucosa to DEP increased the IgE response to a common inhaled allergen in sensitized patients. In addition, they demonstrated that DEP facilitated the IgE-mediated sensitization to a new allergen in atopic subjects. In healthy volunteers, DEP induced an increase in neutrophils with induction of the IL-6, IL-8 and GM-CSF genes expression in IS and bronchial biopsies, but without alteration of the respiratory function.[74] In moderate asthmatics, exposure to DEP increased the non-specific bronchial hyperresponsiveness induced by metacholine.[75]

The mechanism of action of DEP in triggering asthma symptoms is unknown. In ex-vivo experiments, we have shown that exposure of PBMC from asthmatics to DEP induced the increase of both Th1 and Th2 cytokine production, without allergen stimulation.[76] Importantly, this effect was significantly higher in patients displaying exacerbations. Indeed, the basal level of Th1 and Th2 cytokine production by T cells was higher in exacerbated patients compared to controlled asthmatics, but after DEP stimulation, the difference in cytokine production was dramatically increased in exacerbating patients. These findings are concordant with previous results obtained in guinea pigs, which clearly showed that DEP exacerbate allergen-induced airway responses.[77] There is therefore a non-specific effect of DEP, depending on the basal state of T cell activation. Pollutants can therefore non-specifically amplify the ongoing bronchial inflammation. An interesting finding relevant to the synergy between pollutants and allergens is that DEP can bind some allergens such as pollen major allergens.[78]

Regarding the effect of passive exposure to tobacco smoke, less data are paradoxically available, and essentially epidemiological studies demonstrate an effect on asthma symptoms. Therefore, it is not possible to determine if this pollutant effectively induces a higher prevalence of asthma or if, like other pollutants, it triggers symptoms in already affected subjects, which is more likely.[79]

Taken together, these data about relationships between pollutants and asthma show that all pollutants are at least able to increase the response to allergens and/or viruses. This interaction between pollutants and allergens is illustrated in an epidemiological study demonstrating that living in a polluted area increases by 3.14 the risk of pollen-induced exacerbations.[80]

The cellular target of pollutants is unknown, but when considering their non-protein composition (ozone, SO_2, NO_2), or conversely the huge amount of organic and non-organic dusts (DEP, tobacco smoke), it is most likely that pollutants act non-specifically on innate immunity. They probably modify the permeability of bronchial epithelium, and trigger activation of both BEC and DCs through PRR stimulation.[81] This action is in keeping with findings indicating that mice exposure to DEP induces the production of various chemokines.[82] Recently, it was showed in a mouse model of ozone exposure that induction of airways hyperresponsiveness by ozone required both NKT and Th17 cells.[83] It must be said that experimental works are needed to confirm this action of pollutants on innate immunity, which are difficult to set up because of the difficulty of usingh these products in conditions sufficiently close to the natural exposure to drive relevant conclusions.

4.6.3 Allergens

Allergens intervene both at the level of inception of asthma, by inducing sensitizations that define atopy, and at that of exacerbations, by triggering symptoms in allergic subjects. Experimental exposure of sensitized patients to allergens induces a bronchial inflammation and a decrease of lung function relevant *a minima* to real allergen-induced exacerbation.[84] Many reports confirm the relationships between sensitization, allergen exposure and the risk of exacerbations. This was clearly showed for cockroach and cat allergens,[85] house dust mites,[86] moistures[87, 88] and also pollens.[89] Although it is clear that indoor allergens are more likely to be associated to asthma than pollens,[90] this difference is unclear with regard to exacerbations. Allergen exposure induces a paradigm Th2 response[91] in conditions of acute massive exposure, but little is known about the immune reaction induced by allergens in usual exposure conditions. During cypress pollen season in the south of France, we observed in rhinitic patients sensitized to cypress an increase in blood Th1 activation with a parallel unexpected decrease of the Th2 activation.[92] During grass pollen season, a decrease in Treg cell activation was observed during rhinitis.[20] However, rhinitis is not asthma and these results cannot be extended to exacerbations of asthma. In addition, as developed above, many cofactors including virus and pollutant effects intervene and modify the course of the immune response due to pollen exposure.

The action of allergens in bronchi at the level of innate immunity is dual, with a classical activation of BEC and DCs through the activation of TLR, but also through their enzymatic activity. The TLR involved in response to allergens are unknown, as PAMPS associated to allergen stimulation are not clearly identified. Lipopolysaccharide can be frequently associated to allergen and stimulate TLR4. The proteolytic activity of allergens is important as it induces both the activation of PAR and the disruption of the epithelial barrier. This enzymatic activity of allergens was recently nicely reviewed.[26] Briefly, Der p 1, a major allergen of house dust mites, spores from *Aspergillus spp*, including the *Aspergillus fumigatus allergens Asp f 5*, ragweed and birch pollen allergens and cockroach allergens display serine and cysteine protease activity that could promote paracellular access to submucosa and subepithelial DCs by cleaving the tight junction occluding proteins, claudin proteins and zonula occludens 1. This non-specific action of allergens of course facilitates the access of allergens themselves to the submucosa, but also of any accompanying inhaled substances, including viruses and pollutants. This mechanism could therefore be relevant for the synergic action of allergens with the other triggers of asthma exacerbations.

4.7 Concluding remarks: at least two synergistic inflammatory processes are required to induce asthma exacerbations

Asthma exacerbations result from the activation of BEC and DCs, These cells then produce cytokines and chemokines attracting and activating T cells, eosinophils and neutrophils which in turn injure the epithelium and amplify the inflammatory process (Figure 4.3).

We have largely developed above the theory that asthma exacerbations are related to a proper inflammatory response, differing from the ongoing chronic inflammation related to asthma itself. It is nevertheless clear that this first chronic inflammatory step is necessary, as neither viruses, pollutants nor allergens induce exacerbation in non-asthmatic patients, and as exacerbations are efficiently prevented by inhaled corticosteroids in most patients. Indeed, inhaled steroids clear this chronic inflammation. In atopics, allergens are considered as responsible for this first chronic inflammatory step. In non-atopic asthma, the chronic inflammation is similar but the trigger is unknown. However, whatever the atopic status, an intrinsic chronic inflammation is found in asthmatic patients.

What, therefore, is the role of allergens, if any, in the first step of inflammation? It was indeed demonstrated recently that innate cells,

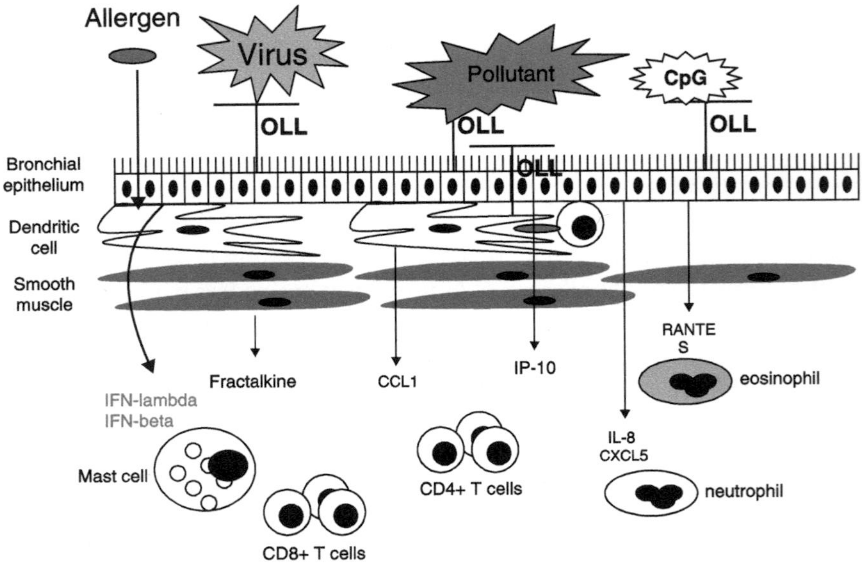

Figure 4.3 Immunopathology of asthma exacerbations. Upon allergen, virus or pollutant stimulation, bronchial epithelial cells and dendritic cells are activated via pattern recognition receptors to produce cytokines and chemokines and express membrane molecules that will attract and activate T cells, eosinophils, mast cells and neutrophils.

eosinophils, were required for the recruitment of T cells in tissues and induce an allergic pulmonary inflammation, indicating that an inflammatory trigger, not necessarily antigen-specific, is necessary for the specific T cell response.[(59)] Therefore, any trigger leading to specific or non-specific chronic inflammation in predisposed subjects could create the conditions of asthma exacerbations. In the case of atopy, for instance, allergens would be able, in atopic subjects, to induce the chronic inflammation necessary for the recruitment of other allergen-, virus- or pollutant-associated protein-specific T cells in case of exposure to the respective pathogen.

Conversely, could viruses or pollutants create the conditions of the chronic first step of inflammation? With regard to viruses and other microbial agents, both epidemiological and experimental findings suggest that it could be the case. Indeed, latent bronchial infection by adenoviruses causes the eosinophilic component of an allergic response to become steroid-resistant;[(93)] more recently, it was shown that IL-13-secreting NKT cells recruited and activated during a respiratory viral infection induce bronchial lesions reminiscent of those found in asthma through interaction with IL-13-producing macrophages. In such a model, a subsequent allergic sensitization would probably exacerbate the observed phenotype.[94]

What about pollutants? The evidence is probably smaller, and the question of the ability of pollutants to induce a chronic inflammation able to create the conditions for exacerbations is open. A recent epidemiological survey of 9,651 adults randomly selected from the general population followed up at ten years elegantly demonstrated that reduced exposure to PM10 attenuated age-related decline in lung function, independently of the presence of asthma, which suggests PM10 is able to induce inflammation *per se.*[95]

In conclusion, innate immunity is the core of asthmatic inflammation, creating the conditions of adaptive immunity to express itself as a disease. We hypothesize that innate immunity is pivotal in the chronic asthmatic inflammation required as a first step of the disease and in the second step leading to symptom occurrence and exacerbations. In both steps, allergens, viruses and inhaled pollutants are triggering factors activating innate immune cells (Figure 4.4). It therefore appears that treatment

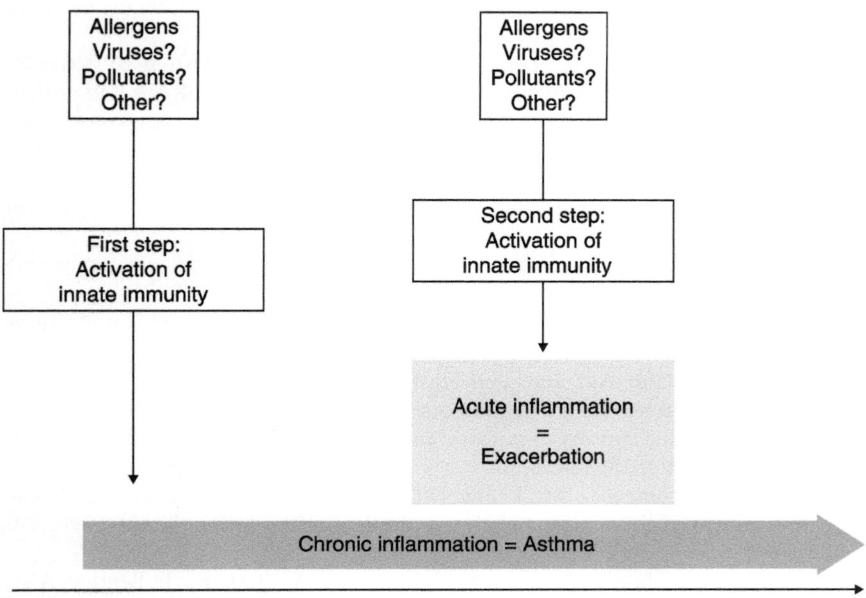

Figure 4.4 Hypothesis.

Exacerbations of asthma result from the addition of two inflammatory responses in which allergens, pollutants and viruses are involved. The first is chronic and defines the disease itself. The second occurs in case of acute exposure to triggers.

strategies aiming to modify innate cell activation in association or not to antigen-specific immunotherapy could prevent both the disease and its exacerbations.

References

1 GINA. NIH Publication 02-3659. www.ginasthma.org.

2 Humbert M, Beasley R, Ayres J, Slavin R, Hébert J, Bousquet J, Beeh KM, Ramos S, Canonica GW, Hedgecock S, Fox H, Blogg M, Surrey K. Benefits of omalizumab as add-on therapy in patients with severe persistent asthma who are inadequately controlled despite best available therapy (GINA 2002 step 4 treatment): INNOVATE. *Allergy* 2005, 60: 309.

3 Leckie MJ, ten Brinke A, Khan J, Diamant Z, O'Connor BJ, Walls CM, Mathur AK, Cowley HC, Chung KF, Djukanovic R, Hansel TT, Holgate ST, Sterk PJ, Barnes PJ. Effects of an interleukin-5 blocking monoclonal antibody on eosinophils, airway hyper-responsiveness, and the late asthmatic response. *Lancet* 2000, 356: 2144–8.

4 Brightling C, Berry M, Amrani Y. Targeting TNF-alpha: a novel therapeutic approach for asthma. *J Allergy Clin Immunol* 2008, 121: 5.

5 Nieves A, Magnan A, Boniface S, Proudhon H, Lanteaume A, Romanet S, Vervloet D, Godard P. ARIA. Phenotypes of asthma revisited upon the presence of atopy. *Respir Med* 2005, 99: 347–54.

6 Humbert M, Durham SR, Ying S, Kimmitt P, Barkans J, Assoufi B, Pfister R, Menz G, Robinson DS, Kay AB, Corrigan CJ. IL-4 and IL-5 mRNA and protein in bronchial biopsies from patients with atopic and nonatopic asthma: evidence against "intrinsic" asthma being a distinct immunopathologic entity. *Am J Respir Crit Care Med* 1996, 154: 1497–504.

7 Vercelli D. Advances in asthma and allergy genetics in 2007. *J Allergy Clin Immunol* 2008, 122: 267–71.

8 Strachan DP. Family size, infection and atopy: the first decade of the "hygiene hypothesis". *Thorax* 2000, 55 Suppl 1: S2–10.

9 Mosmann T, Coffman R. Two types of mouse helper T-cell clone. Implications for immune regulation. *Immunology Today* 1987, 8: 223–7.

10 Tang MLK, Kemp AS, and Thorburn J, and Hill DJ. Reduced Interferon-#t12 secretion in neonates and subsequent atopy. *Lancet* 1994, 344: 983–5.

11 Durham SR. Mechanisms of mucosal inflammation in the nose and lungs. *Clin Exp Allergy* 1998, 28: 11–16.

12 Hamid Q, Boguniewicz M, Leung DYM. Differential in situ cytokine gene expression in acute versus chronic atopic dermatitis. *J Clin Invest* 1994, 94: 870–6.

13 Robinson DS, Hamid Q, Ying S, Tsicopoulos A, Barkans J, Bentley AM, Corrigan C, Durham SR, and Kay AB. Predominant TH2-like bronchoalveolar T-lymphocyte population in atopic asthma. *N Engl J Med* 1992, 326: 298–304.

14 El Biaze M, Boniface S, Koscher V, Mamessier E, Dupuy P, Milhe F, Ramadour M, Vervloet D, Magnan A. T cell activation, from atopy to asthma: More a paradox than a paradigm. *Allergy* 2003, 58: 844–53.

15 Magnan A, Mély L, Camilla CA, Badier M, Bongrand P, Vervloet D. Assessment of the TH1/TH2 paradigm in whole blood in atopy and Asthma: increased IFN-gamma-producing CD8+ T cells in asthma. *Am J Respir Crit Care Med* 2000, 161: 1790–6.
16 Krug N, Madden J, Redington AE, Lackie P, Djukanovic R, Schauer U, et al. T-cell cytokine profile evaluated at the single cell level in BAL and blood in allergic asthma. *Am J Respir Cell Mol Biol* 1996, 14: 319–26.
17 Boniface S, Koscher V, Mamessier E, El Biaze M, Dupuy P, Lorec AM, Guillot C, Badier M, Bongrand P, Vervloet D, Magnan A. Assessment of T lymphocyte cytokine production in induced sputum from asthmatics: a flow cytometry study. *Clin Exp Allergy* 2003, 33: 1238–43.
18 Liu W, Putnam AL, Xu-Yu Z, Lee MR, Zhu S, Gottlieb PA, Kapranov P, Gingeras TR, Fazekas de St Groth B, Clayberger C, Soper DM, Ziegler SF, Bluestone JA. CD127 expression inversely correlates with FoxP3 and suppressive function of human CD4+ T reg cells. *J Exp Med* 2006, 203: 1701–11.
19 Akdis M, Verhagen J, Taylor A, Karamloo F, Karagiannidis C, Crameri R, Thunberg S, Deniz G, Valenta R, Fiebig H, Kegel C, Disch R, Schmidt-Weber CB, Blaser K, Akdis CA. Immune Responses in Healthy and Allergic Individuals Are Characterized by a Fine Balance between Allergen-specific T Regulatory 1 and T Helper 2 Cells. *J Exp Med* 2004, 199: 1567–75.
20 Ling EM, Smith T, Nguyen XD, Pridgeon C, Dallman M, Arbery J, Carr VA, Robinson DS. Relation of CD4+CD25+ regulatory T-cell suppression of allergen-driven T-cell activation to atopic status and expression of allergic disease. *Lancet* 2004, 363: 608–15.
21 Mamessier E, Nieves A, Lorec AM, Dupuy P, Pinot D, Pinet C, Vervloet D, Magnan A. T cell activation during exacerbations: a longitudinal study in refractory asthma. *Allergy* 2008, 63: 1202–10.
22 Botturi K, Lacoeuille Y, Cavailles A. Pinot D, Nieves A, Lorec AM. European Respiratory Society Conference, Berlin 2008.
23 Mamessier E, Birnbaum J, Dupuy P, Vervloet D, Magnan A. Ultra-rush VIT induces differential T cell activation and regulatory patterns according to the severity of allergy. *Clin Exp Allergy* 2006, 36: 704–13.
24 Botturi K, Vervloet D, Magnan A. T cells and allergens relationships: are they that specific? *Clin Exp Allergy* 2007, 37: 1121–3.
25 Des Roches A, Paradis L, Menardo JL, Bouges S, Daurés JP, Bousquet J. Immunotherapy with a standardized Dermatophagoides pteronyssinus extract. VI. Specific immunotherapy prevents the onset of new sensitizations in children. *J Allergy Clin Immunol* 1997, 99: 450–3.
26 Hammad H, Lambrecht BN. Dendritic cells and epithelial cells: linking innate and adaptive immunity in asthma. *Nat Rev Immunol* 2008, 8: 193–204.
27 Runswick S, Mitchell T, Davies P, Robinson C, Garrod DR. Pollen proteolytic enzymes degrade tight junctions. *Respirology* 2007, 12: 834–42.
28 Magnan A, Frachon I, Rain B, Peuchmaur M, Monti G, Lenot B, Fattal M, Simonneau G, Galanaud P, Emilie D. Transforming Growth Factor-beta in normal human lung: preferential location in bronchial epithelial cells. *Thorax* 1994, 49: 789–92.

29 Magnan A, Retornaz F, Tsicopoulos A, Brisse J, Van Pee D, Gosset P, Chamlian A, Tonnel AB, Vervloet D. Altered compartimentalization of TGFß in asthmatic airways. *Clin Exp Allergy* 1997, 27: 389–95.
30 Hammad H, Smits HH, Ratajczak C, Nithiananthan A, Wierenga EA, Stewart GA, Jacquet A, Tonnel AB, Pestel J. Monocyte-derived dendritic cells exposed to Der p 1 allergen enhance the recruitment of Th2 cells: major involvement of the chemokines TARC/CCL17 and MDC/CCL22. *Eur Cytokine Netw* 2003, 14: 219–28.
31 Sung SS, Fu SM, Rose CE Jr, Rose CE Jr, Gaskin F, Ju ST, Beaty SR. A major lung CD103 (alphaE)-beta7 integrin-positive epithelial dendritic cell population expressing Langerin and tight junction proteins. *J Immunol* 2006, 176: 2161–72.
32 Akbari O, Freeman GJ, Meyer EH, Greenfield EA, Chang TT, Sharpe AH, Berry G, DeKruyff RH, Umetsu DT. Antigen-specific regulatory T cells develop via the ICOS-ICOS-ligand pathway and inhibit allergen-induced airway hyperreactivity. *Nat Med* 2002, 8: 1024.
33 Lohning M, Hutloff A, Kallinich T Mages HW, Bonhagen K, Radbruch A, Hamelmann E, Kroczek RA. Expression of ICOS in vivo defines CD4+ effector T cells with high inflammatory potential and a strong bias for secretion of interleukin 10. *J Exp Med* 2003, 197: 181–93.
34 Harrington LE, Hatton RD, Mangan PR, Turner H, Murphy TL, Murphy KM, Weaver CT. Interleukin 17-producing CD4+ effector T cells develop via a lineage distinct from the T helper type 1 and 2 lineages. *Nat Immunol* 2005, 6: 1123.
35 Smit LA, Bongers SI, Ruven HJ Rijkers GT, Wouters IM, Heederik D, Omland Ø, Sigsgaard T. Atopy and new-onset asthma in young Danish farmers and CD14, TLR2, and TLR4 genetic polymorphisms: a nested case-control study. *Clin Exp Allergy* 2007, 37: 1602–8.
36 Magnan A, Mély L, Romagné F, Camilla C, Necker A, Bongrand P, Casano P, Pratop S, Fert V, Montero-Jullian F, Malissen B, Vervloet D. Relationships between natural T cells, atopy, IgE levels and IL-4 production. *Allergy* 2000, 55: 286–90.
37 Akbari O, Stock P, Meyer E, Kronenberg M, Sidobre S, Nakayama T, Taniguchi M, Grusby MJ, DeKruyff RH, Umetsu DT. Essential role of NKT cells producing IL-4 and IL-13 in the development of allergen-induced airway hyperreactivity. *Nat Med* 2003, 9: 582–8.
38 Lisbonne Diem S, de Castro Keller A, Lefort J, Araujo LM, Hachem P, Fourneau JM, Sidobre S, Kronenberg M, Taniguchi M, Van Endert P, Dy M, Askenase P, Russo M, Vargaftig BB, Herbelin A, Leite-de-Moraes MC. Cutting edge: invariant V alpha 14 NKT cells are required for allergen-induced airway inflammation and hyperreactivity in an experimental asthma model. *J Immunol* 2003, 171: 1637–41.
39 Hachem A Lisbonne M, Michel ML, Diem S, Roongapinun S, Lefort J, Marchal G, Herbelin A, Askenase PW, Dy M, Leite-de-Moraes MC. Alpha-galactosylceramide-induced iNKT cells suppress experimental allergic asthma in sensitized mice: role of IFN-gamma. *Eur J Immunol* 2005, 35: 2793–802.
40 Pham-Thi N, de Blic J, Le Bourgeois M, Dy M, Scheinmann P, Leite-de-Moraes MC. Enhanced frequency of immunoregulatory invariant natural killer T cells

in the airways of children with asthma. *J Allergy Clin Immunol* 2006, 117: 217–18.

41 Akbari O, Faul JL, Hoyte EG, Berry GJ, Wahlström J, Kronenberg M, DeKruyff RH, Umetsu DT. CD4+ invariant T-cell-receptor+ natural killer T cells in bronchial asthma. *N Engl J Med* 2006, 354, 11: 1117–29.

42 Vijayanand P, Seumois G, Pickard C, Powell RM, Angco G, Sammut D, Gadola SD, Friedmann PS, Djukanovic R. Invariant natural killer T cells in asthma and chronic obstructive pulmonary disease. *N Engl J Med* 2007, 356: 1410–22.

43 Holz O, Kips J, Magnussen H. Update on sputum methodology. *Eur Respir J* 2000, 2: 355–9.

44 Jatakanon A, Lim S, Barnes PJ. Changes in sputum eosinophils predict loss of asthma control. *Am J Respir Crit Care Med* 2000, 161: 64–72.

45 Green RH, Brightling CE, McKenna S, Hargadon B, Parker D, Bradding P, Wardlaw AJ, Pavord ID. Asthma exacerbations and sputum eosinophil counts: a randomised controlled trial. *Lancet* 2002, 360: 1715–21.

46 Petsky HL, Kynaston JA, Turner C, Li AM, Cates CJ, Lasserson TJ, Chang AB. Tailored interventions based on sputum eosinophils versus clinical symptoms for asthma in children and adults. *Cochrane Database Syst Rev* 2007, 2: CD005603.

47 Pinot D, Nieves A, Lorec AM. European Respiratory Society Conference, Berlin 2008.

48 in't Veen J, Smits HH, Hiemstra PS, Zwinderman AE, Sterk PJ, Bel EH. Lung function and sputum characteristics of patients with severe asthma during an induced exacerbation by double-blind steroid withdrawal. *Am J Respir Crit Care Med* 1999, 160: 93–9.

49 Jatakanon A, Uasuf C, Maziak W. Lim S, Chung KF, Barnes PJ. Neutrophilic inflammation in severe persistent asthma. *Am J Respir Crit Care Med* 1999, 160: 1532–9.

50 Norzila MZ, Fakes K, Henry RL, Simpson J, Gibson PG. Interleukin-8 secretion and neutrophil recruitment accompanies induced sputum eosinophil activation in children with acute asthma. *Am J Respir Crit Care Med* 2000, 161: 769–74.

51 Qiu Y, Zhu J, Bandi V, Guntupalli KK, Jeffery PK. Bronchial mucosal inflammation and upregulation of CXC chemoattractants and receptors in severe exacerbations of asthma. *Thorax* 2007, 62: 475–82.

52 Bullens DM, Truyen E, Coteur L, Dilissen E, Hellings PW, Dupont LJ, Ceuppens JL. IL-17 mRNA in sputum of asthmatic patients: linking T cell driven inflammation and granulocytic influx? *Respir Res* 2006, 7: 135.

53 Johnston NW, Sears MR. Asthma exacerbations 1: epidemiology. *Thorax* 2006, 61: 722–8.

54 Papadopoulos NG, Xepapadaki P, Mallia P, Brusselle G, Watelet JB, Xatzipsalti M, Foteinos G, van Drunen CM, Fokkens WJ, D'Ambrosio C, Bonini S, Bossios A, Lötvall J, van Cauwenberge P, Holgate ST, Canonica GW, Szczeklik A, Rohde G, Kimpen J, Pitkäranta A, Mäkelä M, Chanez P, Ring J, Johnston SL. Mechanisms of virus-induced asthma exacerbations: state-of-the-art. A GA2LEN and InterAirways document. *Allergy* 2007, 62: 457–72.

55 Xepapadaki P, papadopoulos NG, Bossios A, Manoussakis E, Manousakas T, Saxoni-Papageorgiou P. Duration of postviral airway hyperresponsiveness in children with asthma: effect of atopy. *J Allergy Clin Immunol* 2005, 116: 299–304.

56 Wark PA, Johnston SL, Bucchieri F, Powell R, Puddicombe S, Laza-Stanca V, Holgate ST, Davies DE. Asthmatic bronchial epithelial cells have a deficient innate immune response to infection with rhinovirus. *J Exp Med* 2005, 201: 937–47.
57 Contoli M, Message SD, Laza-Stanca V, Edwards MR, Wark PA, Bartlett NW, Kebadze T, Mallia P, Stanciu LA, Parker HL, Slater L, Lewis-Antes A, Kon OM, Holgate ST, Davies DE, Kotenko SV, Papi A, Johnston SL. Role of deficient type III interferon-lambda production in asthma exacerbations. *Nat Med* 2006, 12: 1023–6.
58 Papadopoulos NG, Stanciu LA, Papi A, Holgate ST, Johnston SL. A defective type 1 response to rhinovirus in atopic asthma. *Thorax* 2002, 57: 328–32.
59 Jacobsen EA, Ochkur SI, Pero RS, Taranova AG, Protheroe CA, Colbert DC, Lee NA, Lee JJ. Allergic pulmonary inflammation in mice is dependent on eosinophil-induced recruitment of effector T cells. *J Exp Med* 2008, 205: 699–710.
60 Wark PA, Bucchieri F, Johnston SL, Gibson PG, Hamilton L, Mimica J, Zummo G, Holgate ST, Attia J, Thakkinstian A, Davies DE. IFN-gamma-induced protein 10 is a novel biomarker of rhinovirus-induced asthma exacerbations. *J Allergy Clin Immunol* 2007, 120: 586–93.
61 O'Sullivan S, Cormican L, Faul JL, Ichinohe S, Johnston SL, Burke CM, Poulter LW. Activated, cytotoxic CD8(+) T lymphocytes contribute to the pathology of asthma death. *Am J Respir Crit Care Med* 2001, 164: 560–4.
62 Bartlett NW, Walton RP, Edwards MR, Aniscenko J, Caramori G, Zhu J, Glanville N, Choy KJ, Jourdan P, Burnet J, Tuthill TJ, Pedrick MS, Hurle MJ, Plumpton C, Sharp NA, Bussell JN, Swallow DM, Schwarze J, Guy B, Almond JW, Jeffery PK, Lloyd CM, Papi A, Killington RA, Rowlands DJ, Blair ED, Clarke NJ, Johnston SL. Mouse models of rhinovirus-induced disease and exacerbation of allergic airway inflammation. *Nature Med* 2008, 14: 199–204.
63 Coyle AJ, Erard F, Bertrand C, Walti S, Pircher H, Le Gros G. Virus-specific CD8+ cells can switch to interleukin 5 production and induce airway eosinophilia. *J Exp Med* 1995, 181: 1229–33.
64 Lemanske RF, Dick EC, Swenson CA, Vrtis RF, Busse WW. Rhinovirus upper respiratory infection increases airway hyperreactivity and late asthmatic reactions. *J Clin Invest* 1989, 83: 1.
65 Barends M, Van Oosten M, De Rond CG, Dormans JA, Osterhaus AD, Neijens HJ, Kimman TG. Timing of infection and prior immunization with respiratory syncytial virus (RSV) in RSV-enhanced allergic inflammation. *J Infect Dis* 2004, 189: 1866–72.
66 Folkerts G, Busse WW, Nijkamp FP, Sorkness R, Gern JE. Virus-induced airway hyperresponsiveness and asthma. *Am J Respir Crit Care Med* 1998, 157: 1708–20.
67 Murray CS, Poletti G, Kebadze T, Morris J, Woodcock A, Johnston SL, Custovic A. Study of modifiable risk factors for asthma exacerbations: virus infection and allergen exposure increase the risk of asthma hospital admissions in children. *Thorax* 2006, 61: 376–82.
68 McCreanor J, Cullinan P, Nieuwenhuijsen MJ, Stewart-Evans J, Malliarou E, Jarup L, Harrington R, Svartengren M, Han IK, Ohman-Strickland P, Chung KF, Zhang J. Respiratory effects of exposure to diesel traffic in persons with asthma. *N Engl J Med* 2007, 357: 2348–58.

69 Koren HS, Devlin RB, Graham DE, Mann R, McGee MP, Horstman DH, et al. Ozone-induced inflammation in the lower airways of human subjects. *Am Rev Respir Dis* 1989, 139: 407–15.
70 Vagaggini B, Carnevali S, Macchioni P, et al. Airway inflammatory response to ozone in subjects with different asthma severity. *Eur Respir J* 1999, 13: 274–80.
71 Horstman DH, Folinsbee LJ. Sulfur dioxide-induced bronchoconstriction in asthmatics exposed for short durations under controlled conditions: a selected review. In: Utell MJ, Frank R, eds. *Susceptibility to inhaled pollutants*. Philadelphia: American Society for Testing and Materials, 1989.
72 Sandstrom T, Stjernberg N, Eklund A, Ledin MC, Bjermer L, Kolmodin-Hedman B, et al. Inflammatory cell response in bronchoalveolar lavage fluid after nitrogen dioxide exposure of healthy subjects: a dose-response study. *Eur Respir J* 1991, 4: 332–9.
73 Diaz Sanchez D, Garcia MP, Wang M, Jyrala M, Saxon A. Nasal challenge with diesel exhaust particles can induce sensitization to a neoallergen in the human mucosa. *J Allergy Clin Immunol* 1999, 104: 1183–8.
74 Yanagisawa R, Takano H, Inoue KI, Ichinose T, Sadakane K, Yoshino S, Yamaki K, Yoshikawa T, Hayakawa K. Components of diesel exhaust particles differentially affect Th1/Th2 response in a murine model of allergic airway inflammation. *Clin Exp Allergy* 2006, 36: 386–95.
75 Nordenhall C, Pourazar J, Ledin MC, Levin JO, Sandström T, Adelroth E. Diesel exhaust enhances airway responsiveness in asthmatic subjects. *Eur Respir J* 2001, 17: 909–15.
76 Mamessier M, Nieves A, Vervloet D, Magnan A. Diesel exhaust particles enhance T cell activation in severe asthmatics. *Allergy* 2006, 61: 581–8.
77 Hashimoto K, Ishii Y, Uchida Y, Masuyama K, Morishima Y, Hirano K, Nomura A, Sakamoto T, Takano H, Sagai M, Sekizawa K.. Exposure to diesel exhaust exacerbates allergen-induced airway responses in guinea pigs. *Am J Respir Crit Care Med* 2001, 164: 1957–63.
78 Knox RB, Suphioglu C, Taylor P, Desai R, Watson HC, Peng JL, Bursill LA. Major grass pollen allergen Lol p 1 binds to diesel exhaust particles: implications for asthma and air pollution. *Clin Exp Allergy* 1997, 27: 246–51.
79 Vork KL, Broadwin RL, Blaisdell RJ. Developing asthma in childhood from exposure to secondhand tobacco smoke: insights from a meta-regression. *Environ Health Perspect* 2007, 115: 1394–400.
80 Mur Gimeno P, Feo Brito F, Martínez C, Tobías A, Suárez L, Guerra F, Galindo PA, Gómez E. Decompensation of pollen-induced asthma in two towns with different pollution levels in La Mancha, Spain. *Clin Exp Allergy* 2007, 37: 558–63.
81 Baulig A, Sourdeval M, Meyer M, Marano F, Baeza-Squiban A. Biological effects of atmospheric particles on human bronchial epithelial cells. Comparison with diesel exhaust particles. *Toxicol In Vitro* 2003, 17: 567–73.
82 Senechal S, de Nadai P, Ralainirina N, Scherpereel A, Vorng H, Lassalle P, Tonnel AB, Tsicopoulos A, Wallaert B. Effect of diesel on chemokines and chemokine receptors involved in helper T cell type 1/type 2 recruitment in patients with asthma. *Am J Respir Crit Care Med* 2003, 168: 215–21.

83 Pichavant M, Goya S, Meyer EH, Johnston RA, Kim HY, Matangkasombut P, Zhu M, Iwakura Y, Savage PB, DeKruyff RH, Shore SA, Umetsu DT. Ozone exposure in a mouse model induces airway hyperreactivity that requires the presence of natural killer T cells and IL-17. *J Exp Med* 2008, 205: 385–93.
84 Moore WC, Hasday JD, Meltzer SS, Wisnewski PL, White B, Bleecker ER. Subjects with mild and moderate asthma respond to segmental allergen challenge with similar, reproducible, allergen-specific inflammation. *J Allergy Clin Immunol* 2001: 108: 908–14.
85 Lewis SA, Weiss ST, Platts-Mills TA, Burge H, Gold DR. The role of indoor allergen sensitization and exposure in causing morbidity in women with asthma. *Am J Respir Crit Care Med* 2002, 165: 961–6.
86 Gehring U, Bischof W, Fahlbusch B, Wichmann HE, Heinrich J. House dust endotoxin and allergic sensitization in children. *Am J Respir Crit Care Med* 2002, 166: 939–44.
87 Dales RE, Cakmak S, Judek S, Dann T, Coates F, Brook JR, Burnett RT. Influence of outdoor aeroallergens on hospitalization for asthma in Canada. *J Allergy Clin Immunol* 2004, 113: 303–6.
88 Matheson MC, Abramson MJ, Dharmage SC, Forbes AB, Raven JM, Thien FC, Walters EH. Changes in indoor allergen and fungal levels predict changes in asthma activity among young adults. *Clin Exp Allergy* 2005, 35: 907–13.
89 Tobias A, Galan I, Banegas JR. Non-linear short-term effects of airborne pollen levels with allergenic capacity on asthma emergency room admissions in Madrid, Spain. *Clin Exp Allergy* 2004, 34: 871–8.
90 Magnan A, Fourré-Julian C, Jullian H, Badier M, Lanteaume A, Vervloet D, Charpin D. Rhinitis alone or rhinitis plus asthma: What makes the difference? *Eur Respir J* 1998, 12: 1073–8.
91 Wark PA, Simpson J, Hensley MJ, Gibson PG. Airway inflammation in thunderstorm asthma. *Clin Exp Allergy* 2002, 32: 1750–6.
92 Koscher V, Milhe F, El Biaze M, Vervloet D, Magnan A. Variation of T cell activation in allergic subjects during natural pollen exposure. *Allergy* 2006, 61: 35–42.
93 Yamada K, Elliott WM, Hayashi S, Brattsand R, Roberts C, Vitalis TZ, Hogg JC. Latent adenoviral infection modifies the steroid response in allergic lung inflammation. *J Allergy Clin Immunol* 2000, 106: 844–51.
94 Kim EY, Battaile JT, Patel AC, You Y, Agapov E, Grayson MH, Benoit LA, Byers DE, Alevy Y, Tucker J, Swanson S, Tidwell R, Tyner JW, Morton JD, Castro M, Polineni D, Patterson GA, Schwendener RA, Allard JD, Peltz G, Holtzman MJ. Persistent activation of an innate immune response translates respiratory viral infection into chronic lung disease. *Nat Med* 2008, 14: 633–40.
95 Downs SH, Schindler C, Liu LJ, Keidel D, Bayer-Oglesby L, Brutsche MH, Gerbase MW, Keller R, Künzli N, Leuenberger P, Probst-Hensch NM, Tschopp JM, Zellweger JP, Rochat T, Schwartz J, Ackermann-Liebrich U; SAPALDIA Team. Reduced exposure to PM10 and attenuated age-related decline in lung function. *N Engl J Med* 2007, 357: 2338–47.

5

Bronchial hyperresponsiveness and lung inflammation induced by allergic immune response and oxidative stress: role of innate and adaptive immune responses

Kian Fan Chung and Alison S. Williams

Abstract. Airway response to the external environment forms the basis for many airway/lung diseases such as asthma and chronic obstructive airways disease (COPD) which are characterized by chronic airflow obstruction, chronic airway inflammation and tissue remodeling. Allergic inflammation and oxidative stress contribute to airways dysfunction and direct effects of these processes have been demonstrated in human and animal models. Airway responses to allergens and to environmental pollution such as ozone represent a mixture of innate and adaptive immune responses. Through the release of inflammatory cytokines and expression of co-stimulatory molecules, and antigen presentation, innate immune cells such as dendritic cells can interact with CD4 T-cells and direct their maturation program. The oxidant, ozone, can also utilize innate immune recognition pathways through toll-like receptors and activate a range of innate immune cells including dendritic cells (DCs), macrophages, and immune responses. Cross-talk between these two responses is likely to be common occurrence as exposure to oxidants is unavoidable in urban environments with high levels of pollution and allergic inflammation is a potential source of oxidants. The interaction of ozone and allergen offers interesting perspectives in unraveling further the interactions of innate and adaptive responses that could form the basis of chronic airway diseases of chronic airflow obstruction and inflammation.

Keywords: airway hyper-responsiveness, airway inflammation, chronic obstructive airways disease, allergic inflammation, oxidative stress, dendritic cells, innate immune response, ozone, particulate matter, allergen, pattern recognition receptors

5.1 Introduction

Understanding the response of the airways to its external environment may provide clues to the pathogenesis of several airway conditions underlying chronic airflow obstruction including asthma and chronic obstructive pulmonary disease (COPD). The influence of the external environment is well recognized from observations that exposure of human beings to pollutants such as ozone or particulates or to allergen (in sensitized subjects) induces changes in pulmonary function and airway inflammatory responses that often mimic the abnormalities observed in established disease. From the clinical viewpoint, chronic airflow obstruction constitutes a heterogeneous group of conditions that may be characterized by different inflammatory profiles and possibly different clinical outcomes. One of the potential explanations for heterogeneity of presentation could be the differential contributions of the innate and acquired immune responses to the external environment, responses that could be determined by genetic influences.

The recent rise in the incidence of allergies and of asthma in industrialized countries indicates that environmental factors may be important in the induction of these conditions, among which environmental pollution and infections may be important. The concept underlying these interactions is that the organism's response to environmental pollution and infections may interact and modify the allergic response. One hypothesis is that improved hygiene standards associated with a rise in living standards and less frequent microbial infections or direct exposure to microbial constituents may skew the immune response towards the T-helper T cells (Th-2) phenotype, thus increasing the risk of developing asthma and other atopic diseases.[1] Conversely, a skewing towards a Th-1 response in response to microbial invasion protects against asthma.[2] This hypothesis, although still under debate, has focused on the interactions between innate and adaptive immunity as the basis for asthma development. This has also led to a renewed interest in the effects of environmental pollutants on the immune response.

Asthma has been very much considered as primarily a disease occurring on the basis of an allergic response, while the disease that comes under the umbrella of COPD, a disease resulting from a direct response to constituents of tobacco smoke, is perhaps mediated largely through an acute on chronic inflammatory response. There is now, however, evidence for a role for immunological pathways involving dendritic cell activation and CD8+ T cells.[3] The response of the airways to ozone and allergens has been studied in humans and in animal rodent models, and to some extent there is good understanding of the chronic inflammatory pathways activated. The link between the inflammatory response and the airway smooth muscle (ASM) response in terms of chronic airway narrowing and airways hyperesponsiveness (AHR) in these models has been emphasized, but more important are the contributions of innate and acquired immune responses exhibited in these models, that can both in turn be modeled in chronic airways disease.

The innate immune response is a critical interface between the environment and adaptive responses, and provides the first-line defence against potential pathogens,[4] consisting of physical, chemical and cellular aspects of detection of pathogens by sensors such as toll-like receptors (TLRs), and of activation of effector functions such as production of antibacterial peptides such as defensins and activation of macrophages. Through the release of inflammatory cytokines and the expression of co-stimulatory molecules and activation of immune cells including dendritic cells, these may interact with CD4 T-cells, which can differentiate along certain specific pathways, illustrating a common example of innate and adaptive immune interactions.

In this chapter, we have chosen to focus on ozone as a component of environmental pollution, while cognisant of the fact that there are also other important constituents such as the particulate fraction and allergen exposure, which is a known trigger of asthmatic episodes in patients with asthma. Both have been extensively studied in both humans and animals, and the information available in both humans and rodents will be used, with data from animals providing mechanistic pathways. The potential interactions between the responses to allergen and to ozone will be discussed.

5.2 Airway responses to allergens

The allergic response is an important fundamental part of the pathophysiology of asthma, and an important supporting observation is that exposure of sensitized human asthmatics to aerosols of allergens to which they are sensitized reproduces many features of chronic asthma. Under experimental conditions in the laboratory, exposure to allergen results in an acute bronchoconstrictor response that is over within an hour (the early response) and is often followed by the development of a second wave of airway narrowing occurring four to eight hours later that is more gradual and prolonged, lasting for a few hours, referred to as the late response. The early response to allergen exposure results from the bronchoconstrictor effect via the acute release of mediators such as histamine and cysteinyl-leukotrienes from mast cells on airway smooth muscle.[5] The late response is the result of the inflammatory consequences of mediators and of cellular mechanisms leading to more prolonged airway narrowing and airway hyperresponsiveness (AHR). The allergen exposure model has been used extensively to understand the pathophysiologic inflammatory processes involved in chronic asthma, as this represents a mirror of chronic asthma.

Both the late asthmatic response and the increased airways responsiveness are associated with increases in airway inflammation, particularly characterized by an influx of eosinophils and increased amounts of eosinophil cationic protein in sputum supernatants.[6–8] That allergen challenge may represent a worsening of baseline asthma is supported by further increased expression of cytokines already expressed at baseline in mild asthmatic patients. These include the Th2 cytokines IL-4 and IL-5, the chemokines RANTES and eotaxin, and GM-CSF.[7, 9–12] Features of airway wall remodeling can be observed after single allergen challenge such as an increase in procollagen and tenascin in the sub-basement membrane.[13] Certain features of remodeling following single allergen challenge persist for up to seven days, including the increase in sub-basement membrane procollagen III expression, procollagen I, a smooth muscle actin, and the disappearance of inflammatory cells but persistence of AHR.[14]

5.2.1 Regulation of the immune response to allergens

The response to allergen observed in allergic asthmatics has been reproduced in many animal species, particularly in rodents. Current studies are mainly focused on mice strains because of the availability of genetically-engineered mice, but initial studies in a bigger rodent, the rat, have established some of the adaptive immune responses of the model. Thus, many of the characteristics of the allergen response including the late phase response and AHR have been shown in the Brown-Norway rat model.[15, 16] AHR can be induced by allergen challenge of rats that are sensitized by the adoptive transfer of CD4+ T cells from sensitized donors.[17, 18] CD8+ T cells can exert a protective effect since depletion of these cells augments allergen-induced AHR.[19] There is significant correlation between airway responsiveness and eosinophil numbers in BAL flowing allergen challenge.[20] AHR is associated with the expression of Th2 cytokines, and adoptive transfer of Th2 cells and subsequent allergen challenge causes AHR.[19] Transfer of Th1 cells in conjunction with Th2 cells prevents the development of AHR.

The roles of specific Th2 cytokines have been probed, using genetically-engineered mice. The role of the Th2 cytokine, IL-13, in allergen-induced

AHR has been established using IL-13$^{-/-}$ mice, in which AHR, eosinophilic inflammation and increased ASM in the airways induced by chronic allergen exposure were abolished. Similar results were obtained in a mouse knock-out of the Th2 cytokines, IL-4, IL-5, IL-9 and IL-13; a "quadruple" knock-out mouse.[(21)] IL-13 is mainly responsible for AHR, ASM hyperplasia and increases in IgE, while IL-4, -5 and -9 may contribute to goblet cell hyperplasia and eosinophilic inflammation induced by chronic allergen exposure. IL-5 was the most important of the Th2 cytokines in inducing eosinophilia caused by allergen, as demonstrated in IL-5$^{-/-}$ mice.[(22, 23)] While in IL-4$^{-/-}$ and IL-9$^{-/-}$ mice, allergen-induced eosinophilia was not inhibited.[(24, 25)] Allergen-induced AHR and airway wall remodeling were unaffected in IL-9$^{-/-}$ mice. Therefore IL-5 appears to be a major contributor of allergen-induced eosinophilia, with some contribution from IL-13. IL-13 may contribute to airway wall remodeling in the mouse. CC10-driven over-expression of IL-13 in the lungs causes eosinophilic and mononuclear inflammation with goblet cell hyperplasia, subepithelial fibrosis, airway obstruction, and AHR.[(26)] Dual IL-9 and IL-5 overexpression also caused subepithelial fibrosis and AHR.

5.2.2 AHR and airway smooth muscle

The link between AHR and abnormal ASM contractile responses continues to be studied. The fact that allergen challenge can provoke a transient episode of AHR indicates that factors released or induced by allergen challenge can lead to transient changes in intrinsic ASM contractility or that the contractile response may be amplified by factors outside the ASM. Several mechanisms may be implicated. An increase in ASM mass could be associated with a greater contractile effect for the same stimulus after allergen exposure, and there could be changes in the cytoskeletal composition of ASM such as an increase in the filamentous-actin content in relation to the globular actin component.[(27)] Change in myosin light chain kinase phosphorylation is increased in contracting ASM from hyperresponsive ragweed pollen-sensitized dogs and is associated with a faster shortening velocity and increased shortening capacity.[(28)] Changes in the extracellular matrix proteins can be observed within 24 hours of allergen challenge, such as an increase in fibronectin or collagen, and this may change the interaction between ASM and its surrounding matrix. Alteration of mechanical impedances to airway narrowing such as the lung parenchymal elastic properties or local changes in the parenchyma near the airways may cause mechanical uncoupling.[(29)]

Another possibility is that the ASM acquires a secretory pro-inflammatory role during allergic airway inflammation.[30, 31] Certainly, ASM cells in culture have the capacity to release many cytokines and chemokines, an effect dependent upon the stimulatory signal.[32] Constitutive CCL5/RANTES and CCL11/eotaxin expression in ASM is increased in asthma.[33, 34] Expression of the TGFβ protein is also increased in ASM cells from asthmatic bronchi,[35] which may stimulate ASM proliferation and hypertrophy. ASM cells can release CCL11/eotaxin,[34, 36] CXCL10/IP-10,[37] stem cell factor,[38] and CX3CL1/fractalkine.[39] Increased release of CXCL10/IP-10 has been reported from asthmatic ASM cells,[37] which may mediate lung mast cell migration into the ASM bundle. The potential for autocrine effects of the released chemokines/cytokines is illustrated by the production of CXCL8/IL-8 by ASM cells, which can interact with CXCR1 and CXCR2 receptors on ASM cells to induce ASM contraction and migration.[40] How these secretory patterns of ASM cells in asthma or during an episode of airway allergic inflammation influence the functional aspects of airway smooth muscle remains to be determined.[41]

5.2.3 Dendritic cells and Th2 responses

Dendritic cells (DCs) are important in both the primary immune response to inhaled allergens, and also in the effector phase of the asthmatic inflammation. DCs migrate to mediastidanal lymph nodes to present antigen to T cells.[42] Intratracheal transfer of bone-marrow-derived DCs pulsed ex-vivo with ovalbumin sensitizes mice towards ovalbumin, leading to airway inflammation and acute bronchoconstriction with ovalbumin challenge. DCs which migrate to the lung during asthmatic inflammation also play a role in induction of allergic inflammation after allergen re-exposure.[43] Lung DCs are thus necessary for induction of tolerance to inhaled antigens, and for the induction of Th2 sensitization that leads to the priming of Th2 effector cells. Depletion of myeloid DCs at the time of allergen challenge can lead to the prevention of allergic airway inflammation, goblet cell hyperplasia and AHR,[44] but is restored by administration of GM-CSF-cultured CD11b+ CD11c+ myeloid DCs. DCs can also present antigen during the effector phase of airway inflammation.[45] DCs may produce the inflammatory cytokines CCL17 and CCL22, which attract Th2 cells to the airways and may induce eosinophil-selective chemokines.

The innate immune system provides the earliest response to infectious agents and can modulate Th2 cell activity. In the ovalbumin-sensitized mouse model, lipopolysaccharide (LPS), which activates toll-like receptor (TLR) -4, is required for CD4+ T cell priming and Th2 lung inflammatory responses to inhaled allergens.[46, 47] However, this effect is largely dependent on the various aspects of LPS including dosing. High doses of LPS are associated with immunity of Th1 type, and low doses with Th2 responses.[46] Transfer of in vitro LPS-stimulated DCs causes a reduced Th2 and an increased Th1 response in vivo.[48] These observations serve as a backdrop to the ongoing hygiene hypothesis regarding the potential protective effect of exposure to bacterial infections in allergy. Therefore, the relationship between LPS exposure and asthma is complex; LPS may provoke Th-1 or Th-2 responses depending on the strength of the activation, which depends on the level of exposure to LPS and on the genetic variability of the host.[49] The innate immune system may direct Th2 differentiation through modulation of DCs or differential activation of intracellular adaptor molecules after TLR ligation. In the mouse model of allergic Th2 response to intranasal antigen, innate control of adaptive Th2 immunity is MyD88-dependent.[50] This activation of Th2 responses by LPS which usually induces a Th-1 inflammatory response is therefore surprising, but this phenomenon may be restricted to the immune response of the lung.

5.3 Ozone and lung disease

Ozone is an urban air pollutant produced from the action of sunlight on hydrocarbons and nitrogen oxides produced by combustion of fuels. Ozone exposure is associated with worsening athletic performance, a decrease in lung function, shortness of breath, chest pain, wheezing and coughing. Ozone can contribute to increased morbidity and mortality.[51, 52, 53] In the Air Pollution and Health: A European Approach (APHEA2) project, of 23 European cities, an increase in one-hour ozone concentration by 10 $\mu g/m^3$ during the summer months (levels ranging from 32 to 166 $\mu g/m^3$) was associated with a 0.33 percent increase in total daily number of deaths, and a 1.13 percent increase in the number of respiratory deaths.[51] A 4 percent increase in overall mortality can be detected with a greater, 50 $\mu g/m^3$ rise in ozone. The EPA has advocated a reduction in ambient ozone concentration from 120 to 80 ppb. Such a reduction is predicted to prevent 800 premature deaths, 4,500 hospital admissions, 900,000 school absences and more than one million minor restricted activity days across three years.[54] During the warm season, the two-day cumulative effect of 5 ppb increase in ozone was a 0.27 percent increase in admissions for COPD and a 0.41 percent increase in pneumonia admissions, with a similar association found for PM10 (55).

5.3.1 Controlled exposure of humans to ozone

Studies of the effects of ozone in humans will be reviewed first and studies in animals second. Animal studies are included to reflect on potential mechanisms of ozone action. In all species studied, exposure to ozone induces a concentration-dependent deterioration in lung function, some degree of AHR, and evidence of inflammation. In humans, the maximum level of exposure has been 400 ppb, while in rodents up to 3 ppm exposure levels have been used.

5.3.1.1 Lung function changes

In the majority of studies conducted in non-smoking normal volunteers, 10 to 20 percent respond to ozone exposure with a decrease in FEV_1, while others are insensitive.[56, 57] Part of this response may be related to genetic susceptibilities such as polymorphisms of oxidative stress genes, eg NQO1, GSTM1 or GSTP1. Various groups may be more prone to the effects of ozone, such as obese versus non-obese, and those with airway hyperresponsiveness versus non-hyperresponsiveness.[58] The elderly are less sensitive to reductions in lung function after ozone exposure although they are more vulnerable to death related to ozone.[59] Interestingly, studies in asthmatics and atopics do not report increased susceptibility to ozone.[60, 60–62] However, these studies do not match cohort studies in children that show associations between acute ozone exposure and occurrence of asthma deterioration or exacerbations.[63, 64] COPD patients showed no changes in lung function when exposed to ozone, although there was some significant decrease in oxygen saturation.[65]

5.3.1.2 Inflammatory responses in humans

Many studies have examined the effect of ozone at ambient concentrations ranging from 0.2 to 0.4 ppm, usually for a couple of hours, while the subject is exercising in order to increase minute ventilation and therefore exposure of the lungs. Consistently, there is an increase in neutrophil numbers measured in bronchoalveolar lavage (BAL) fluid or sputum,[66–70] observed as early as one hour after cessation of exposure,[71] lasting up to 24 hours. The increase in neutrophils is a function of the level of ozone.[72] Other features of BAL fluid include increased levels of prostaglandin E2 and F2, IL-6, IL-8, GROα and Clara cell protein[73,74] and increased myeloperoxidase and decreased ascorbate.[75] Depletion of ascorbate levels in BAL at six hours indicates an interaction of ozone with ascorbic acid, that may lead to the production of an ascorbate ozonide, which can generate cytotoxic free radicals in vivo.[76] Thus, the oxidant effects of ozone may occur at the level of the surface epithelium.

There is less evidence for neutrophilic inflammation in airway biopsies, although increased submucosal mast cells, with increased vascular endothelial P-selectin and ICAM-1, and increased expression of HLA-DR in alveolar macrophages has been reported.[77] Increased CD14 expression in sputum macrophages is also described.[78] Clara cell 16 protein, a marker of lung epithelial cell injury, is increased in serum following exposure to ozone.[79] These studies provide evidence for the activation of a wide range of cells, other than the neutrophil.

Asthmatics develop similar degrees of FEV_1 fall and neutrophilic responses in BAL or sputum compared to normal subjects when exposed to ozone.[80] However, significant increase in IL-5, GM-CSF, ENA-78 and IL-8 in the airway epithelium was reported in asthmatics exposed to ozone versus normals,[81] indicating that the allergic state of the asthmatic epithelium may prime the response to ozone. Repeated exposures to ozone led to an attenuation of the spirometric response, and also attenuated the neutrophilic response in BAL,[82, 83] but increased BAL macrophage numbers.[84] However, other aspects of inflammation were still increased such as BAL protein levels of IL-6, IL-8, reduced glutathione, and also neutrophil and lymphocytes in the biopsies.[83]

5.3.2 Mechanisms of AHR induced by ozone

The mechanisms of AHR after ozone exposure remain unclear and many mechanisms are possible. Inflammatory factors induced by the oxidative stress effects of ozone exposure may directly change the responsiveness of ASM. Maximal isometric contractile response of ex-vivo bronchi to acetylcholine obtained from ozone-exposed mice is increased, concomitant with AHR. Pretreatment with the antioxidant N-acetylcysteine abolishes these effects (Blanc, Leung and Chung, *unpublished*), indicating a potential direct effect of oxidants on ASM. Similarly, there is attenuation of the proliferative activity of the airway epithelium with antioxidant treatment

(85). How oxidant stress can directly increase ASM contractility is unclear. Consistent with an oxidative stress response involvement, inhibitors of p38 mitogen-activated protein kinase (MAPK) and c-jun N-terminal kinase (JNK) inhibit AHR and neutrophilic inflammation of ozone;[86] in addition, activation of NF-κB is a feature of ozone-exposed lungs.[87, 88] Microchip gene array of lungs exposed to acute ozone shows up-regulated expression of inflammatory genes that are involved with inflammatory cell chemotaxis and recruitment, including *CXCL1* (*KC*), *CXCL2* (*MIP-2*), *CCL2*, eotaxin, *MMP-8, ADAMTS4*, and metalloproteinases *MT-1* and *MT-2*,[86, 89, 90] with *IL-6* being the most highly regulated.[91] *IL-6* may be important for the induction of ozone-induced neutrophilia but not of AHR. It can cause the induction of neutrophilic chemokines, such as *MIP-2*.[92] CINC-2, another neutrophil chemoattractant, has also been implicated in ozone-induced AHR. Previous studies have indicated that neutrophils could be responsible for the AHR component.[93, 94] Therefore, the paradigm of neutrophilic cytokines directly inducing AHR is a possibility worth exploring.

5.3.3 Role of innate immunity in ozone responses

Using inbred strains of mice derived from ozone-susceptible and ozone-resistant progenitors, Kleeberger and colleagues found that TLR4 was differentially expressed between these mice after exposure to ozone in terms of lung permeabilitry responses.[95] Hollingsworth et al. found that $TLR4^{-/-}$ mice did not develop AHR after ozone exposure but still exhibited a neutrophilic inflammatory response to ozone.[96] We found that TLR2, TLR4 and MyD88 were involved in the development of AHR after ozone, and MyD88 was particularly most important in regulating ozone-induced neutrophil recruitment (Figure 5.1).[97] This indicates that ozone, via lipid ozonation products, may activate the TLR system. Interestingly, ASM express TLR4 that can be regulated by LPS, a mechanism by which oxidative stress may activate these cells.[98]

TLR4 may modulate responses to ozone through the scavenger receptor, macrophage receptor with collagenous structure (Marco), interfering with ozone-induced and surfactant-derived oxidized lipid (eg beta-epoxide and PON-GPC)-induced inflammation.[99] Other effects of ozone on the innate immune system include impairment of airway epithelial permeability,[100] impairment of macrophage phagocytosis, superoxide production and increased cytokine release,[101] and also impaired phagocytic function,[102, 103] which could influence the outcome of AHR. Ozone can also prime the pulmonary innate response, as demonstrated by the effect of ozone in

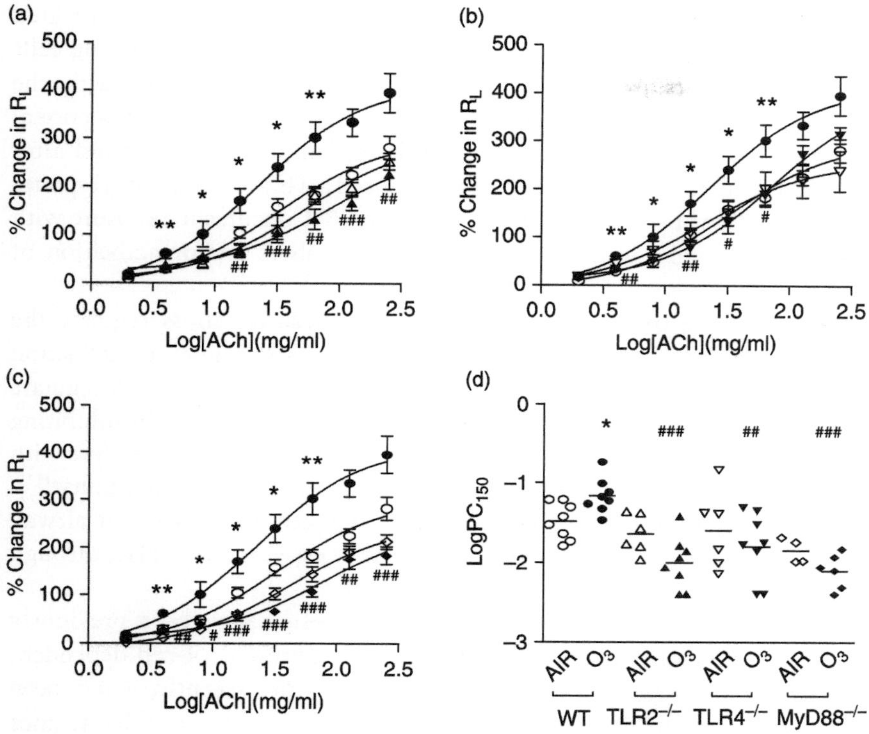

Figure 5.1 Concentration-response curves to acetylcholine (ACh) of TLR2$^{-/-}$ (Δ, ▲) (Panel A), TLR4$^{-/-}$ (∇,▼) (Panel B), MyD88$^{-/-}$ (◊, ◆) (Panel C) and Wt (o, ●) (all Panels) mice exposed to air (open symbols) or to ozone (closed symbols). -log PC_{150} (panel D). Data shown as mean±SEM. *P<0.05; ** P<0.01, compared to air-exposed WT mice. # P<0.05; ## P<0.01; ### P<0.001, compared to ozone-exposed WT mice. Reproduced with permission from Reference 85.

enhancing LPS-induced AHR, pro-inflammatory cytokine release and increased systemic inflammatory response, caused by increased surface expression of TLR4 receptors on macrophages.[104]

Pulmonary surfactant protein-D (SP-D), a member of the collectin family of soluble innate host-defence molecules, modulates immune and inflammatory responses in the lung. Absence or low levels of SP-D predisposes to enhanced inflammatory changes in the lung following ozone exposure.[105] The Th2 cytokines, IL-4 and IL-13 induces SP-D protein that can act as a negative feedback to prevent further activation of sensitized T cells.[106]

Direct activation of DCs by oxidative stress has been demonstrated following exposure to ozone. The antigen-presenting activity of lung cells and DCs of rats exposed to ozone was increased, together with the expression of Ia and costimulatory molecules, B7.1 and B7.2.[107] Functional stimulation of lymphocytes from mediastinal lymph nodes occurred after ozone exposure.[108] Exposure to ozone induced a Th2-like immune response (with increases in serum IgE, IL-4 and IL-5).[109] Concurrent exposure with ozone and allergen leads to an increase in numbers and/or activation of DCs in the airways.[110]

Thus, reactive oxygen species (ROS) and oxidative stress regulate the induction of the immune response by controlling signal transduction pathways in antigen-presenting cells and in lymphocytes.[111] ROS regulate T cell activation and favours Th2 skewing of immune responses by inhibiting Th1 differentiation. Glutathione depletion has been shown to interfere with LPS-induced DC maturation with down-regulation of Th1 immunity.[112] Repeated exposure of mice to ozone also induced an increase in airway natural killer (NK) -T cells, which appear to be essential for AHR, through the production of IL-17.[113]

Adaptive immune responses after ozone exposure have been previously studied. Smaller lymphoid organs, and suppressed T-cell-dependent immunological responses are reported.[114–116] More recently, it has been shown that the Th2 cytokine, IL-13, may interact with ozone effects, since IL-13$^{-/-}$ mice demonstrate an attenuated AHR following ozone exposure; similar attenuated responses were shown in the double IL-4 and IL-13 knock-out mice (Fig. 5.2).[117] Conversely, IL-13 overexpressing mice showed an enhancement of the airway response. Wild-type mice exposed to ozone release high levels of IL-13 and IL-17 in the airways, indicating that the release of IL-17 induced by ozone may be an important mediator of the neutrophilic inflammation and AHR. In addition, ozone caused an increased expression of MIP-3α/CCL20 in the lung and these were inhibited in IL-13$^{-/-}$ mice, indicating that DC migration could be under control of IL-13. The release of IL-17 indicates the possibility that Th17 cells may be involved in the induction of AHR and airway neutrophilia.[118] IL-25 of the IL-17 family promotes Th2 responses[119] and regulates the inflammation mediated by Th17 T-cells.[120]

5.3.4 Interactions between allergen and ozone

Low-level exposure to ozone does not potentiate the immediate or late bronchoconstrictor response after allergen exposure in mild atopic

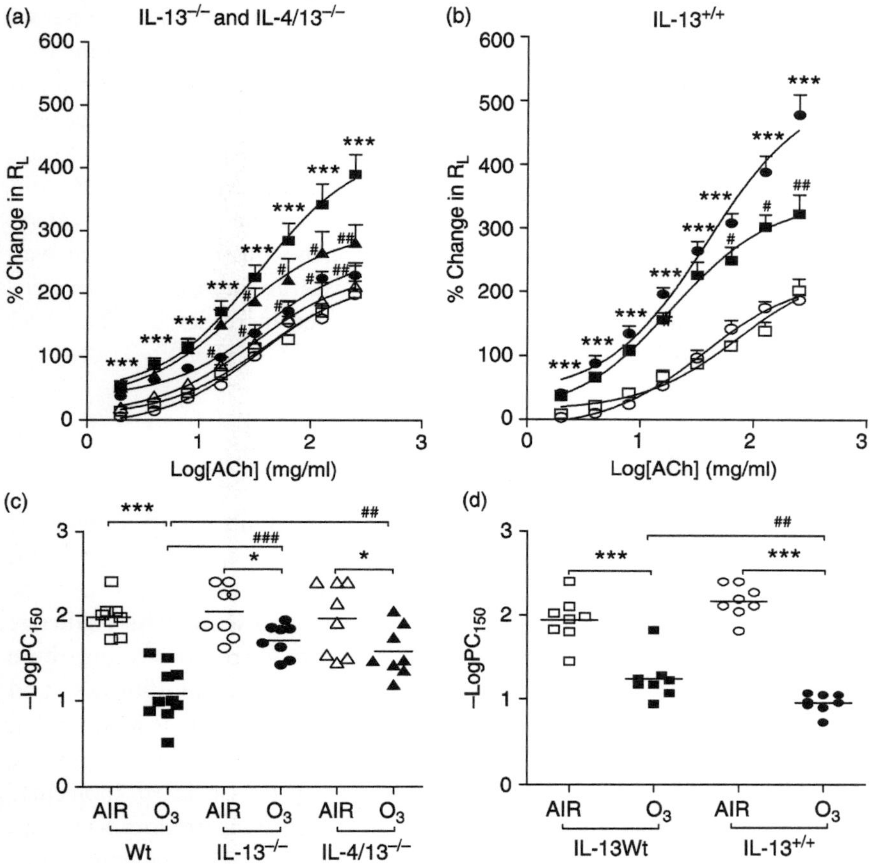

Figure 5.2 Concentration-response curves to acetylcholine (ACh) (panel A) and -log PC_{150} (panel C) of IL-$13^{-/-}$ (o, ●) and IL-4/IL-$13^{-/-}$ (Δ, ▲) and Wt (□, ■) mice exposed to air or to ozone. Panels B and D are for IL-$13^{+/+}$ (o, ●) and IL-13Wt mice (□, ■). Data shown as mean ±SEM. *P<0.05, **P<0.01, ***P<0.001 compared to air-exposed of same strain; #P<0.05, ##P<0.01 compared to ozone-exposed Wt mice. Reproduced with permission from reference 105.

asthmatics,[121, 122] while in asthmatics, ozone exposure for one hour (0.12 ppm) increased the bronchial response to inhaled allergen.[123] Another study using 0.25 ppm ozone exposure for three hours demonstrated a small increase in the responsiveness of the lower airways to allergen.[124] The effect on inflammation is less conclusive. However, an increase in BAL eosinophil numbers is seen after allergic asthmatics are exposed to ozone, and exposure to ozone 24 hours after allergen challenge potentiated eosinophilic inflammatory response in mild atopic asthmatics.[125] In mild asthmatics exposed to 0.12 ppm ozone before allergen challenge by bronchial instillation, no difference in inflammatory cells in biopsies was seen compared to air challenge.(126) There is a priming effect of ozone on allergen-induced responses with an increase in late phase responses and eosinophil cationic protein levels intrinsic inflammatory responses in nasal airways of allergic asthmatics.(127) Ozone exposure augments allergen-induced AHR and eosinophilic inflammation(128) and repeated ozone exposure causes persistent neutrophilic lung inflammation, bronchoconstriction and airway remodeling.(129, 130) Ozone exposure also causes an increase in allergen-induced AHR in mice, accompanied by further increases in eosinophil survival and increased levels of IL-5, GM-CSF and G-CSF.(131)

5.4 Conclusions

Studying the innate and adaptive immune responses and how they interact when the airways and lungs are exposed to external environmental factors such as allergens and environmental pollutants will provide valuable insights into the pathogenesis of airways disease. The challenge is to understand how these innate and adaptive immune responses contribute to functional abnormalities such as AHR, increased fibrosis and airway smooth muscle, and contractility in conditions such as asthma and COPD. Such studies may also pinpoint some new approaches to treating these diseases. For example, the use of pathogen-associated molecular patterns to promote Th1 responses to counterbalance the predominant Th2 responses seen in allergic diseases was derived from the hygiene hypothesis. Other approaches based on innate immune responses include the use of TLR9-based allergen-specific immunotherapy, an approach effective in animal models in ameliorating or reversing allergic inflammation.(132) Although not discussed here, another possible means of innate immune therapy is the modulation of regulatory T-cell function.(133) Harnessing innate immune mechanisms may provide ways of modulating the detrimental airway responses following exposures to allergen and ozone, and those observed in chronic airways diseases such as asthma and COPD.

Acknowledgements

Work by the authors has been supported by the UK Wellcome Trust. We are grateful to Dr A.McKenzie of the MRC Molecular Biology Laboratory, Cambridge, UK for his collaboration and support.

References

1 Strachan DP. Hay fever, hygiene, and household size. *Br. Med. J.* 1989; 299: 1259–60.
2 von Mutius E. The environmental predictors of allergic disease. *J. Allergy Clin. Immunol.* 2000; 105: 9–19.
3 Chung KF, Adcock IM. Multifaceted mechanisms in COPD: inflammation, immunity, and tissue repair and destruction. *Eur. Respir. J.* 2008; 31: 1334–56.
4 Janeway CA, Jr., Medzhitov R. Innate immune recognition. *Annu.Rev.Immunol.* 2002; 20: 197–216.
5 Manning PJ, Rokach J, Malo JL, et al. Urinary leukotriene E4 levels during early and late asthmatic responses. *J. Allergy Clin. Immunol.* 1990; 86: 211–20.
6 Pin I, Freitag AP, O'Byrne PM et al. Changes in the cellular profile of induced sputum after allergen-induced asthmatic responses. *Am. Rev. Respir. Dis.* 1992; 145: 1265–9.
7 Gauvreau GM, Watson RM, O'Byrne PM. Kinetics of allergen-induced airway eosinophilic cytokine production and airway inflammation. *Am J Respir Crit Care Med* 1999; 160: 640–7.
8 Sulakvelidze I, Inman MD, Rerecich T, O'Byrne PM. Increases in airway eosinophils and interleukin-5 with minimal bronchoconstriction during repeated low-dose allergen challenge in atopic asthmatics. *Eur. Respir. J.* 1998; 11: 821–7.
9 Woolley KL, Adelroth E, Woolley MJ, Ellis R, Jordana M, O'Byrne PM. Effects of allergen challenge on eosinophils, eosinophil cationic protein, and granulocyte-macrophage colony-stimulating factor in mild asthma. *Am. J. Respir. Crit.Care Med.* 1995; 151: 1915–24.
10 Bentley AM, Meng Q, Robinson DS, Hamid Q, Kay AB, Durham SR. Increases in activated T lymphocytes, eosinophils, and cytokine mRNA expression for interleukin-5 and granulocyte/macrophage colony-stimulating factor in bronchial biopsies after allergen inhalation challenge in atopic asthmatics. *ajrcmb* 1993; 8: 35–42.
11 Robinson D, Hamid Q, Bentley A, Ying S, Kay AB, Durham SR. Activation of CD4+ T cells, increased TH2-type cytokine mRNA expression, and eosinophil recruitment in bronchoalveolar lavage after allergen inhalation challenge in patients with atopic asthma. *J. Allergy Clin. Immunol.* 1993; 92: 313–24.
12 Hallden G, Hellman C, Gronneberg R, Lundahl J. Increased levels of IL-5 positive peripheral blood eosinophils and lymphocytes in mild asthmatics after allergen inhalation provocation. *Clin. Exp. Allergy* 1999; 29: 595–603.
13 Torrego A, Hew M, Oates T, Sukkar M, Fan CK. Expression and activation of TGF-β isoforms in acute allergen-induced remodelling in asthma. *Thorax* 2007; 62: 307–13.
14 Kariyawasam HH, Aizen M, Barkans J, Robinson DS, Kay AB. Remodeling and airway hyperresponsiveness but not cellular inflammation persist after allergen challenge in asthma. *Am. J. Respir. Crit Care Med.* 2007; 175: 896–904.
15 Martin JG, Tamaoka M. Rat models of asthma and chronic obstructive lung disease. *Pulm. Pharmacol. Ther.* 2006; 19: 377–85.
16 Groneberg DA, Chung KF. Models of chronic obstructive pulmonary disease. *Respir Res.* 2004; 5: 18.

17 Mishima H, Hojo M, Watanabe A, Hamid QA, Martin JG. CD4+ T cells can induce airway hyperresponsiveness to allergen challenge in the brown Norway rat. *Am. J. Respir. Crit. Care Med.* 1998; 158: 1863–70.
18 Haczku A, MacAry P, Huang TJ, et al. Adoptive transfer of allergen-specific CD4+ T cells induces airway inflammation and hyperresponsiveness in brown Norway rats. *Immunol* 1997; 91: 176–85.
19 Huang TJ, Macary PA, Eynott P, et al. Allergen-specific Th1 cells counteract efferent Th2 cell-dependent bronchial hyperresponsiveness and eosinophilic inflammation partly via IFN-gamma. *J.Immunol.* 2001; 166: 207–17.
20 Elwood W, Barnes PJ, Chung KF. Airway hyperresponsiveness is associated with inflammatory cell infiltration in allergic Brown Norway rats. *International Archives of Allergy and Immunology* 1992; 99: 91–7.
21 Nath P, Yee LS, Williams AS, et al. Complete inhibition of allergic airway inflammation and remodelling in quadruple IL-4/5/9/13–/– mice. *Clin. Exp. Allergy.* 2007; 37: 1427–35.
22 Wang J, Palmer K, Lotvall J, et al. Circulating, but not local lung, IL-5 is required for the development of antigen-induced airways eosinophilia. *J. Clin. Invest.* 1998; 102: 1132–41.
23 Tanaka H, Komai M, Nagao K, et al. Role of interleukin-5 and eosinophils in allergen-induced airway remodeling in mice. *Am. J. Respir. Cell Mol. Biol.* 2004; 31: 62–8.
24 Walter DM, McIntire JJ, Berry G, et al. Critical role for IL-13 in the development of allergen-induced airway hyperreactivity. *J. Immunol* 2001; 167: 4668–75.
25 McMillan SJ, Bishop B, Townsend MJ, McKenzie AN, Lloyd CM. The absence of interleukin 9 does not affect the development of allergen-induced pulmonary inflammation nor airway hyperreactivity. *J. Exp. Med.* 2002; 195: 51–7.
26 Zhu Z, Homer RJ, Wang Z, et al. Pulmonary expression of interleukin-13 causes inflammation, mucus hypersecretion, subepithelial fibrosis, physiologic abnormalities, and eotaxin production. *J. Clin. Invest.* 1999; 103: 779–88.
27 McVicker CG, Leung SY, Kanabar V, et al. Repeated Allergen Inhalation Induces Cytoskeletal Remodeling in Smooth Muscle from Rat Bronchioles. *Am. J. Respir. Cell Mol. Biol.* 2007; 36: 721–7.
28 Jiang H, Rao K, Halayko AJ, Liu X, Stephens NL. Ragweed sensitization-induced increase of myosin light chain kinase content in canine airway smooth muscle. *Ajrcmb* 1992; 7: 567–73.
29 Macklem PT. A theoretical analysis of the effect of airway smooth muscle load on airway narrowing. *Am. J. Respir. Crit. Care Med.* 1996; 153: 83–9.
30 Chung KF. Airway smooth muscle cells: contributing to and regulating airway mucosal inflammation? *Eur. Respir. J.* 2000; 15: 961–8.
31 Chung, K. F. Should treatments for asthma be aimed at the airway smooth muscle? *Expert. Rev. Respir. Med.* 2007; 1: 209–18.
32 Jarai G, Sukkar M, Garrett S, et al. Effects of interleukin-1beta, interleukin-13 and transforming growth factor-beta on gene expression in human airway smooth muscle using gene microarrays. *Eur. J. Pharmacol.* 2004; 497: 255–65.
33 Berkman N, Krishnan VL, Gilbey T, et al. Expression of RANTES mRNA and protein in airways of patients with mild asthma. *Am. J. Resp. Crit. Care Med.* 1996; 154: 1804–11.

34 Ghaffar O, Hamid Q, Renzi PM et al. Constitutive and cytokine-stimulated expression of eotaxin by human airway smooth muscle cells. *Am. J. Respir. Crit. Care Med.* 1999; 159: 1933–42.
35 Xie S, Sukkar MB, Issa R, Khorasani NM, Chung KF. Mechanisms of induction of airway smooth muscle hyperplasia by transforming growth factor-beta. *Am. J. Physiol Lung Cell Mol.Physiol.* 2007; 293: L245–L253.
36 Chung KF, Patel HJ, Fadlon EJ, et al. Induction of eotaxin expression and release from human airway smooth muscle cells by IL-1beta and TNFalpha: effects of IL-10 and corticosteroids. *Br. J. Pharmacol.* 1999; 127: 1145–50.
37 Hardaker EL, Bacon AM, Carlson K et al. Regulation of TNF-alpha- and IFN-gamma-induced CXCL10 expression: participation of the airway smooth muscle in the pulmonary inflammatory response in chronic obstructive pulmonary disease. *FASEB J.* 2004; 18: 191–3.
38 Kassel O, Schmidlin F, Duvernelle C, Gasser B, Massard G, Frossard N. Human bronchial smooth muscle cells in culture produce stem cell factor. *Eur. Respir. J.* 1999; 13: 951–4.
39 Sukkar MB, Issa R, Xie S, Oltmanns U, Newton R, Chung KF. Fractalkine/CX3CL1 production by human airway smooth muscle cells: induction by IFN-gamma and TNF-alpha and regulation by TGF-beta and corticosteroids. *Am. J. Physiol Lung Cell Mol. Physiol* 2004; 287: L1230–L1240.
40 Govindaraju V, Michoud MC, Al Chalabi M, Ferraro P, Powell WS, Martin JG. Interleukin-8: novel roles in human airway smooth muscle cell contraction and migration. *Am.J.Physiol Cell Physiol.* 2006; 291: C957–C965.
41 Chung KF.Ed. *Airway smooth muscle in asthma and COPD*. Wiley; 2008.
42 Lambrecht BN, De Veerman M, Coyle AJ, Gutierrez-Ramos JC, Thielemans K, Pauwels RA. Myeloid dendritic cells induce Th2 responses to inhaled antigen, leading to eosinophilic airway inflammation. *J. Clin. Invest* 2000; 106: 551–9.
43 van Rijt LS, Prins JB, Leenen PJ et al. Allergen-induced accumulation of airway dendritic cells is supported by an increase in CD31(hi)Ly-6C(neg) bone marrow precursors in a mouse model of asthma. *Blood* 2002; 100: 3663–71.
44 van Rijt LS, Jung S, Kleinjan A, et al. In vivo depletion of lung CD11c+ dendritic cells during allergen challenge abrogates the characteristic features of asthma. *J. Exp. Med.* 2005; 201: 981–91.
45 Huh JC, Strickland DH, Jahnsen FL, et al. Bidirectional interactions between antigen-bearing respiratory tract dendritic cells (DCs) and T cells precede the late phase reaction in experimental asthma: DC activation occurs in the airway mucosa but not in the lung parenchyma. *J. Exp. Med.* 2003; 198: 19–30.
46 Eisenbarth SC, Piggott DA, Huleatt JW, Visintin I, Herrick CA, Bottomly K. Lipopolysaccharide-enhanced, Toll-like receptor 4-dependent T helper cell type 2 responses to inhaled antigen. *J. Exp. Med.* 2002; 196: 1645–51.
47 Dabbagh K, Dahl ME, Stepick-Biek P, Lewis DB. Toll-like receptor 4 is required for optimal development of Th2 immune responses: role of dendritic cells. *J. Immunol.* 2002; 168: 4524–30.
48 Kuipers H, Hijdra D, De Vries VC, et al. Lipopolysaccharide-induced suppression of airway Th2 responses does not require IL-12 production by dendritic cells. *J. Immunol.* 2003; 171: 3645–54.
49 Vercelli D. Innate immunity: sensing the environment and regulating the regulators. *Curr. Opin. Allergy Clin. Immunol.* 2003; 3: 343–6.

50 Piggott DA, Eisenbarth SC, Xu L, et al. MyD88-dependent induction of allergic Th2 responses to intranasal antigen. *J.Clin.Invest* 2005; 115: 459–67.
51 Gryparis A, Forsberg B, Katsouyanni K, et al. Acute effects of ozone on mortality from the "air pollution and health: a European approach" project. *Am. J. Respir. Crit. Care Med.* 2004; 170: 1080–7.
52 Bell ML, McDermott A, Zeger SL, Samet JM, Dominici F. Ozone and short-term mortality in 95 US urban communities, 1987–2000. *JAMA* 2004; 292: 2372–8.
53 Katsouyanni K, Zmirou D, Spix C et al. Short-term effects of air pollution on health: a European approach using epidemiological time-series data. The APHEA project: background, objectives, design. *Eur. Respir. J.* 1995; 8: 1030–8.
54 Hubbell BJ, Hallberg A, McCubbin DR, Post E. Health-related benefits of attaining the 8-hr ozone standard. *Environ.Health Perspect.* 2005; 113: 73–82.
55 Medina-Ramon M, Zanobetti A, Schwartz J. The effect of ozone and PM10 on hospital admissions for pneumonia and chronic obstructive pulmonary disease: a national multicity study. *Am. J. Epidemiol.* 2006; 163: 579–88.
56 Hazucha MJ, Folinsbee LJ, Bromberg PA. Distribution and reproducibility of spirometric response to ozone by gender and age. *J. Appl. Physiol.* 2003; 95: 1917–25.
57 Horstman DH, Folinsbee LJ, Ives PJ, Abdul-Salaam S, McDonnell MF. Ozone concentration and pulmonary response relationships for a 6.6-hour exposure with five hours of moderate exercise to 0.08, 0.1, and 0.12 ppm. *Am. Rev. Respir. Dis.* 1990; 142: 1158–63.
58 Alexeeff SE, Litonjua AA, Suh H, Sparrow D, Vokonas PS, Schwartz J. Ozone exposure and lung function: effect modified by obesity and airways hyperresponsiveness in the VA normative aging study. *Chest* 2007; 132: 1890–7.
59 Medina-Ramon M, Schwartz J. Who is More Vulnerable to Die From Ozone Air Pollution? *Epidemiology* 2008.
60 Linn WS, Jones MP, Bachmayer EA, et al. Short-term respiratory effects of polluted ambient air: a laboratory study of volunteers in a high-oxidant community. *Am. Rev. Respir. Dis.* 1980; 121: 243–52.
61 Koenig JQ, Covert DS, Marshall SG, Van Belle G, Pierson WE. The effects of ozone and nitrogen dioxide on pulmonary function in healthy and in asthmatic adolescents. *Am. Rev. Respir. Dis.* 1987; 136: 1152–7.
62 Holtzman MJ, Cunningham JH, Sheller JR, Irsigler GB, Nadel JA, Boushey HA. Effect of ozone on bronchial reactivity in atopic and nonatopic subjects. *Am. Rev. Respir. Dis.* 1979; 120: 1059–67.
63 Thurston GD, Lippmann M, Scott MB, Fine JM. Summertime haze air pollution and children with asthma. *Am. J. Respir. Crit. Care Med.* 1997; 155: 654–60.
64 Just J, Segala C, Sahraoui F, Priol G, Grimfeld A, Neukirch F. Short-term health effects of particulate and photochemical air pollution in asthmatic children. *Eur. Respir. J.* 2002; 20: 899–906.
65 Gong H, Jr., Shamoo DA, Anderson KR, Linn WS. Responses of older men with and without chronic obstructive pulmonary disease to prolonged ozone exposure. *Arch. Environ. Health* 1997; 52: 18–25.
66 Seltzer J, Bigby BG, Stulborg M, Holtzman MJ, Nadel JA. O_3-induced charge in bronchial reactivity to methacholine and airway inflammation in humans. *J. Appl. Physiol.* 1986; 60: 1321–6.

67 Koren HS, Devlin RB, Graham DE. Ozone-induced inflammation in the lower airways of human subjects. *Am. Rev. Respir. Dis.* 1989; 139: 407–15.
68 Devlin RB, McDonnell WF, Mann R, et al. Exposure of humans to ambient levels of ozone for 6.6 hours causes cellular and biochemical changes in the lung. *American Journal of Respiratory Cell & Molecular Biology* 1991; 4: 72–81.
69 Nightingale JA, Rogers DF, Barnes PJ. Effect of inhaled ozone on exhaled nitric oxide, pulmonary function, and induced sputum in normal and asthmatic subjects. *Thorax* 1999; 54: 1061–9.
70 Krishna MT, Madden J, Teran LM, et al. Effects of 0.2 ppm ozone on biomarkers of inflammation in bronchoalveolar lavage fluid and bronchial mucosa of healthy subjects. *Eur. Respir. J.* 1998; 11: 1294–300.
71 Koren HS, Devlin RB, Becker S, Perez R, McDonnell WF. Time-dependent changes of markers associated with inflammation in the lungs of humans exposed to ambient levels of ozone. *Toxicol. Pathol.* 1991; 19: 406–11.
72 Mudway IS, Kelly FJ. An investigation of inhaled ozone dose and the magnitude of airway inflammation in healthy adults. *Am. J. Respir. Crit. Care Med.* 2004; 169: 1089–95.
73 Devlin RB, McKinnon KP, Noah T, Becker S, Koren HS. Ozone-induced release of cytokines and fibronectin by alveolar macrophages and airway epithelial cells. *Am. J. Physiol.* 1994; 266: L612–L619.
74 Aris RM, Christian D, Hearne PQ, Kerr K, Finkbeiner WE, Balmes JR. Ozone-induced airway inflammation in human subjects as determined by airway lavage and biopsy. *Am. Rev. Respir. Dis.* 1993; 148: 1363–72.
75 Mudway IS, Krishna MT, Frew AJ, et al. Compromised concentrations of ascorbate in fluid lining the respiratory tract in human subjects after exposure to ozone. *Occup. Environ. Med.* 1999; 56: 473–81.
76 Enami S, Hoffmann MR, Colussi AJ. Acidity enhances the formation of a persistent ozonide at aqueous ascorbate/ozone gas interfaces. *Proc. Natl. Acad. Sci. U.S.A.* 2008; 105: 7365–9.
77 Blomberg A, Mudway IS, Nordenhall C, et al. Ozone-induced lung function decrements do not correlate with early airway inflammatory or antioxidant responses. *Eur. Respir. J.* 1999; 13: 1418–28.
78 Alexis NE, Becker S, Bromberg PA, Devlin R, Peden DB. Circulating CD11b expression correlates with the neutrophil response and airway mCD14 expression is enhanced following ozone exposure in humans. *Clin. Immunol.* 2004; 111: 126–31.
79 Blomberg A, Mudway I, Svensson M, et al. Clara cell protein as a biomarker for ozone-induced lung injury in humans. *Eur. Respir. J.* 2003; 22: 883–8.
80 Stenfors N, Pourazar J, Blomberg A, et al. Effect of ozone on bronchial mucosal inflammation in asthmatic and healthy subjects. *Respir. Med.* 2002; 96: 352–8.
81 Bosson J, Stenfors N, Bucht A, et al. Ozone-induced bronchial epithelial cytokine expression differs between healthy and asthmatic subjects. *Clin. Exp. Allergy.* 2003; 33: 777–82.
82 Christian DL, Chen LL, Scannell CH, Ferrando RE, Welch BS, Balmes JR. Ozone-induced inflammation is attenuated with multiday exposure. *Am. J. Respir. Crit. Care Med.* 1998; 158: 532–7.

83 Jorres RA, Holz O, Zachgo W, et al. The effect of repeated ozone exposures on inflammatory markers in bronchoalveolar lavage fluid and mucosal biopsies. *Am. J. Respir. Crit. Care Med.* 2000; 161: 1855–61.
84 Arjomandi M, Witten A, Abbritti E, et al. Repeated exposure to ozone increases alveolar macrophage recruitment into asthmatic airways. *Am. J. Respir. Crit. Care Med.* 2005; 172: 427–32.
85 Salmon M, Koto H, Lynch OT, et al. Proliferation of airway epithelium after ozone exposure: effect of apocynin and dexamethasone. *Am. J. Respir. Crit. Care Med.* 1998; 157: 970–7.
86 Williams AS, Issa R, Leung SY, et al. Attenuation of ozone-induced airway inflammation and hyper-responsiveness by c-Jun NH2 terminal kinase inhibitor SP600125. *J. Pharmacol. Exp. Ther.* 2007; 322: 351–9.
87 Haddad, E.-B., Salmon, M., Koto, H., Barnes, P. J., Adcock, I., and Chung, K. F. Ozone induction of cytokine-induced neutrophil chemoattractant (CINC) and nuclear factor-kB in rat lung: inhibition by corticosteroids. *FEBS Letts* 1996; 379: 265–268.
88 Fakhrzadeh L, Laskin JD, Laskin DL. Regulation of caveolin-1 expression, nitric oxide production and tissue injury by tumor necrosis factor-alpha following ozone inhalation. *Toxicol. Appl. Pharmacol.* 2008; 227: 380–9.
89 Bhalla DK, Reinhart PG, Bai C, Gupta SK. Amelioration of ozone-induced lung injury by anti-tumor necrosis factor-alpha. *Toxicol. Sci.* 2002; 69: 400–8.
90 Gohil K, Cross CE, Last JA. Ozone-induced disruptions of lung transcriptomes. *Biochem. Biophys. Res. Commun.* 2003; 305: 719–28.
91 Johnston CJ, Stripp BR, Reynolds SD, Avissar NE, Reed CK, Finkelstein JN. Inflammatory and antioxidant gene expression in C57BL/6J mice after lethal and sublethal ozone exposures. *Exp. Lung Res.* 1999; 25: 81–97.
92 Johnston RA, Schwartzman IN, Flynt L, Shore SA. Role of interleukin-6 in murine airway responses to ozone. *Am. J. Physiol Lung Cell Mol. Physiol.* 2005; 288: L390–L397.
93 Holtzman MJ, Fabbri LM, O'Byrne PM, et al. Importance of airway inflammation for hyperresponsiveness induced by ozone. *Am. Rev. Respir. Dis.* 1983; 127: 686–90.
94 O'Byrne PM, Walters EH, Gold BD, et al. Neutrophil depletion inhibits airway hyperresponsiveness induced by ozone exposure. *Am. Rev. Respir. Dis.* 1984; 130: 214–9.
95 Kleeberger SR, Reddy S, Zhang LY, Jedlicka AE. Genetic susceptibility to ozone-induced lung hyperpermeability: role of Toll-like receptor 4. *ajrcmb* 2000; 22: 620–7.
96 Hollingsworth JW, Cook DN, Brass DM, et al. The role of Toll-like receptor 4 in environmental airway injury in mice. *Am. J. Respir. Crit. Care Med.* 2004; 170: 126–32.
97 Williams AS, Leung SY, Nath P, et al. Role of TLR2, TLR4, and MyD88 in murine ozone-induced airway hyperresponsiveness and neutrophilia. *J. Appl. Physiol.* 2007; 103: 1189–95.
98 Sukkar MB, Xie S, Khorasani NM, et al. Toll-like receptor 2, 3, and 4 expression and function in human airway smooth muscle. *J. Allergy Clin. Immunol.* 2006; 118: 641–8.

99 Dahl M, vestbo J, Lange P, Bojesen SE, Tybjaerg-Hansen A, Nordestgaard BG. C-reactive protein as a predictor of prognosis in chronic obstructive pulmonary disease. *Am. J. Respir. Crit Care Med.* 2007; 175: 250–5.
100 Kehrl HR, Vincent LM, Kowalsky RJ, et al. Ozone exposure increases respiratory epithelial permeability in humans. *Am. Rev. Respir. Dis.* 1987; 135: 1124–8.
101 Becker S, Madden MC, Newman SL, Devlin RB, Koren HS. Modulation of human alveolar macrophage properties by ozone exposure in vitro. *Toxicol. Appl. Pharmacol.* 1991; 110: 403–15.
102 Gilmour MI, Hmieleski RR, Stafford EA, Jakab GJ. Suppression and recovery of the alveolar macrophage phagocytic system during continuous exposure to 0.5 ppm ozone. *Exp. Lung Res.* 1991; 17: 547–58.
103 Gilmour MI, Park P, Doerfler D, Selgrade MK. Factors that influence the suppression of pulmonary antibacterial defenses in mice exposed to ozone. *Exp. Lung Res.* 1993; 19: 299–314.
104 Hollingsworth JW, Maruoka S, Li Z, et al. Ambient ozone primes pulmonary innate immunity in mice. *J. Immunol.* 2007; 179: 4367–75.
105 Kierstein S, Poulain FR, Cao Y, et al. Susceptibility to ozone-induced airway inflammation is associated with decreased levels of surfactant protein D. *Respir. Res.* 2006; 7: 85.
106 Haczku A, Cao Y, Vass G, et al. IL-4 and IL-13 form a negative feedback circuit with surfactant protein-D in the allergic airway response. *J. Immunol.* 2006; 176: 3557–65.
107 Koike E, Watanabe H, Kobayashi T. Exposure to ozone enhances antigen-presenting activity concentration dependently in rats. *Toxicology* 2004; 197: 37–46.
108 Dziedzic D, White HJ. T-cell activation in pulmonary lymph nodes of mice exposed to ozone. *Environ. Res.* 1986; 41: 610–22.
109 Neuhaus-Steinmetz U, Uffhausen F, Herz U, Renz H. Priming of allergic immune responses by repeated ozone exposure in mice. *Am. J. Respir Cell Mol. Biol.* 2000; 23: 228–33.
110 Depuydt PO, Lambrecht BN, Joos GF, Pauwels RA. Effect of ozone exposure on allergic sensitization and airway inflammation induced by dendritic cells. *Clin. Exp. Allergy.* 2002; 32: 391–6.
111 Peterson JD, Herzenberg LA, Vasquez K, Waltenbaugh C. Glutathione levels in antigen-presenting cells modulate Th1 versus Th2 response patterns. *Proc. Natl. Acad. Sci. U.S.A.* 1998; 95: 3071–6.
112 Kim HJ, Barajas B, Chan RC, Nel AE. Glutathione depletion inhibits dendritic cell maturation and delayed-type hypersensitivity: implications for systemic disease and immunosenescence. *J. Allergy Clin. Immunol.* 2007; 119: 1225–33.
113 Pichavant M, Goya S, Meyer EH, et al. Ozone exposure in a mouse model induces airway hyperreactivity that requires the presence of natural killer T cells and IL-17. *J. Exp. Med.* 2008; 205: 385–93.
114 Fujimaki H, Ozawa M, Imai T, Shimizu F. Effect of short-term exposure to O3 on antibody response in mice. *Environ. Res.* 1984; 35: 490–6.
115 Dziedzic D, White HJ. Thymus and pulmonary lymph node response to acute and subchronic ozone inhalation in the mouse. *Environ. Res.* 1986; 41: 598–609.
116 Fujimaki H, Shiraishi F, Ashikawa T, Murakami M. Changes in delayed hypersensitivity reaction in mice exposed to O3. *Environ. Res.* 1987; 43: 186–90.

117 Williams AS, Nath P, Leung SY, et al. Modulation of ozone-induced airways hyperresponsiveness and inflammation by IL-13. *Eur. Respir. J.* 2008.
118 Umetsu DT, Meyer EH, DeKruyff RH. Natural killer T cells regulate the development of asthma. *Int. Rev. Immunol* 2007; 26: 121–40.
119 Ballantyne SJ, Barlow JL, Jolin HE, et al. Blocking IL-25 prevents airway hyperresponsiveness in allergic asthma. *J. Allergy Clin. Immunol.* 2007; 120: 1324–31.
120 Kleinschek MA, Owyang AM, Joyce-Shaikh B, et al. IL-25 regulates Th17 function in autoimmune inflammation. *J. Exp. Med.* 2007; 204: 161–70.
121 Ball BA, Folinsbee LJ, Peden DB, Kehrl HR. Allergen bronchoprovocation of patients with mild allergic asthma after ozone exposure. *J. Allergy Clin. Immunol.* 1996; 98: 563–72.
122 Chen LL, Tager IB, Peden DB, et al. Effect of ozone exposure on airway responses to inhaled allergen in asthmatic subjects. *Chest* 2004; 125: 2328–35.
123 Molfino NA, Wright SC, Katz I, et al. Effect of low concentrations of ozone on inhaled allergen responses in asthmatic subjects. *Lancet* 1991; 338: 199–203.
124 Jorres R, Nowak D, Magnussen H. The effect of ozone exposure on allergen responsiveness in subjects with asthma or rhinitis. *Am. J. Respir. Crit. Care Med.* 1996; 153: 56–64.
125 Vagaggini B, Taccola M, Cianchetti S, et al. Ozone exposure increases eosinophilic airway response induced by previous allergen challenge. *Am. J. Respir. Crit. Care Med.* 2002; 166: 1073–7.
126 Rusznak C, Devalia JL, Davies RJ. Airway response of asthmatic subjects to inhaled allergen after exposure to pollutants. *Thorax* 1996; 51: 1105–8.
127 Peden DB, Setzer RW, Jr., Devlin RB. Ozone exposure has both a priming effect on allergen-induced responses and an intrinsic inflammatory action in the nasal airways of perennially allergic asthmatics. *Am. J. Respir. Crit. Care Med.* 1995; 151: 1336–45.
128 Sun J, Koto H, Chung KF. Interaction of ozone and allergen challenges on bronchial responsiveness and inflammation in sensitised guinea pigs. *Int. Arch. Allergy Immunol.* 1997; 112: 191–5.
129 Sun J, Chung KF. Airway inflammation despite loss of bronchial hyperresponsiveness after multiple ozone exposures. *Respir. Med.* 1997; 91: 47–55.
130 Jang AS, Choi IS, Lee JH, Park CS, Park CS. Prolonged ozone exposure in a murine model of asthma: adaptation of airway responsiveness and airway remodeling. *Respir. Res.* 2006; 7: 24.
131 Kierstein S, Krytska K, Sharma S, et al. Ozone inhalation induces exacerbation of eosinophilic airway inflammation and hyperresponsiveness in allergen-sensitized mice. *Allergy* 2008; 63: 438–46.
132 Hayashi T, Raz E. TLR9-based immunotherapy for allergic disease. *Am. J. Med.* 2006; 119: 897–6.
133 Caramalho I, Lopes-Carvalho T, Ostler D, Zelenay S, Haury M, Demengeot J. Regulatory T cells selectively express Toll-like receptors and are activated by lipopolysaccharide. *J. Exp. Med.* 2003; 197: 403–11.

6

Effects of air pollutants on allergic sensitization through the airway

Donald N. Cook and Hideki Nakano

Abstract. Allergic asthma is a widespread disease that exacts a tremendous burden on health and on health care systems. The increased prevalence of this disease in the developed world over the last several decades suggests that a changing environment is affecting the initiation or progression of allergic asthma. The focus of this chapter is on how various components of air pollution might impact allergic sensitization through the airway, the presumptive initial event in asthma. More specifically, the impact of pollutants on pulmonary dendritic cells and their subsequent interactions with naïve T cells will be discussed. It is hoped that an improved understanding of these interactions will help to identify individuals that are at increased risk for developing asthma and will lead to improved strategies to treat this disease.

Keywords: allergic asthma, airway hyperresponsiveness, particulate matter, diesel exhaust particulate matter, air pollution, allergic sensitization, pulmonary immunology, immune adjuvant, T helper cells, pattern-recognition receptors, dendritic cells, immune tolerance, co-stimulation, immunological synapse, animal models of allergic disease

6.1 Introduction

Allergic asthma is characterized by inflammation in and around the airway, mucus production, and reversible airway hyperresponsiveness (AHR).[1] According to World Health Organization estimates, approximately 300 million people suffer from asthma, with a large proportion of them being children. Unlike many diseases, the prevalence of allergic respiratory diseases such as asthma has been increasing over the last several decades, especially in industrialized countries. The relatively short time span over which this increase has occurred suggests that it results from a changing environment, rather than from genetic changes in the population. Indeed, epidemiologic studies show that asthma exacerbations correlate with the proximity to high levels of vehicle traffic. The principal components of air pollution in urban areas with high traffic volumes include particulate matter (PM),[2–5] nitrogen dioxide and ozone.[6–8] These components likely increase the incidence of asthma in two different ways; by exacerbating existing asthma, and by creating new cases of asthma by promoting allergic sensitization to otherwise innocuous airborne antigens. The latter hypothesis is supported by animal studies in which various components of air pollution can act as adjuvants.[9–12] Unfortunately, the mechanisms by which air pollution promotes allergic sensitization remain largely unidentified. Significant progress in this area will require a more complete understanding of the molecular and cellular mechanisms that normally lead to immunotolerance or allergic sensitization following antigen inhalation. The purpose of this chapter is to summarize the state of knowledge in this area, and describe animal-based studies that have begun to address mechanisms whereby air pollution might contribute to allergic sensitization.

6.2 Adjuvants

The ability of air pollution to promote allergic sensitization to otherwise harmless antigens is a property shared by a family of compounds known as adjuvants. On their own, adjuvants are not immunogenic, but they can nonetheless enhance immune responses to co-administered antigens. The most commonly-used adjuvants in human vaccines are the inorganic salts, aluminum phosphate and aluminum hydroxide (alum). The mechanisms of action for these salts are only now beginning to be understood,[13–15] but alum has been widely used for many years in animal studies because of its ability to promote very strong, T helper (Th)2 cell-mediated immune responses. In many studies, ovalbumin (OVA) is used as the provoking antigen for reasons discussed below. Typically, OVA is mixed with alum, and introduced to the animal by intra-peritoneal (i.p.) injections. Adjuvants are generally thought to function by activating one or more innate immune signaling pathways triggered by germline-encoded, pattern recognition receptors (PRRs), such as the toll-like receptors (TLRs) or NOD-like receptors. The function of PRRs is to sense and initiate immune responses to pathogens by recognizing so-called pathogen-associated molecular patterns (PAMPs). These PAMPs are structures that are essential for the survival of the infecting pathogen and have therefore been conserved through evolution.[16] By directly recognizing such PAMPS, PRRs initiate brisk innate immune responses to pathogens and thereby limit the spread of the infection. In addition, PRRs also trigger adaptive immune responses, which are more slow developing, but also more specific. Some examples of PAMPs are lipopolysaccharide (LPS), components of bacterial cell walls, double-stranded RNA, single-stranded DNA, and unmethylated CpG dinucleotide-containing DNA. It is likely that different PAMPs induce specific types of immune responses that are particularly well suited to clear the invading pathogen. The elucidation of these differences and the discovery of the underlying mechanisms involved represent exciting new areas of immunologic research. Although the adjuvant activities inherent in PAMPs have made them very useful as components in vaccines, these same adjuvant activities can also be detrimental to human health because they can provoke inappropriate immune responses to otherwise harmless airborne antigens. The ability of air pollution to provoke allergic sensitization might well have an enormous, but unappreciated, impact on the number of individuals that will ultimately develop allergic asthma. An improved understanding the mechanisms underlying this phenomenon might therefore have the potential to prevent millions of people from developing asthma.

6.3 Dendritic cells

The primary cell type impacted by adjuvants is the mature dendritic cell (DC). The primary purpose of DCs is to process and present antigen to antigen-specific, naïve T cells, and thereby initiate adaptive immune responses. DCs are strategically located in tissues that are exposed to the environment and therefore likely to encounter invading pathogens. Such tissues include the skin and the mucosal epithelia of the gut and airway.[17, 18] Most of the DCs residing in these tissues are in an intermediate state of differentiation. Unlike their blood-borne precursors, these DCs are highly efficient at taking up and processing antigens, but have a limited ability to migrate. Following antigen uptake, DCs undergo a maturation step that includes a reduced capacity to take up antigen, but an increased ability to migrate to draining lymph nodes. This DC migration event is necessary because naïve T cells are not present at high levels within peripheral tissues and instead circulate continuously between the blood and secondary lymphoid tissues such as the spleen and lymph nodes. Unique architectural features and chemical signals within the lymph nodes appear to facilitate interactions between allergen-bearing DCs and rare antigen-specific lymphocytes.[19] Naïve T cells that fail to recognize presented antigen interact only briefly with allergen-bearing DC, and then resume their search for cognate antigen. By contrast, antigen-specific T cells have a much more sustained contact with antigen-bearing DCs. This interaction, which involves docking of multiple receptors with their cognate counter-receptors, is sometimes referred to as the "immunological synapse". Following this encounter with DCs, naïve T cells differentiate and undergo proliferation.[20] The immunologic consequences of this interaction depend on the activation state of antigen-bearing DC and on the specific cytokines they produce. In the setting of inflammation, DCs activate effector or helper T cells, which perform adaptive immune functions.[21] For example, in the presence of IL-4, T cells differentiate into Th2 cells, which are important for allergic responses. In the presence of IL-12, DCs induce Th1 cells, which are not associated with asthma, but may negatively regulate the actions or development of Th2 cells. The cytokines IL-6 and TGF-β promote the differentiation of a more recently described cell type, the Th17 cell. An increasing body of evidence suggests that these cells might be relevant to human asthma. However, effector immune responses such as these are not the usual response to antigen presentation. Rather, during steady-state conditions, meaning in the absence of inflammation, DCs tend to induce regulatory T (Treg) cells, which confer immunotolerance.[22, 23] It is likely that air pollution can induce low levels of pulmonary inflammation that activates pulmonary DCs, which in turn promotes allergic sensitization to innocuous antigens, rather than antigen specific immunotolerance.

6.3.1 Effect of air pollution on DCs in vitro

Allergic responses to inhaled allergens result from complex interactions between the allergen, non-allergenic components of the environment, epithelial cells, DCs, lymphocytes, macrophages and a host of bioactive molecules produced by these various cell types. To reduce the complexity of these interactions, some investigators have studied the impact of various components of air pollution on DCs that have been prepared and cultured in vitro. In general, human DCs have been cultured from monocytes, whereas murine DCs are usually cultured from bone marrow. The results of these experiments have been mixed. In three reports,[24–26] diesel exhaust particles (DEP) or ambient air pollutant particles were found to directly activate DCs.[24–26] A different group failed to see direct activation, but found that DEP-treated epithelial cells could activate DCs.[27] It is possible that the extent to which DEPs activate DCs in vitro depends on the source of these particles and the methods used to collect them. The source of DCs might also impact the outcome of such experiments. In principal, such in vitro approaches will prove to be very helpful in identifying specific molecular pathways in DCs that can be affected by pollutants. However, it remains to be demonstrated that such in vitro responses accurately reflect responses that pulmonary DCs undergo following exposure to such pollutants in vivo. A second disadvantage of in vitro studies is they cannot be used to study the effects of air pollution on pulmonary DC localization in the lung, or the migration of these cells to draining lymph nodes. Rather, whole animal studies will be necessary to confirm and extend findings from in vitro studies.

6.3.2 Pulmonary dendritic cells

The airway is continuously exposed to a wide variety of airborne particles that have the potential for immunoreactivity. Most such particles are harmless, and immune responses to them would be at best unnecessary, and at worst potentially lethal to the host. However, the host must remain vigilant to the presence of inhaled pathogens that could, if left unchecked, initiate life-threatening infections. It is therefore absolutely critical to effectively distinguish between these types of agents, and respond accordingly. This "decision" is made largely by pulmonary DC that are strategically positioned within, and directly beneath, the pulmonary epithelium. Like DCs within the intestinal epithelium,[(28)] pulmonary DCs lying beneath the epithelium also extend projections into the lumen of the airway,[(29)] presumably as a means to capture antigen within the airway. Like their counterparts in other tissues, pulmonary DCs typically display the cell surface molecule, CD11c. However, analysis of pulmonary DCs is complicated by the fact that alveolar macrophages also display CD11c, although alveolar macrophages can be identified by their autofluorescence.[(30)] The DC population within the airway mucosa is not homogeneous, but can be subdivided into multiple groups, based on display levels of multiple cell surface markers, including CD11b, CD4, CD8, CD205 and CD103. A large proportion of pulmonary DC display the myeloid cell marker, CD11b, and these cells tend to induce Th2 responses.[(31)] Plasmacytoid DCs (pDCs) represent another class of DC that are present in several organs, including the lung. Cell surface display of B220 and Gr-1 distinguishes pDCs from other $CD11c^+$ DCs. One of the main functions of pDCs is to produce high amounts of type I interferons (IFN) during viral infection. In addition to this function, pDCs might also function to confer immunotolerance to inhaled antigens.[32] The impact of air pollution components on these various DC subsets in the lung has not yet been studied in any detail.

6.4 Immunotolerance to inhaled antigens

Mice that are exposed to aerosolized OVA do not become sensitized to this protein. Similarly, mice receiving intra-nasal (i.n.) applications of OVA containing sufficiently low levels of LPS also fail to become sensitized. This lack of sensitization can be demonstrated by their inability to develop pulmonary inflammation upon subsequent OVA challenge. However, the absence of a detectable response to allergen challenge does not indicate that these mice have not responded immunologically to the first antigen exposure. These animals do indeed generate immune responses, but the responses are tolerogenic, meaning that these animals are resistant to further attempts to sensitize them, even when a powerful adjuvant, such as alum, is used. This phenomenon, known as immunotolerance, is currently a subject of considerable interest because it holds enormous potential as a means to prevent, or even reverse, inappropriate immune responses. Immunotolerance is mediated by cells known as suppressor or regulatory T cells (Tregs). Treg cells that develop in the thymus function to inhibit the actions of self-antigen-specific T cells that have escape clonal deletion in the thymus. Treg cells are usually identified based on their expression of the forkhead transcription factor, Foxp3, and on their high cell surface levels of CD25. This molecule is the a-chain of the IL-2 receptor, and its high display levels on Tregs probably function to sequester extracellular IL-2, which is required for the proliferation of newly differentiated T cells.

Tregs can also arise in the periphery. These cells recognize exogenous antigens and function to prevent or limit unnecessary immune responses to exogenous, but innocuous antigens. Not all T cells with a regulatory function display CD25. Some Tregs inhibit effector T cells by producing the anti-inflammatory cytokines, IL-10 or TGF-β, or both. Paradoxically, some regulatory T cells, now termed T_{R1} cells, produce IL-10 in addition to effector cytokines, such as IFN-γ or IL-5.[33] The biology of Tregs is a rapidly evolving field, and it is not yet known which of these cell types will emerge as having the greatest therapeutic use.[34] Because immunotolerance and allergic sensitization are the alternative immunologic outcomes stemming from antigen inhalation, it seems likely that some components of air pollution can augment sensitization by inhibiting the development or actions of one or more Treg subsets. This will likely be an area of intense interest in the near future as mechanisms that give rise to Treg induction and regulation become better understood.

6.4.1 Mechanisms of dendritic cell-mediated immunotolerance

Just as several subsets of regulatory T cells have been identified, more than one subset of DCs has been implicated in immunotolerance. One such subset is the IL-10-producing DC, which are required for the development of OVA-specific tolerance following i.n. exposure to OVA.[35] Interestingly, these IL-10-producing DCs display high levels of the co-stimulatory molecules B7-1 (CD80) and B7-2 (CD86), and induce the proliferation of T cells displaying CD69, an early activation marker of T cells. Thus, the induction of immunotolerance by IL-10-producing DCs is associated with active T cell proliferation, rather than with a simple unresponsiveness to the inhaled antigen.

A second cell type associated with immunotolerance is the macrophage. It has been known for about 30 years that alveolar macrophages have immunosuppressive activities,[36] which are probably mediated by their production of TGF-β. Thus, the ability of alveolar macrophages to inhibit DC-mediated proliferation of T cells is blocked by antibodies against TGF-β.[37] Because alveolar macrophages are the predominant cell type in the non-inflamed airway, these cells likely suppress the activation of pulmonary DCs. Recent evidence suggests that this suppression involves the transcription factor, Runx3. Runx3 is expressed in mature DCs and mediates their response to TGF-β. *Runx3*$^{-/-}$ mice develop spontaneous eosinophilic lung inflammation, mucus hypersecretion, and airway remodeling.[38]

These findings might be relevant to human asthma because human RUNX3 resides in a region of chromosome 1p36 that contains susceptibility genes for asthma and hypersensitivity. In addition to their asthma-like phenotype, *Runx3*$^{-/-}$ mice have increased levels of the chemokine receptor, CCR7, on pulmonary DCs, which undergo increased migration to lung-draining lymph nodes. These associations suggest that increased CCR7-dependent pulmonary DC migration might lead to enhanced allergic sensitization in the *Runx3*$^{-/-}$ mice. However, Hintzen and co-workers have shown that the migration of tolerance-inducing DCs to draining lymph nodes is also dependent on CCR7.[39] Under these conditions, tolerance was associated with the migration of CCR7$^+$ DCs bearing the α_E integrin (CD103) surface marker, suggesting that CD103$^+$ pulmonary DCs can promote tolerance. If both tolerogenic and immunogenic DCs depend on CCR7 for their migration to draining lymph nodes, which DC subset is dominant? Based on findings with *Runx3*$^{-/-}$ mice, it seems likely that immunogenic DCs are dominant, but this has not yet been directly demonstrated experimentally.

Yet another cell type associated with tolerance to inhaled antigens is the pDC. Antibody-mediated depletion of pDCs impairs the ability of mice to develop tolerance, and adoptive transfer of pDCs together with allergen prevented disease in am alum/OVA mouse model of allergic sensitization.[32] Interestingly, despite their impaired ability to become tolerized to inhaled antigen, *Ccr7*$^{-/-}$ mice did not display decreased migration of pDCs from the lung to draining lymph nodes. The ability of different DC subsets to induce immunotolerance to inhaled OVA in these different studies raises the following question: what is the primary DC subset in the lung that gives rise to antigen-specific immunotolerance? Is it the IL-10-producing DC, the CD103$^+$ DC, or the pDC? The answer to this question might depend on the experimental conditions used in the study. It is also possible that each of these DC subsets co-operates to promote tolerance because in general, disrupting the function of a single DC subset did not completely block tolerance. Clearly, additional experiments will be determined to compare the relative importance of these subsets under different conditions. More to the point of this chapter, it will be interesting to learn whether one or more of these subsets are specifically impacted by different components of air pollution.

6.5 Animal models of air pollution-enhanced allergic sensitization

In theory, the mechanisms by which various components of air pollution promote allergic sensitization to otherwise innocuous inhaled antigens can be studied in whole animal experiments. To date, virtually all of these studies have employed OVA as the provoking antigen. Although OVA is not a clinically relevant antigen, there are several excellent reasons for using it in these types of studies. First, it can be commercially obtained in a fluorescently-tagged form, which allows the migration patterns of allergen-bearing DCs to be tracked in experimental animals. For example, it will be helpful to determine whether air pollution components increase the migration of pulmonary DC to draining lymph nodes, and if so, whether such an increase is functionally relevant to air pollution-enhanced allergic sensitization through the airway. Detection of fluorescent OVA-bearing

DCs in the lymph node does not, however, necessarily mean that these cells originated in the lung because OVA can be passively carried to the draining lymph nodes in lymph fluid, and taken up by DCs residing there. One approach to address this complication is to selectively label DCs residing in the airway at the time of allergen transfer. Such studies have been done by delivering the fluorescent dye, carboxyfluoroscein succinimidyl ester (CFSE), to the airways of experimental mice.[40] Allergen-bearing DCs migrating from the lung to draining lymph nodes can be subsequently identified by virtue of their staining for both CFSE and fluorescently-tagged OVA.

A second reason for using OVA as an antigen is the availability of transgenic mouse strains in which the entire repertoire of T cells recognizes OVA. These stains are useful because antigen-specific T cells in wild type mice are very rare and difficult to follow in vivo. This difficulty has been surmounted by the creation of mice in which every T cell can recognize OVA. To generate these animals, DNA encoding the alpha-chain and beta-chain of the T-cell receptor from a T-cell hybridoma recognizing OVA was used as a transgene. Mice of this sort are available on the MHC class II (I-A^d)-restricted background (the DO11.10 strain) and on the I-A^b-restricted background (the OT-II strain), and correspond to two of the most commonly used mouse strains, Balb/c and C57BL/6, respectively. One drawback of using these mice is that their immune responses do not accurately mimic those of wild type mice in all situations. For this reason, T cells from OT-II or DO11.10 mice are sometimes adoptively transferred to wild type mice, where from OVA-specific T cells can be followed in a mouse having normal immune responses.

Another advantage of using OVA to study allergic sensitization is that when obtained in a relatively pure form, this protein is not immunogenic. This lack of immunogenicity in OVA is useful because it can be used together with various components of air pollution to test for associated adjuvant activities. For example, LPS, DEP, (ozone) O_3 and NO_2 have all been shown to promote allergic sensitization to OVA. These studies have shed light on potential mechanisms related to air pollution-enhanced, allergic sensitization through the airway.

6.5.1 LPS-mediated allergic sensitization

LPS is a component of the outer membrane of Gram-negative bacteria. The potent inflammatory activity associated with this molecule is referred to as endotoxin. Thus, LPS is measured in units of weight, whereas endotoxin is measured in units of activity. Due to the ubiquity of Gram-negative bacteria, LPS is commonly found in dust from many domestic and occupational sources[41] and can therefore be reasonably used as a surrogate of air pollution in studies of air pollution-enhanced allergic sensitization. Eisenbarth et al. have shown that when OVA is introduced into the airway together with low levels of LPS, recipient mice develop OVA-specific Th2 responses.[42] Interestingly, the adaptor protein, MyD88, is required for OVA sensitization through the airway when LPS is used as an adjuvant, but not for sensitization through the peritoneum when alum is used as an adjuvant.[43] This differential requirement of MyD88 is not due solely to the different adjuvants used because MyD88 is required for LPS-mediated upregulation of MHC class II and B7 in pulmonary DCs, but not in spleen- or bone marrow-derived DCs.[44, 45] Unlike most TLRs, TLR4 can signal either through MyD88 or through an alternative adaptor protein, the TIR domain-containing adaptor inducing IFN-γ (TRIF).[46, 47] Although there is some redundancy between these two pathways, there are also some differences. For example, the TRIF-dependent pathway is required for LPS-induced production of IFN-#δυβ.[46] Piggott and colleagues took advantage of this property to show that engagement of the TRIF-dependent pathway is defective in pulmonary DCs.[43] As a result, signaling responses to LPS are completely dependent on MyD88 and therefore defective in MyD88-deficient mice. These findings underscore the notion that pulmonary DCs are fundamentally different, at least in some ways, from their counterparts in other tissues. Piggott et al. also showed that the requirement of MyD88 could be bypassed by instilling exogenous TNF-α into the airway together with OVA. This finding is consistent with previous results showing that production of TNF-α, but not signaling responses to it, are dependent on MyD88. Taken together, these results suggest that LPS functions as an adjuvant by inducing the production of TNF-α through a MyD88-dependent pathway. The consequences of this TNF-α production, and the extent to which this pathway is also involved in allergic sensitization mediated by other air pollutants, remains to be determined.

6.5.2 NO_2-mediated allergic sensitization

NO_2 is a toxic gas formed in internal combustion engines when atmospheric nitrogen combines with oxygen. This free radical gas is highly reactive and has been implicated in the exacerbation of asthma, particularly in children. Brown Norway rats exposed to NO_2 prior to OVA exposure had increased OVA-specific IgE, IgA, and IgG compared to mice receiving OVA, but not

NO_2.[48] More recently, mice were also shown to develop allergic sensitization to OVA following exposure to as little as ten parts per million (ppm) NO_2.[49] After being sensitized twice in this way, and challenged on three occasions with OVA, these mice developed pulmonary eosinophilia, mucus cell metaplasia, Th2-biased $CD4^+$ T cell responses, and airway hyperreactivity (AHR). These findings are reminiscent of the ability of LPS to promote allergic sensitization. However, the timing of OVA administrations relative to NO_2 exposures was critical. Thus, NO_2 could promote allergic sensitization when given up to two days prior to OVA administration, but when the order of these exposures was reversed, sensitization was not achieved. In fact, sensitization failed to occur when mice were exposed to NO_2 as little as one hour after OVA. The mechanism of sensitization might involve NF-kB because exposure to NO_2 induced localization of this important transcription factor to the nucleus. As was seen previously with LPS, NO_2-mediated sensitization required the adaptor protein, MyD88. This suggests that MyD88 might be required for allergic sensitization through the airway, regardless of which adjuvant is used. Just as LPS-mediated allergic sensitization requires TLR4, NO_2-mediated sensitization requires TLR2. However, whereas LPS is a ligand of the TLR4 receptor complex, NO_2 is not a "ligand" of TLR2. It remains to be seen whether NO_2 induces the production of endogenous factors that signal through TLR2, or whether NO_2 can directly modify the structure of this receptor, and thereby promote its signaling.

6.5.3 Ozone-mediated allergic sensitization

Ozone is a highly reactive component of air pollution formed by the combination of sunlight, nitrous oxides, volatile organic compounds and oxygen. The biologic properties of ozone likely stem from its ability to form highly reactive oxygen species, which can damage cells and trigger the release of proinflammatory mediators. Interestingly, at least some of the biologic and physiologic responses to ozone are dependent on the 4 TLR4, a molecule best known for its role in signaling responses to LPS. It has been known for several years that exposure to ozone not only exacerbates existing asthma, but, at least in animal models, can also promote allergic sensitization to inhaled OVA.[50, 51] Despite this long-standing observation, the mechanism by which ozone gives rise to allergic sensitization is very poorly understood. One might anticipate that exposure to ozone activates DC, thereby promoting allergic sensitization. However, exposure to ozone does not affect the ability of OVA-pulsed

DCs to sensitize mice receiving these cells by intratracheal instillation.[52] One interpretation of this result is that ozone does not affect DC function. However, another interpretation is that bone marrow-derived DCs cultured in the presence of growth factors are already sufficiently activated to promote allergic sensitization, and that ozone does not further enhance this capacity. By contrast, pulmonary DCs are, in the absence of an additional stimulus, normally immunoregulatory. A third possibility is that ozone activates cells indirectly, for example by damaging epithelial cells. Additional studies will be required to address these questions.

6.5.4 DEP-mediated allergic sensitization

It has been known for more than twenty years that DEP can act as an adjuvant to promote allergic sensitization.[53] In general these types of studies have used OVA as the allergen.[9, 12, 53] Although OVA is a useful allergen for reasons described above, until recently, most preparations of OVA have been contaminated with LPS.[54, 55] This might be relevant to experimental results with DEP because LPS and DEP can synergize to aggravate acute lung injury and promote free radical generation.[56–58] Their ability to synergize for free radical formation suggests that these two agents might also synergize to promote allergic sensitization. Indeed, reactive oxygen species (ROS) appear to contribute significantly to the adjuvant effects of DEP because two different thiol antioxidants can protect cells from protein and lipid oxidation, and inhibit the adjuvant effects of DEP.[59] It will be informative to learn whether DEP will have similar effects when OVA (that is essentially free of LPS) is used as an adjuvant. Recent studies have shown that TNF-α is induced by diesel exhaust[60] although it is not yet clear whether the production of this cytokine is dependent on the oxidizing activity of DEP. Regardless of the order of events, DEP-mediated production of TNF-α might be relevant to the adjuvant activities associated with these particles because TNF-α can promote allergic sensitization through the airway, even in the absence of other adjuvants.[61]

6.6 Mechanisms of air pollution-enhanced allergic sensitization

Although a comprehensive understanding of the impact of air pollution on allergic sensitization is not yet at hand, some general conclusions can be tentatively drawn. The bulk of evidence emerging from the above-described experiments suggests that mechanisms giving rise to allergic sensitization through the airway are substantially different from those at play in other tissues. For example, MyD88, an adaptor molecule involved in the TLR and IL-1 signaling pathways, is generally dispensable for the induction of Th2 responses, whereas it was required for both LPS- and for N_2-mediated sensitization through the airway.[43, 49] In both studies, MyD88 was shown to be dispensable for allergic sensitization using alum as an adjuvant, demonstrating that MyD88 is indeed required during the sensitization phase and not the challenge phase. Although its production in all experimental models has not been reported, increasing evidence suggests that TNF-α is an important molecule in air pollution-mediated allergic sensitization. It is unclear, however, which cells must respond to TNF-α to effect allergic sensitization. The observed differences in molecular requirements for the activation of pulmonary DC and bone marrow-derived DC suggest that there is a limit to what we can learn about allergic sensitization through the airway by studying bone marrow- or blood cell-derived DCs. On the other hand, the lengthy procedures that must currently be used to prepare pulmonary DCs might limit the type of experiments that can be done, and perhaps more importantly, might affect the responses of these cells to antigens or adjuvants. New tools that permit the rapid isolation of different subsets of DCs should prove very useful in this regard. Meanwhile, our understanding of air pollution-mediated sensitization through the airway will improve based on both in vitro models and analyses of immune responses in intact animals.

References

1 Cohn, L., J.A. Elias, and G.L. Chupp. 2004. Asthma: mechanisms of disease persistence and progression. *Annual Review of Immunology* 22: 789–815.
2 Carbajal-Arroyo, L., A. Barraza-Villarreal, R. Durand-Pardo, H. Moreno-Macias, R. Espinoza-Lain, P. Chiarella-Ortigosa, and I. Romieu. 2007. Impact of traffic flow on the asthma prevalence among school children in Lima, Peru. *J Asthma* 44: 197–202.
3 McCreanor, J., P. Cullinan, M.J. Nieuwenhuijsen, J. Stewart-Evans, E. Malliarou, L. Jarup, R. Harrington, M. Svartengren, I.K. Han, P. Ohman-Strickland, K.F. Chung, and J. Zhang. 2007. Respiratory effects of exposure to diesel traffic in persons with asthma. *N Engl J Med* 357: 2348–2358.
4 Morgenstern, V., A. Zutavern, J. Cyrys, I. Brockow, U. Gehring, S. Koletzko, C.P. Bauer, D. Reinhardt, H.E. Wichmann, and J. Heinrich. 2007. Respiratory health and individual estimated exposure to traffic-related air pollutants in a cohort of young children. *Occup Environ Med* 64: 8–16.

5 von Klot, S., G. Wolke, T. Tuch, J. Heinrich, D.W. Dockery, J. Schwartz, W.G. Kreyling, H.E. Wichmann, and A. Peters. 2002. Increased asthma medication use in association with ambient fine and ultrafine particles. *Eur Respir J* 20: 691–702.
6 Bates, D.V., and R. Sizto. 1983. Relationship between air pollutant levels and hospital admissions in Southern Ontario. *Canadian Journal of Public Health* 74: 117–122.
7 White, M.C., R.A. Etzel, W.D. Wilcox, and C. Lloyd. 1994. Exacerbations of childhood asthma and ozone pollution in Atlanta. *Environmental Research* 65: 56–68.
8 Whittemore, A.S., and E.L. Korn. 1980. Asthma and air pollution in the Los Angeles area. *American Journal of Public Health* 70: 687–696.
9 Fujimaki, H., O. Nohara, T. Ichinose, N. Watanabe, and S. Saito. 1994. IL-4 production in mediastinal lymph node cells in mice intratracheally instilled with diesel exhaust particulates and antigen. *Toxicology* 92: 261–268.
10 Miyabara, Y., T. Ichinose, H. Takano, H.B. Lim, and M. Sagai. 1998. Effects of diesel exhaust on allergic airway inflammation in mice. *J Allergy Clin Immunol* 102: 805–812.
11 Muranaka, M., S. Suzuki, K. Koizumi, S. Takafuji, T. Miyamoto, R. Ikemori, and H. Tokiwa. 1986. Adjuvant activity of diesel-exhaust particulates for the production of IgE antibody in mice. *J Allergy Clin Immunol* 77: 616–623.
12 Steerenberg, P.A., C.E. Withagen, J.A. Dormans, W.J. van Dalen, H. van Loveren, and F.R. Casee. 2003. Adjuvant activity of various diesel exhaust and ambient particles in two allergic models. *J Toxicol Environ Health A* 66: 1421–1439.
13 Franchi, L., and G. Nunez. 2008. The Nlrp3 inflammasome is critical for aluminium hydroxide-mediated IL-1beta secretion but dispensable for adjuvant activity. *European Journal of Immunology* 38: 2085–2089.
14 Kool, M., V. Petrilli, T. De Smedt, A. Rolaz, H. Hammad, M. van Nimwegen, I.M. Bergen, R. Castillo, B.N. Lambrecht, and J. Tschopp. 2008. Cutting Edge: alum adjuvant stimulates inflammatory dendritic cells through activation of the NALP3 inflammasome. *J Immunol* 181: 3755–3759.
15 Kool, M., T. Soullie, M. van Nimwegen, M.A. Willart, F. Muskens, S. Jung, H.C. Hoogsteden, H. Hammad, and B.N. Lambrecht. 2008. Alum adjuvant boosts adaptive immunity by inducing uric acid and activating inflammatory dendritic cells. *The Journal of Experimental Medicine* 205: 869–882.
16 Medzhitov, R. 2007. Recognition of microorganisms and activation of the immune response. *Nature* 449: 819–826.
17 Banchereau, J., R.M. Steinman, I. Mellman, and R.M. Steinman. 1998. Dendritic cells and the control of immunity. Dendritic cells: specialized and regulated antigen processing machines. *Nature* 392: 245–252.
18 Mellman, I., and R.M. Steinman. 2001. Dendritic cells: specialized and regulated antigen processing machines. *Cell* 106: 255–258.
19 Bajenoff, M., J.G. Egen, H. Qi, A.Y. Huang, F. Castellino, and R.N. Germain. 2007. Highways, byways and breadcrumbs: directing lymphocyte traffic in the lymph node. *Trends in Immunology* 28: 346–352.

20 Mempel, T.R., S.E. Henrickson, and U.H. Von Andrian. 2004. T-cell priming by dendritic cells in lymph nodes occurs in three distinct phases. *Nature* 427: 154–159.
21 Medzhitov, R. 2007. Recognition of microorganisms and activation of the immune response. *Nature* 449: 819–826.
22 Bonifaz, L., D. Bonnyay, K. Mahnke, M. Rivera, M.C. Nussenzweig, and R.M. Steinman. 2002. Efficient targeting of protein antigen to the dendritic cell receptor DEC-205 in the steady state leads to antigen presentation on major histocompatibility complex class I products and peripheral CD8+ T cell tolerance. *J Exp Med* 196: 1627–1638.
23 Hawiger, D., K. Inaba, Y. Dorsett, M. Guo, K. Mahnke, M. Rivera, J.V. Ravetch, R.M. Steinman, and M.C. Nussenzweig. 2001. Dendritic cells induce peripheral T cell unresponsiveness under steady state conditions in vivo. *J Exp Med* 194: 769–779.
24 Chan, R.C., M. Wang, N. Li, Y. Yanagawa, K. Onoe, J.J. Lee, and A.E. Nel. 2006. Pro-oxidative diesel exhaust particle chemicals inhibit LPS-induced dendritic cell responses involved in T-helper differentiation. *The Journal of Allergy and Clinical Immunology* 118: 455–465.
25 Porter, M., M. Karp, S. Killedar, S.M. Bauer, J. Guo, D. Williams, P. Breysse, S.N. Georas, and M.A. Williams. 2007. Diesel-enriched particulate matter functionally activates human dendritic cells. *American Journal of Respiratory Cell and Molecular Biology* 37: 706–719.
26 Williams, M.A., M. Porter, J. Roman, P. Breysse, D. Williams, and S.N. Georas. 2007. Ambient Baltimore particulate matter directs non-classical immune activation of human myeloid dendritic cells. *The Journal of Allergy and Clinical Immunology* 119: 488–97.
27 Bleck, B., D.B. Tse, I. Jaspers, M.A. Curotto de Lafaille, and J. Reibman. 2006. Diesel exhaust particle-exposed human bronchial epithelial cells induce dendritic cell maturation. *J Immunol* 176: 7431–7437.
28 Niess, J.H., S. Brand, X. Gu, L. Landsman, S. Jung, B.A. McCormick, J.M. Vyas, M. Boes, H.L. Ploegh, J.G. Fox, D.R. Littman, and H.C. Reinecker. 2005. CX3CR1-mediated dendritic cell access to the intestinal lumen and bacterial clearance. *Science (New York, NY)* 307: 254–258.
29 Jahnsen, F.L., D.H. Strickland, J.A. Thomas, I.T. Tobagus, S. Napoli, G.R. Zosky, D.J. Turner, P.D. Sly, P.A. Stumbles, and P.G. Holt. 2006. Accelerated antigen sampling and transport by airway mucosal dendritic cells following inhalation of a bacterial stimulus. *J Immunol* 177: 5861–5867.
30 Vermaelen, K., and R. Pauwels. 2004. Accurate and simple discrimination of mouse pulmonary dendritic cell and macrophage populations by flow cytometry: methodology and new insights. *Cytometry A* 61: 170–177.
31 Stumbles, P.A., J.A. Thomas, C.L. Pimm, P.T. Lee, T.J. Venaille, S. Proksch, and P.G. Holt. 1998. Resting respiratory tract dendritic cells preferentially stimulate T helper cell type 2 (Th2) responses and require obligatory cytokine signals for induction of Th1 immunity. *The Journal of Experimental Medicine* 188: 2019–2031.
32 de Heer, H.J., H. Hammad, T. Soullie, D. Hijdra, N. Vos, M.A. Willart, H.C. Hoogsteden, and B.N. Lambrecht. 2004. Essential role of lung plasmacytoid

dendritic cells in preventing asthmatic reactions to harmless inhaled antigen. *The Journal of Experimental Medicine* 200: 89–98.

33 Groux, H., A. O'Garra, M. Bigler, M. Rouleau, S. Antonenko, J.E. de Vries, and M.G. Roncarolo. 1997. A CD4+ T-cell subset inhibits antigen-specific T-cell responses and prevents colitis. *Nature* 389: 737–742.

34 Hawrylowicz, C.M., and A. O'Garra. 2005. Potential role of interleukin-10-secreting regulatory T cells in allergy and asthma. *Nature Reviews* 5: 271–283.

35 Akbari, O., R.H. DeKruyff, and D.T. Umetsu. 2001. Pulmonary dendritic cells producing IL-10 mediate tolerance induced by respiratory exposure to antigen. *Nature Immunology* 2: 725–731.

36 Holt, P.G. 1978. Inhibitory activity of unstimulated alveolar macrophages on T-lymphocyte blastogenic response. *The American Review of Respiratory Disease* 118: 791–793.

37 Lipscomb, M.F., A.M. Pollard, and J.L. Yates. 1993. A role for TGF-beta in the suppression by murine bronchoalveolar cells of lung dendritic cell initiated immune responses. *Regional Immunology* 5: 151–157.

38 Fainaru, O., E. Woolf, J. Lotem, M. Yarmus, O. Brenner, D. Goldenberg, V. Negreanu, Y. Bernstein, D. Levanon, S. Jung, and Y. Groner. 2004. Runx3 regulates mouse TGF-beta-mediated dendritic cell function and its absence results in airway inflammation. *The EMBO journal* 23: 969–979.

39 Hintzen, G., L. Ohl, M.L. del Rio, J.I. Rodriguez-Barbosa, O. Pabst, J.R. Kocks, J. Krege, S. Hardtke, and R. Forster. 2006. Induction of tolerance to innocuous inhaled antigen relies on a CCR7-dependent dendritic cell-mediated antigen transport to the bronchial lymph node. *J Immunol* 177: 7346–7354.

40 Legge, K.L., and T.J. Braciale. 2003. Accelerated migration of respiratory dendritic cells to the regional lymph nodes is limited to the early phase of pulmonary infection. *Immunity* 18: 265–277.

41 Thorne, P.S., K. Kulhankova, M. Yin, R. Cohn, S.J. Arbes, Jr., and D.C. Zeldin. 2005. Endotoxin exposure is a risk factor for asthma: the national survey of endotoxin in United States housing. *American Journal of Respiratory and Critical Care Medicine* 172: 1371–1377.

42 Eisenbarth, S.C., D.A. Piggott, J.W. Huleatt, I. Visintin, C.A. Herrick, and K. Bottomly. 2002. Lipopolysaccharide-enhanced, toll-like receptor 4-dependent T helper cell type 2 responses to inhaled antigen. *The Journal of Experimental Medicine* 196: 1645–1651.

43 Piggott, D.A., S.C. Eisenbarth, L. Xu, S.L. Constant, J.W. Huleatt, C.A. Herrick, and K. Bottomly. 2005. MyD88-dependent induction of allergic Th2 responses to intranasal antigen. *The Journal of Clinical Investigation* 115: 459–467.

44 Kaisho, T., K. Hoshino, T. Iwabe, O. Takeuchi, T. Yasui, and S. Akira. 2002. Endotoxin can induce MyD88-deficient dendritic cells to support T(h)2 cell differentiation. *International Immunology* 14: 695–700.

45 Kaisho, T., O. Takeuchi, T. Kawai, K. Hoshino, and S. Akira. 2001. Endotoxin-induced maturation of MyD88-deficient dendritic cells. *J Immunol* 166: 5688–5694.

46 Hoebe, K., E.M. Janssen, S.O. Kim, L. Alexopoulou, R.A. Flavell, J. Han, and B. Beutler. 2003. Upregulation of costimulatory molecules induced by

lipopolysaccharide and double-stranded RNA occurs by Trif-dependent and Trif-independent pathways. *Nature Immunology* 4: 1223–1229.
47 Yamamoto, M., S. Sato, H. Hemmi, K. Hoshino, T. Kaisho, H. Sanjo, O. Takeuchi, M. Sugiyama, M. Okabe, K. Takeda, and S. Akira. 2003. Role of adaptor TRIF in the MyD88-independent toll-like receptor signaling pathway. *Science* 301: 640–643.
48 Siegel, P.D., N.H. Al-Humadi, E.R. Nelson, D.M. Lewis, and A.F. Hubbs. 1997. Adjuvant effect of respiratory irritation on pulmonary allergic sensitization: time and site dependency. *Toxicology and Applied Pharmacology* 144: 356–362.
49 Bevelander, M., J. Mayette, L.A. Whittaker, S.A. Paveglio, C.C. Jones, J. Robbins, D. Hemenway, S. Akira, S. Uematsu, and M.E. Poynter. 2007. Nitrogen dioxide promotes allergic sensitization to inhaled antigen. *J Immunol* 179: 3680–3688.
50 Gershwin, L.J., J.W. Osebold, and Y.C. Zee. 1981. Immunoglobulin E-containing cells in mouse lung following allergen inhalation and ozone exposure. *International Archives of Allergy and Applied Immunology* 65: 266–277.
51 Osebold, J.W., L.J. Gershwin, and Y.C. Zee. 1980. Studies on the enhancement of allergic lung sensitization by inhalation of ozone and sulfuric acid aerosol. *Journal of Environmental Pathology and Toxicology* 3: 221–234.
52 Depuydt, P.O., B.N. Lambrecht, G.F. Joos, and R.A. Pauwels. 2002. Effect of ozone exposure on allergic sensitization and airway inflammation induced by dendritic cells. *Clin Exp Allergy* 32: 391–396.
53 Takafuji, S., S. Suzuki, K. Koizumi, K. Tadokoro, T. Miyamoto, R. Ikemori, and M. Muranaka. 1987. Diesel-exhaust particulates inoculated by the intranasal route have an adjuvant activity for IgE production in mice. *Journal of Allergy and Clinical Immunology* 79: 639–645.
54 Hollingsworth, J.W., G.S. Whitehead, K.L. Lin, H. Nakano, M.D. Gunn, D.A. Schwartz, and D.N. Cook. 2006. TLR4 signaling attenuates ongoing allergic inflammation. *J Immunol* 176: 5856–5862.
55 Watanabe, J., Y. Miyazaki, G.A. Zimmerman, K.H. Albertine, and T.M. McIntyre. 2003. Endotoxin contamination of ovalbumin suppresses murine immunologic responses and development of airway hyper-reactivity. *J Biol Chem* 278: 42361–42368. Epub 42003 Aug 42368.
56 Arimoto, T., M.B. Kadiiska, K. Sato, J. Corbett, and R.P. Mason. 2005. Synergistic production of lung free radicals by diesel exhaust particles and endotoxin. *Am J Respir Crit Care Med* 171: 379–387.
57 Verstraelen, S., R. Van Den Heuvel, I. Nelissen, H. Witters, G. Verheyen, and G. Schoeters. 2005. Flow cytometric characterisation of antigen presenting dendritic cells after in vitro exposure to diesel exhaust particles. *Toxicol In Vitro* 19: 903–907.
58 Yanagisawa, R., H. Takano, K. Inoue, T. Ichinose, K. Sadakane, S. Yoshino, K. Yamaki, Y. Kumagai, K. Uchiyama, T. Yoshikawa, and M. Morita. 2003. Enhancement of acute lung injury related to bacterial endotoxin by components of diesel exhaust particles. *Thorax* 58: 605–612.
59 Whitekus, M.J., N. Li, M. Zhang, M. Wang, M.A. Horwitz, S.K. Nelson, L.D. Horwitz, N. Brechun, D. Diaz-Sanchez, and A.E. Nel. 2002. Thiol antioxidants inhibit the adjuvant effects of aerosolized diesel exhaust particles in a murine model for ovalbumin sensitization. *J Immunol* 168: 2560–2567.

60 Gowdy, K., Q.T. Krantz, M. Daniels, W.P. Linak, I. Jaspers, and M.I. Gilmour. 2008. Modulation of pulmonary inflammatory responses and antimicrobial defenses in mice exposed to diesel exhaust. *Toxicol Appl Pharmacol* 229(3): 310–319. Epub 2008 Feb 15.
61 Lambert, A.L., M.K. Selgrade, D.W. Winsett, and M.I. Gilmour. 2001. TNF–alpha enhanced allergic sensitization to house dust mite in brown Norway rats. *Exp Lung Res* 27: 617–635.

7

Particulate matter and oxidative stress: dangerous partners in inflammation, vascular dysfunction and innate immunity

Steve N. Georas and Mark W. Frampton

Abstract. Exposure to inhaled particulate matter (PM) is associated with adverse health outcomes including asthma, chronic obstructive pulmonary disease (COPD), respiratory infections, and cardiovascular morbidity and mortality. In the case of asthma, exposure to pollutants including PM is now known to be associated with both an increased incidence of disease as well as asthma exacerbations and reduced lung function. PM exposure is also associated with heart attacks, arrhythmias, heart failure, and stroke. Studies by many investigators have determined that PM from different sources, including ambient PM and diesel exhaust particles (DEP), can activate epithelial cells and other cells in the respiratory tract. Ultrafine or nanoparticles may cross the epithelium and enter the vascular space. Although the literature in this field is rapidly expanding, a common finding is that PM exposed cells produce chemokines, cytokines and other mediators that cause local and systemic inflammation. The molecular mechanisms by which PM activates target cells are beginning to be understood, and a recurring theme in PM research is that oxidative stress is a major intermediary. Here we review current knowledge and propose a model in which PM-induced oxidative stress initiates innate immune and inflammatory responses that result in pulmonary and systemic vascular dysfunction. These effects may lead to acute exacerbation of disease following acute exposures, and initiate disease with long-term exposure.

Keywords: allergic inflammation, allergic asthma, pulmonary immunity, particulate pollution, diesel exhaust particulate matter, oxidative stress, genetic susceptibility, gene polymorphisms, ultrafine particulate matter, toll-like receptor pathways, innate immunity, dendritic cells

7.1 Introduction

Exposure to inhaled particulate matter (PM) is associated with adverse pulmonary and cardiovascular outcomes, including asthma exacerbations, respiratory infections, acute myocardial infarction, and mortality. In the case of asthma, exposure to pollutants including PM is associated with an increased incidence of disease, exacerbations, and reduced lung function.[1, 2] Important studies by many investigators have determined that PM from different sources, including ambient PM and diesel exhaust particles (DEP), can activate epithelial cells and other cells in the respiratory tract. Although the literature in this field is vast and expanding, a common finding is that PM exposed cells produce chemokines, cytokines and other mediators that cause local and systemic inflammation.[3–7] Systemic and cardiovascular effects may result from local airway effects or from translocation of particles or their components out of the lung to the blood and other organs.

The molecular mechanisms by which PM activates target cells are beginning to be understood, and involve the mitogen activated protein kinases and other signaling pathways that activate different transcription factor families. A common theme in PM related research is that oxidative stress is a major intermediary, which in the case of sterile particles (i.e. free of contaminating biological material) may involve mitochondrial dysfunction.[8] Supporting this concept is the observation that genetic polymorphisms that confer impaired defense against oxidative stress are associated with increased susceptibility to the pulmonary and cardiovascular effects of PM. For example, glutathione transferase M1 (GSTM1) is a critical enzyme in cellular defense against reactive oxygen species, and a common polymorphism in this enzyme markedly reduces its function (GSTM1 null). Smokers who are GSTM1 null are at increased risk for coronary artery disease compared with other GST genotypes.[9] Schwartz et al. found that a 10 $\mu g/m^3$ increase in PM2.5 was associated with a 34 percent decrease in high-frequency heart rate variability, but only in people that were GSTM1 null, with no effects in GSTM1+ subjects.[10] Among asthmatic children living in Mexico City, those who were GSTM1 null showed greater ozone-related decrements in small airways function, and greater improvement with antioxidant supplementation, than GSTM1+ children.[11] GSTM1 null subjects showed greater nasal allergic responses in the presence of diesel exhaust particles.[12] These and other studies support the hypothesis that oxidative stress is an important mechanism in the health effects of exposure to PM.

7.2 Role of ultrafine particles

The smallest particles in ambient air, ultrafine particles (UFP, diameter <100 nm), are an important component of combustion-related air pollution, with the potential to contribute to PM health effects, yet current air-pollution monitoring does not routinely measure their presence. UFP possess unique characteristics relevant to pulmonary and cardiovascular effects.[13] First, UFP induce pulmonary inflammation at lower mass concentrations than larger particles.[14, 15] Second, UFP at the same mass concentration in the air have a much higher number concentration and specific surface area than larger particles, which may facilitate delivery of reactive chemical species to the lung and pulmonary endothelium. Third, inhaled UFP have a very high predicted deposition efficiency (see below). Fourth, UFP have enhanced oxidant capacity when compared on a mass basis with larger particles.[16, 17] Fifth, UFP appear able to penetrate the epithelium and move beyond the lung.[18, 19] Although there are relatively few measurements of ambient UFP concentrations, epidemiological evidence links UFP exposure with health effects.[20]

7.2.1 Deposition within the respiratory tract

The factors that determine the dosimetry of inhaled PM in the respiratory tract are complex, and include particle concentration, duration of exposure, volume of air breathed (minute ventilation), sampling efficiency at the nose and mouth, and the fraction of inhaled particles that are deposited.[21] The regional deposition of particulate matter is highly dependent on particle size, and deposition predictions can be calculated based on physical models. Particles larger than 10 μm are mostly filtered out in the upper airway. Ultrafine or nanoparticles between 10 and 100 nm are predicted to have greater deposition efficiency in the tracheobronchial and alveolar regions of the lung, compared with larger particles.

The efficiency of deposition of UFP has been shown to vary with exercise, and with airways disease. Daigle et al. exposed 12 subjects to both 10 and 25 μg/m3 graphitic carbon UFP (mean count median diameter 26 nm, GSD 1.6) and determined the deposition fraction (DF) for both particle number and mass by analyzing the change in the respective particulate number concentrations and particle sizes in the inspired and expired air.[22] Since the particle sizes of the inspired and expired aerosols were measured in 8 particle size ranges that included more than 98 percent of the particles

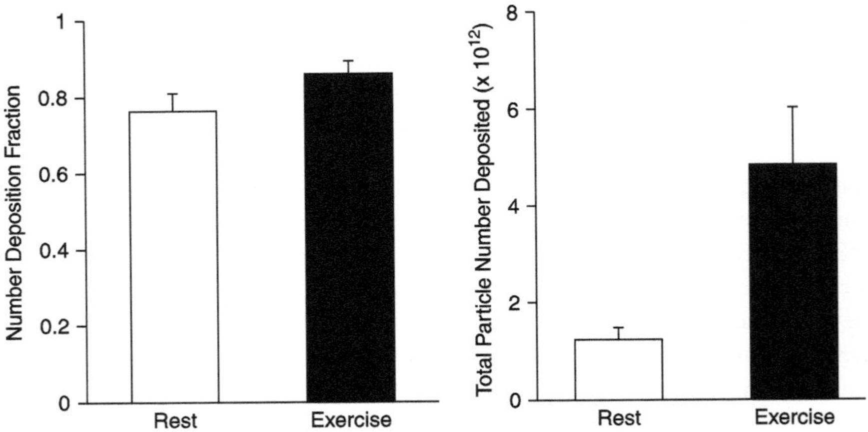

Figure 7.1 Particle number deposition fraction (DF; left panel) and total particle deposition over 1 hour of exposure (right panel) at rest and exercise in 16 subjects with asthma.

(namely from 8.7 to 64.9 nm), a particle size vs DF curve was constructed using the DF values, which ranged from 0.80 for 8.7 nm particles to 0.55 for 64.9 nm particles. The DFs were then compared to theoretical deposition curves for the same size range. The experimental data generally agreed with predicted data under conditions of rest, but DF was found to be significantly greater than predicted under conditions of exercise.[22]

A similar study was conducted in subjects with asthma, allowing a comparison between healthy and asthmatic subjects.[23] The total DFs for healthy subjects were 0.66 ± 0.11 at rest, and 0.83 ± 0.04 during exercise. Asthmatic subjects showed higher respective total DFs, viz., 0.76 ± 0.05 and 0.86 ± 0.04. Moreover, as shown in Figure 7.1, the combination of increased deposition and increased particle intake resulted in a marked increase in total particle deposition during exercise, compared with resting exposure, in subjects with asthma. Thus, with each breath, people with asthma experience increased deposition, and therefore dose, of ultrafine particles, compared with non-asthmatics.

7.3 Dendritic cells as key environmental sensors

After depositing in the airway or respiratory tract, PM will be sensed by the lung's innate immune system as foreign or "dangerous". In contrast to adaptive immune cells, which recognize an extremely broad repertoire of antigens due to genetic recombination of antigen receptor genes, innate immune cells respond to a more limited set of targets via a conserved set of pattern recognition receptors (PRR). Similarly, innate immune cells generally respond quickly to activating signals and have limited capacity for long-term memory. Signals that activate the innate immune system include those encoded by infectious pathogens or produced as a result of tissue injury or inflammation. Thus, one way ambient PM may be sensed as dangerous is by delivering microbial byproducts to the respiratory tract which act on PRRs including Toll-like receptors (TLR's) on target cells (3). In addition, PM-induced airway inflammation could elaborate endogenous danger signals (or "alarmins")[24] that indicate tissue injury and also activate innate immune cells.

Several innate immune cell types can initiate or modulate the immune responses to inhaled PM including dendritic cells, airway epithelial cells, and alveolar macrophages. Dendritic cells (DC) in particular are uniquely poised to respond to tissue injury or infection, and alert adaptive immune cells to dangerous inhaled particles or pathogens.[25] Three features of lung dendritic cells make them uniquely poised to be key environmental sensors. First is their anatomic location within the respiratory epithelium. Certain DC subsets may constitutively sample the airway lumen as part of an immunosurveillance system,[26] whereas other DC reside just below the surface epithelia and come in contact with external particles or antigens that either directly or indirectly disrupt the epithelial barrier. The second key feature of dendritic cells is their ability to respond to diverse environmental cues. This is due to their expression of an array of cell surface and intracellular pattern recognition receptors as well to their enormous capacity for endocytosis. The third key feature of dendritic cells is their ability to intimately interact with antigen specific T cells. This is due not only to migratory properties of these two cell types, which bring them in close contact in secondary lymphoid organs and in tissues, but also to the formation of the intimate DC:T cell synapse that allows a two-way exchange of information. Thus, DC provide a key link between exposures to inhaled PM, generation of inflammation, and development of adaptive immune responses.

7.4 Dangerous properties of PM

Inhaled PM will pose a challenge for the respiratory tract mucosal defense system. First, the delivery of a mix of organic and inorganic compounds coalesced onto a carbon core may overwhelm mucociliary clearance. Second, heavy metals and other compounds coalesced to PM can overwhelm endogenous anti-oxidant defense mechanisms and result in local generation of oxidative stress, which has the potential to disrupt airway epithelial barrier function and allow penetration of PM into subepithelial spaces. By this means, PM and its associated molecules will gain access to the rich network of DC just below the respiratory epithelium. Interestingly, PM exposed epithelial cells secrete the potent DC chemoattractant MIP-3α (or CCL20),[5] and conditioned media from DEP-exposed epithelial cells induce DC maturation.[27] Taken together, these observations suggest that PM can activate, recruit and mature DC within the airway microenvironment, and that DC will be among the first cells in the respiratory tract responding to inhaled ambient particles.

Several PM associated signals have the potential to activate respiratory tract DC. First, via Toll-like receptors activated either by microbial products coalesced to PM or by endogenous TLR ligands induced by PM-associated inflammation, inhaled PM could induce DC maturation similar to what occurs during infections.[28, 29] Although respiratory epithelial cells and other structural lung cells express TLRs, they are generally less responsive to microbial products compared to cells of the myeloid lineage: thus we speculate that respiratory tract DC will be the predominant sensors of TLR ligands associated with PM. After exposure to TLR ligands, DC undergo a complex maturation process involving simultaneous changes in endocytosis, antigen processing and presentation, and secretion of pro-inflammatory and immunoregulatory cytokines and chemokines. DC maturation also results in changes in chemokine receptor expression that facilitate homing to regional lymph nodes where they present peptide antigen in the context of MHC (signal 1) as well as co-stimulatory molecules (signal 2) to naïve T cells. By this means, inhaled PM can act as an adjuvant for inhaled antigens and initiate or influence the development of subsequent adaptive immune responses.

Second, PM-associated polyaromatic hydrocarbons (PAH) can activate the aryl-hydrocarbon receptor (AhR), a nuclear transcription factor expressed by DC and other lung cell types. In contrast to the well-established effects of TLR ligation on DC maturation, less is known about the effects of AhR signaling during DC maturation.[30] Interestingly, emerging evidence indicates that AhR ligands may be involved in promoting Th17-dependent immune responses, which are increasingly associated with allergic airway inflammation,[31] but whether this involves effects on DCs remains to be determined.

7.4.1 PM associated oxidants as danger signals

A third means by which PM may be sensed as dangerous by DC and other innate immune cells involves the induction of oxidative stress. Heavy metals and other molecules associated with PM can induce oxidative stress by overwhelming endogenous anti-oxidant defense mechanisms. Direct evidence that PM associated oxidative stress induces DC maturation and activation was provided by Williams et al., who showed that PM induced oxidative stress in DC, and that PM-dependent DC activation was attenuated by the anti-oxidant N-acetylcysteine (NAC).(32) PM-exposed DC demonstrated enhanced expression of co-stimulatory molecules, cytokines and greater ability to stimulate T cells, resulting in a Th2-like pattern of cytokine secretion. The effects of PM were markedly enhanced using DC derived from mice deficient in nuclear erythroid 2 p45-related factor 2 (Nrf2), a redox-sensitive transcription factor that regulates expression of antioxidant and detoxification genes.(32) Thus, this study demonstrated the importance of robust anti-oxidant defense mechanisms in protecting DC from adverse effects of PM. Studies in other models have demonstrated the importance of oxidative stress in DC maturation. For example, Verhasselt et al. showed that NAC suppressed lipopolysaccharide (LPS)-induced DC maturation,(33) and Kim and colleagues demonstrated that glutathione depletion interfered with DC IL-12 production in a delayed-type hypersensitivity model.(34) The precise mechanism by which an imbalance in oxidants and anti-oxidants regulates DC maturation remains to be determined, but this appears to involve activation of the transcription factor NF-κB.(33, 34)

7.5 Response to inhaled PM

Whether due to direct effects on respiratory tract DC or indirect effects due to local inflammation, inhaled PM including ultrafine particles are now clearly associated with adverse consequences both in epidemiologic association studies as well as in acute exposure models. The physical and chemical characteristics of UFP make them prime candidates for mediating cardiovascular as well as pulmonary effects of particulate air pollution. However, there are very few human inhalation studies of UFP, in part because these same properties make them difficult to study.

A series of studies examined the pulmonary and cardiovascular effects of inhaling laboratory-generated elemental carbon UFP for two hours, at concentrations which have been measured on busy highways (up to 50 μg/m^3 or ~107 particles/cm^3). There were no significant effects on symptoms, pulmonary function, airway inflammation, heart rate, heart rhythm, or heart rate variability.(35, 36) However, small but consistent dose-related decreases were observed in blood monocyte expression of adhesion

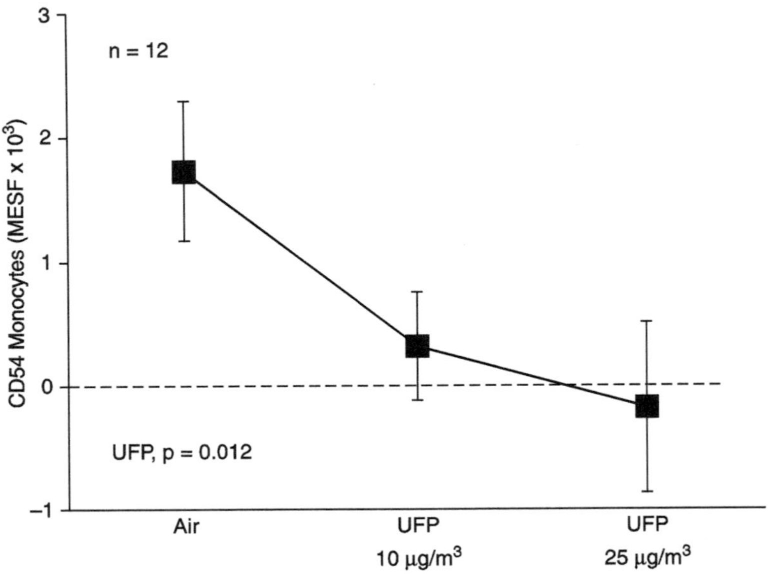

Figure 7.2 Change from pre-exposure in expression of CD54 (ICAM-1) on blood monocytes 3.5 h after exposure to air, 10, and 25 μg/m^3 carbon UFP. MESF: molecules of equivalent soluble fluorochrome.

molecules in the hours following exposure to UFP, occasionally accompanied by small reductions in numbers of monocytes, basophils, and eosinophils.[(37)] Figure 7.2 shows the change in blood monocyte expression of intercellular adhesion molecule-1 (ICAM-1, CD54) from healthy subjects following exposure to air and to two concentrations of UFP. ICAM-1 expression increased following air exposure, which is most likely the result of exercise shortening the transit time through lung capillaries of monocytes that express higher levels of ICAM-1. This exercise effect was blunted and even reversed following UFP exposure. This may reflect an effect of the exposure on pulmonary capillary blood flow or volume, causing the higher CD54-expressing monocytes to be retained longer in the lung.

To test this hypothesis, a subsequent study measured the pulmonary diffusing capacity for carbon monoxide (DLCO) 21 and 45 hours after two-hour exposures to air and 50 μg/m^3 UFP (36). The DLCO is influenced by changes in the pulmonary capillary blood volume. The DLCO decreased 21 hrs after UFP compared with air exposure (Figure 7.3). These findings support the hypothesis that exposure to carbon UFP alters pulmonary vascular hemodynamics, which could affect right and left heart function in people with cardiovascular disease.

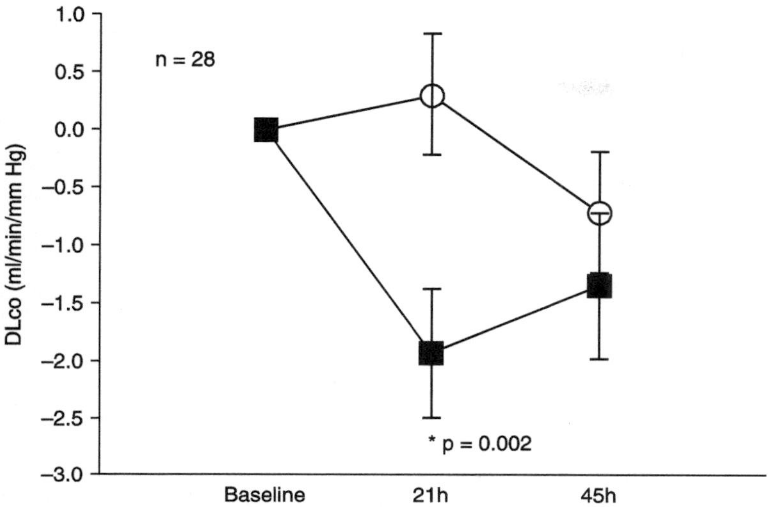

Figure 7.3 Change from pre-exposure in DLCO after exposure to air (circles) and to 50 μg/m³ carbon UFP (squares). From reference 36, with permission.

UFP may also alter systemic vascular function. Using similar exposure protocols, systemic vascular effects were determined by measuring venous occlusion plethysmography and reactive hyperemia (RH) of the forearm, before and up to 45 hours after exposure to 50 μg/m³ UFP. UFP exposure blunted the exercise-related increase in peak forearm blood flow 3.5 hours after exposure (Figure 7.4), and also reduced venous blood nitrite and nitrate levels, suggesting reduced NO production or increased consumption.[38] Impaired forearm RH is associated with endothelial dysfunction in the coronary circulation, and is predictive of cardiovascular disease.

Thus, in these studies, inhalation of carbon UFP, at realistic environmental concentrations, causes subtle alterations in both pulmonary and systemic vascular function, and reduced plasma NO products. These findings support the hypothesis that UFP deliver reactive oxygen species to vascular endothelium, reducing NO bioavailability, and altering vascular responsiveness. While these small changes in vascular responsiveness have no health consequences for healthy individuals, people with severe underlying vascular disease could become more susceptible to acute adverse events. The precise relationship between these systemic effects of inhaled PM and locally induced pulmonary inflammation remains to be determined. Future studies in which local pulmonary immune responses in response to inhaled PM are studied together with systemic side effects should be particularly insightful.

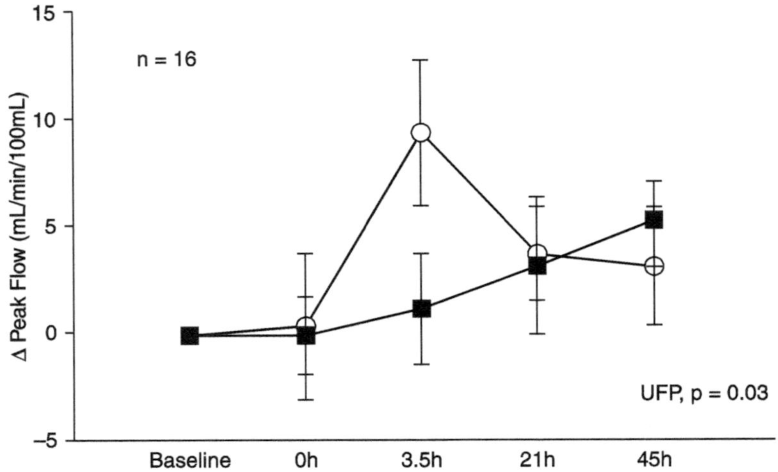

Figure 7.4 Change in peak forearm blood flow after exposure to air (circles) or UFP (squares). From reference 38, with permission.

7.6 Concluding remarks

The human respiratory tract evolved a complex and multifaceted response to inhaled pathogens over hundreds of millions of years. Key features of this response include the sensing of danger by mucosal innate immune cells, and the initiation of a program of pathogen clearance and development of protective adaptive immunity. This response has been subverted by inhaled PM including UFP, resulting in local and systemic inflammation that leads to the adverse health effects of PM. Future studies investigating the innate immune response to inhaled PM (e.g. activation of resident or recruited lung DC subsets), and cross-talk with other leukcoytes and structural cells, should enhance our understanding of the adverse health effects of PM. Understanding how polymorphisms in anti-oxidant (e.g. GSTM1) and other genes confer susceptibility to inhaled PM will facilitate the identification of vulnerable populations and may identify new biomarkers for use in clinical studies.

References

1 Trasande L, Thurston GD. The role of air pollution in asthma and other pediatric morbidities. *J Allergy Clin Immunol* 2005, 115: 689–99.

2 Riedl M, Diaz-Sanchez D. Biology of diesel exhaust effects on respiratory function. *J Allergy Clin Immunol* 2005, 115: 221–8; quiz 229.

3 Becker S, Dailey L, Soukup JM, Silbajoris R, Devlin RB. TLR-2 is involved in airway epithelial cell response to air pollution particles. *Toxicol Appl Pharmacol* 2005, 203: 45–52.

4 Becker S, Fenton MJ, Soukup JM. Involvement of microbial components and Toll-like receptors 2 and 4 in cytokine responses to air pollution particles. *Am J Respir Cell Mol Biol* 2002, 27: 611–8.

5 Reibman J, Hsu Y, Chen LC, Bleck B, Gordon T. Airway epithelial cells release MIP-3alpha/CCL20 in response to cytokines and ambient particulate matter. *Am J Respir Cell Mol Biol* 2003, 28: 648–54.

6 Reibman J, Hsu Y, Chen LC, Kumar A, Su WC, Choy W, et al. Size fractions of ambient particulate matter induce granulocyte macrophage colony-stimulating factor in human bronchial epithelial cells by mitogen-activated protein kinase pathways. *Am J Respir Cell Mol Biol* 2002, 27: 455–62.

7 Nikasinovic L, Just J, Sahraoui F, Seta N, Grimfeld A, Momas I. Nasal inflammation and personal exposure to fine particles PM2.5 in asthmatic children. *J Allergy Clin Immunol* 2006, 117: 1382–8.

8 Li N, Hao M, Phalen RF, Hinds WC, Nel AE. Particulate air pollutants and asthma. A paradigm for the role of oxidative stress in PM-induced adverse health effects. *Clin Immunol* 2003, 109: 250–65.

9 Tamer L, Ercan B, Camsari A, Yildirim H, Cicek D, Sucu N, et al. Glutathione S-transferase gene polymorphism as a susceptibility factor in smoking-related coronary artery disease. *Basic Res Cardiol* 2004, 99: 223–9.

10 Schwartz J, Park SK, O'Neill MS, Vokonas PS, Sparrow D, Weiss S, et al. Glutathione-S-transferase M1, obesity, statins, and autonomic effects of particles: gene-by-drug-by-environment interaction. *Am J Respir Crit Care Med* 2005, 172: 1529–33.

11 Romieu I, Sienra-Monge JJ, Ramirez-Aguilar M, Moreno-Macias H, Reyes-Ruiz NI, Estela del Rio-Navarro B, et al. Genetic polymorphism of GSTM1 and antioxidant supplementation influence lung function in relation to ozone exposure in asthmatic children in Mexico City. *Thorax* 2004, 59: 8–10.

12 Gilliland FD, Li YF, Saxon A, Diaz-Sanchez D. Effect of glutathione-S-transferase M1 and P1 genotypes on xenobiotic enhancement of allergic responses: randomised, placebo-controlled crossover study. *Lancet* 2004, 363: 119–25.

13 Utell MJ, Frampton MW. Acute health effects of ambient air pollution: the ultrafine particle hypothesis. *J Aerosol Med* 2000, 13: 355–59.

14 Oberdorster G, Gelein RM, Ferin J, Weiss B. Association of particulate air pollution and acute mortality: involvement of ultrafine particles? *Inhal Toxicol* 1995, 7: 111–24.

15 Li XY, Brown D, Smith S, MacNee W, Donaldson K. Short-term inflammatory responses following intratracheal instillation of fine and ultrafine carbon black in rats. *Inhal Toxicol* 1999, 11: 709–31.

16 Brown DM, Wilson MR, MacNee W, Stone V, Donaldson K. Size-dependent proinflammatory effects of ultrafine polystyrene particles: a role for surface area and oxidative stress in the enhanced activity of ultrafines. *Toxicol Appl Pharmacol* 2001, 175: 191–9.

17 Li N, Sioutas C, Cho A, Schmitz D, Misra C, Sempf J, et al. Ultrafine particulate pollutants induce oxidative stress and mitochondrial damage. *Environ Health Perspect* 2003, 111: 455–60.
18 Elder A, Oberdorster G. Translocation and effects of ultrafine particles outside of the lung. *Clin Occup Environ Med* 2006, 5: 785–96.
19 Muhlfeld C, Rothen-Rutishauser B, Blank F, Vanhecke D, Ochs M, Gehr P. Interactions of nanoparticles with pulmonary structures and cellular responses. *Am J Physiol Lung Cell Mol Physiol* 2008, 294: L817–29.
20 Wichmann HE, Spix C, Tuch T, Wolke G, Peters A, Heinrich J, et al. Daily mortality and fine and ultrafine particles in Erfurt, Germany part I: role of particle number and particle mass. *Res Rep Health Eff Inst* 2000: 5–86; discussion 87–94.
21 Phalen RF, Oldham MJ. Aerosol dosimetry considerations. *Clin Occup Environ Med* 2006, 5: 773–84.
22 Daigle CC, Chalupa DC, Gibb FR, Morrow PE, Oberdorster G, Utell MJ, et al. Ultrafine particle deposition in humans during rest and exercise. *Inhal Toxicol* 2003, 15: 539–52.
23 Frampton MW, Boscia J, Roberts NJ, Jr., Azadniv M, Torres A, Cox C, et al. Nitrogen dioxide exposure: effects on airway and blood cells. *Am J Physiol Lung Cell Mol Physiol* 2002, 282: L155–65.
24 Bianchi ME. DAMPs, PAMPs and alarmins: all we need to know about danger. *J Leukoc Biol* 2007, 81: 1–5.
25 Hammad H, Lambrecht BN. Dendritic cells and epithelial cells: linking innate and adaptive immunity in asthma. *Nat Rev Immunol* 2008, 8: 193–204.
26 Sung SS, Fu SM, Rose CE, Jr., Gaskin F, Ju ST, Beaty SR. A major lung CD103 (alphaE)-beta7 integrin-positive epithelial dendritic cell population expressing Langerin and tight junction proteins. *J Immunol* 2006, 176: 2161–72.
27 Bleck B, Tse DB, Jaspers I, Curotto de Lafaille MA, Reibman J. Diesel exhaust particle-exposed human bronchial epithelial cells induce dendritic cell maturation. *J Immunol* 2006, 176: 7431–7.
28 Kleeberger SR, Reddy S, Zhang LY, Jedlicka AE. Genetic susceptibility to ozone–induced lung hyperpermeability: role of Toll-like receptor 4. *Am J Respir Cell Mol Biol* 2000, 22: 620–7.
29 Hollingsworth JW, 2nd, Cook DN, Brass DM, Walker JK, Morgan DL, Foster WM, et al. The role of Toll-like receptor 4 in environmental airway injury in mice. *Am J Respir Crit Care Med* 2004, 170: 126–32.
30 Hauben E, Gregori S, Draghici E, Migliavacca B, Olivieri S, Woisetschlager M, et al. Activation of the aryl hydrocarbon receptor promotes allograft-specific tolerance through direct and dendritic cell-mediated effects on regulatory T cells. *Blood* 2008, 112: 1214–22.
31 Veldhoen M, Hirota K, Christensen J, O'Garra A, Stockinger B. Natural agonists for aryl hydrocarbon receptor in culture medium are essential for optimal differentiation of Th17 T cells. *J Exp Med* 2009, 206: 43–9.
32 Williams MA, Rangasamy T, Bauer SM, Killedar S, Karp M, Kensler TW, et al. Disruption of the transcription factor Nrf2 promotes pro-oxidative dendritic cells that stimulate Th2-like immunoresponsiveness upon activation by ambient particulate matter. *J Immunol* 2008, 181: 4545–59.

33 Verhasselt V, Vanden Berghe W, Vanderheyde N, Willems F, Haegeman G, Goldman M. N-acetyl-L-cysteine inhibits primary human T cell responses at the dendritic cell level: association with NF-kappaB inhibition. *J Immunol* 1999, 162: 2569–74.
34 Kim HJ, Barajas B, Chan RC, Nel AE. Glutathione depletion inhibits dendritic cell maturation and delayed-type hypersensitivity: implications for systemic disease and immunosenescence. *J Allergy Clin Immunol* 2007, 119: 1225–33.
35 Frampton MW. Systemic and cardiovascular effects of airway injury and inflammation: ultrafine particle exposure in humans. *Environ Health Perspect* 2001, 109 Suppl 4: 529–32.
36 Pietropaoli AP, Frampton MW, Hyde RW, Morrow PE, Oberdorster G, Cox C, et al. Pulmonary function, diffusing capacity, and inflammation in healthy and asthmatic subjects exposed to ultrafine particles. *Inhal Toxicol* 2004, 16 Suppl 1: 59–72.
37 Frampton MW, Stewart JC, Oberdorster G, Morrow PE, Chalupa D, Pietropaoli AP, et al. Inhalation of ultrafine particles alters blood leukocyte expression of adhesion molecules in humans. *Environ Health Perspect* 2006, 114: 51–8.
38 Shah AP, Pietropaoli AP, Frasier LM, Speers DM, Chalupa DC, Delehanty JM, et al. Effect of inhaled carbon ultrafine particles on reactive hyperemia in healthy human subjects. *Environ Health Perspect* 2008, 116: 375–80.

8

Diesel exhaust particles and the airway epithelial cell–dendritic cell interface in the control of immune homeostasis

Joan Reibman, Bertram Bleck, Doris Tse and Maria Curotto de Lafaille

Abstract. Traffic related air pollution is associated with sensitization to inhaled allergens. Airway epithelial cells are the first targets of airborne pollutants and synthesize and release chemokines and cytokines implicated in local immune responses. Dendritic cells (DC) are abundant in the subepithelial mucosa and rapidly traffic to regional lymph nodes. DC regulate the multiplicity of T cell effector responses that result in the initiation and maintenance of airway inflammation. DC also regulate the less well understood regulatory T cell responses, including the generation of "adaptive" or peripheral T regulatory cells, that result in tolerance to antigens. This chapter will focus on the epithelial cell–dendritic cell interface in the control of effector and regulatory T cell homeostasis of the airway and the disruption of homeostasis by ambient pollutants. The ability of ambient pollutants, specifically diesel exhaust particles (DEP), to modify epithelial cell-derived signals, including CCL20, granulocyte macrophage-colony stimulating factor (CSF2), and thymic stromal lymphopoeitin (TSLP) for recruitment of DC subsets, DC maturation and DC polarization are described.

Keywords: allergic sensitization, allergic inflammation, allergic asthma, immune homeostasis, dendritic cells, T helper cells, airway epithelial cells, ambient pollutants, diesel exhaust particulate matter, oxidative stress, reactive oxygen species, regulatory T cells (Tregs), pattern recognition receptors, cellular trafficking and migration, chemokines, thymic stromal lymphopoietin (TSLP)

8.1 Introduction

Air pollution is linked to an increase in allergic conditions, particularly allergic asthma.[1] Traffic-related air pollution is associated with sensitization to inhaled allergens, as well as wheezing.[2–5] *In vitro* models, animal models, and human observational studies of ambient particulate matter (PM) or diesel exhaust particles (DEP) demonstrate increases in total and specific IgE, induction of Th2 cytokines, as well as airway eosinophilic inflammation and airway hyperresponsiveness.[6] Nasal challenge with DEP in humans results in increased IgE isotype switching and an increase in IgE response to a neoallergen.[7–11] Airway immune homeostasis requires a balance between effector and regulatory T cell responses. Effector and regulatory T cell responses are determined by DC signals, which are in turn governed by the surrounding milieu. Current knowledge about T cell balance and the mechanisms by which traffic-related pollution and DEP alter airway immune responses will be described in this chapter with a focus on epithelial cell–dendritic cell interactions. Data suggesting that ambient PM and DEP upregulate epithelial cell-derived signals for recruitment of dendritic cells (DC), DC maturation and DC polarization will be presented.

8.2 Traffic-related pollution

Ambient PM in urban environments is predominantly derived from mobile sources and almost 90 percent of traffic-generated PM is from diesel exhaust.[12] Compared to gasoline engines, diesel engines emit relatively low concentrations of carbon monoxide and carbon dioxide. However, they can generate more than 100 times the number of particles per distance traveled.[12, 13] Diesel exhaust particles contain a carbon core, which is coated by polyaromatic hydrocarbons, quinones and metals.[6, 14, 15] Diesel exhaust is enriched in ultrafine particles (<0.1 μm in diameter), which are associated with inflammatory responses *in vivo* and *in vitro*.[16–19] The organic and particulate components of DEP differ in their ability to upregulate various inflammatory responses and intact as well as organic extracts of DEP induce oxidative stress with an increase in reactive oxygen species (ROS) in macrophages, epithelial cells and lung microsomes.[6, 20–23] The ability of fine and ultrafine particles to induce ROS is correlated to their polyaromatic hydrocarbon content and volatile organic compounds induce IgE production and T cell polarization.[16, 24, 25] Various DEP may differ in toxicity and immunologic activity depending on the source.[26] The studies described in this chapter use DEP derived from older diesel engines as model particles. Few studies are available on the newer, low-emission diesel engines, although a recent study using human peripheral blood monocyte-derived macrophages suggests that particles from a low-emission DEP (Euro IV diesel engine) are more cytotoxic and inflammatory than those derived from an older European diesel engine.[27] The increase in inflammatory potential of DEP derived from low-emission engines may be due to the irregular surface structure of the DEP, which results in an abundance of chemically reactive structural elements.[27] Ambient PM collected from urban sources consists of a mixture of PM derived from mobile as well as stationary sources and has varied chemical composition depending on the source.

8.3 T cell balance in asthma

Allergic asthma is characterized by elevated levels of allergen-specific IgE antibodies and both allergic and non-allergic asthma are associated with T helper cells that secrete interleukin-4 (IL)-4, IL-5, IL-13 and tumor necrosis factor (TNF-α), a pattern characteristic of T helper 2 (Th2) cells. These cytokines induce recruitment and survival of eosinophils and mast cells with associated goblet-cell hyperplasia and bronchial hyperresponsiveness, the hallmarks of asthma.[28, 29] However, these antigen-specific effector Th2 cells can be suppressed by antigen-specific regulatory T cells (Treg), which induce peripheral tolerance.[30–32] Thus airway homeostasis involves a balance between effector T helper cells and their suppression by regulatory cells. Ambient PM and DEP may disrupt airway homeostasis by promoting recruitment and activation of T helper effector cells. Additionally, ambient PM and DEP may alter the development or persistence of Treg cells and airway tolerance.

To date, most studies, including ours, have focused on the ability of ambient PM and DEP to promote effector T cell functions. As we begin to understand mucosal tolerance, future studies will need to investigate whether ambient PM and DEP also modify the development and persistence of T cell tolerance. The importance of Treg cells in IgE regulation in asthma and allergy has been shown in animal models[31–33] and in human observations, in which an imbalance between Th2 and allergen-specific Treg cells has been described.[34–36] Tolerance can be induced by prolonged inhalation of a specific allergen in the lung.[37–39] Naturally occurring $CD4^+$ Treg cells express IL-2 receptor alpha-chain (CD25), and the transcription factor Foxp3 ($CD4^+$ $CD25^+$ $Foxp3^+$). These cells develop in the thymus and migrate to peripheral lymphoid organs.[40–43] However, $Foxp3^+$ Treg cells that are phenotypically indistinguishable from naturally occurring Treg cells can also be converted from naïve T cells in the periphery under select conditions.[33, 44–46] These cells are called "adaptive" or peripheral Treg cells and may play a critical role in mucosal tolerance. We have studied T-cell differentiation during induction of mucosal tolerance and took advantage of a mouse strain (referred to as T-B monoclonal, or T-Bmc) that has a simplified immune system. T-Bmc mice harbor only non-self reactive monoclonal T and B lymphocytes specific for chicken ovalbumin (OVA) and influenza hemmagglutinin (HA) respectively. Importantly, T-Bmc mice lack naturally-occurring Foxp3$^+$ Treg cells. T-Bmc mice can become sensitized to OVA by immunization and develop a Th2 response, IgE antibodies and allergic inflammation. However, we found that despite the absence of naturally occurring Treg cells, T-Bmc mice develop tolerance to OVA if they are administered OVA by the respiratory or oral routes prior to immunization with antigen in adjuvant. Importantly, tolerance in T-Bmc mice is associated with the differentiation of "adaptive" OVA-specific Foxp3$^+$ Treg cells, i.e. mucosa-induced and immunization-induced Foxp3$^+$ Treg cells.[46, 47] As shown in Figure 8.1, this observation was confirmed in wild type BALB/c mice with the use of chimeric T-Bmc-BALB/c mice that consist of BALB/c mice that received bone marrow cells from naïve T-Bmc mice. These mice were fed OVA in drinking water and subsequently developed Foxp3$^+$CD25$^+$ CD4$^+$ T cells in the mesenteric lymph nodes. The donor origin of these cells was identified by the presence of the anti-DO11.10TCR antibody KJ1-26.[47] These studies demonstrate a role for "adaptive" T reg cells in airway tolerance and tolerance in the absence of naturally occurring Treg cells. To obtain unambiguous information on the role of "adaptive" Treg cells in tolerance and inflammation, we introduced a genetic Foxp3 deficiency (the *scurfy* mutation) into the T-Bmc mice (T-Bmc Foxp3^{sf}). T-Bmc Foxp3^{sf} mice lack both naturally occurring Treg cells (thymus-derived) and the ability to generate "adaptive" Foxp3$^+$ Treg cells. T-Bmc Foxp3^{sf} mice were unable to develop respiratory or oral tolerance to OVA (Figure 8.2). Thus, we concluded that the induction of "adaptive" antigen-specific Foxp3$^+$ Treg cells was essential for mucosal tolerance.

Paradoxically, large numbers of Foxp3$^+$ Treg cells are found at sites of ongoing inflammation.[47–50] This highlights the complexity of Treg cells and raises the question of the role of Treg cells in chronic inflammation as well as in initial sensitization. Several explanations can be proposed, including the possibility that there might be different roles for naturally occurring and "adaptive" Treg cells, that these T cells cannot carry out their function, or that Treg cells are overwhelmed, neutralized, or even pathologic (47). Intriguingly, in our studies, we found that Foxp3$^+$ T cells also developed alongside

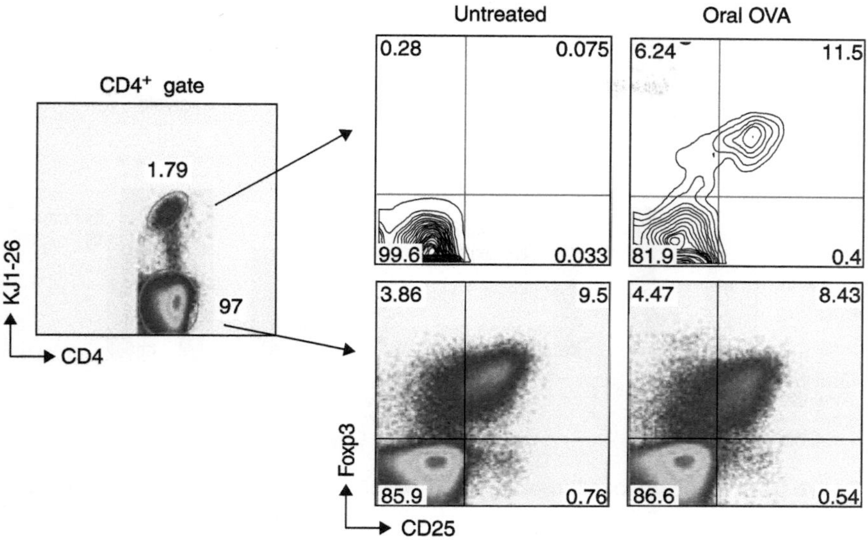

Figure 8.1 Development of "adaptive" Foxp3+ OVA-specific E cells in BALB/c mice. BALB/c mice were "seeded" with a low number of naïve TCR transgenic OVA-specific T cells generated by bone marrow reconstitution. BALB/c mice were irradiated (low dose, 150 rads) and bone marrow cells from naïve T-Bmc mice were transferred. After two months, T-Bmc-BALB/c bone marrow chimeras were fed OVA in drinking water (1%, five days). Mice were sacrificed after 2 weeks and mesenteric LN expression of Foxp3 and CD25 determined in CD4+ cells. CD4+ cells of donor origin were identified with KJ1-26 antibody. Representative dot plots are shown. (Adapted from reference (47).)

Th2 cells after immunization of naïve mice with antigen in adjuvant. However, these cells were unable to prevent sensitization. We speculated that pre-existing antigen-specific Foxp3+ Treg cells were responsible for the complete protection from sensitization in tolerant mice, whereas Foxp3+ Treg cells induced after immunization could play a role in modifying chronic disease. The role of immunization-induced Foxp3+ Treg cells became clear from our study of T-Bmc mice carrying wild type or *scurfy* Foxp3 genes that were immunized and chronically exposed to inhaled antigen.[47] In T-Bmc Foxp3^{wt} mice, Treg cells accumulated in the lungs and over a period of time suppressed Th2 cell-mediated inflammation, lung remodeling and the formation of tertiary lymphoid aggregates in the lungs. In contrast, T-Bmc Foxp3^{sf} mice developed severe inflammation and smooth muscle remodeling, induced lymphoid structures with germinal centers in the lung, and disseminated Th2 inflammation. Thus, "adaptive" allergen-specific Foxp3+ Treg cells can have beneficial effects even after the onset of allergic inflammation.

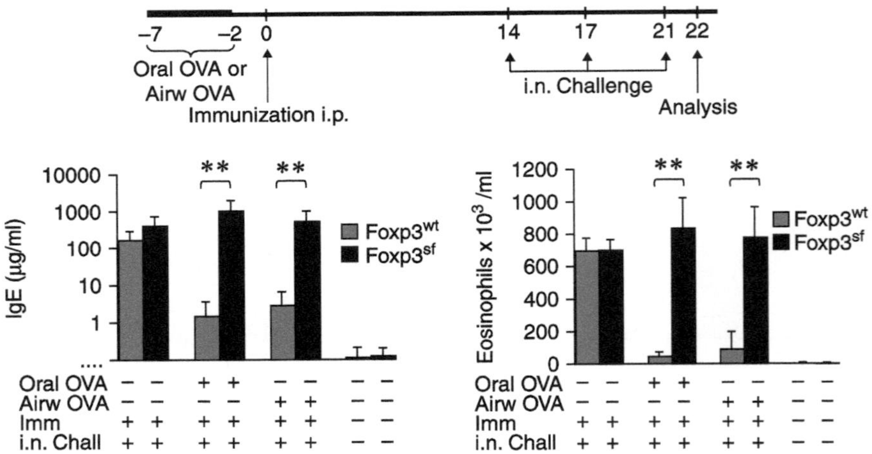

Figure 8.2 Induction of allergen-specific Foxp3+ Tregs is essential for respiratory and oral tolerance. T-Bmc mice carrying wild type (Foxp3wt) or deficient (*scurfy*) Foxp3 genes (Foxp3sf) were treated with OVA by intranasal (airw) or oral routes before being immunization (i.p.) with OVA in alum. Mice were subsequently challenged with OVA by the intranasal (i.n.) route (A). Pretreatment with OVA through mucosal routes prevented development of Th2 mediated IgE production (B) and eosinophilic lung inflammation (C) in Foxp3wt mice. In contrast, Foxp3sf T-Bmc mice were unable to form allergen-specific Tregs in response to mucosal antigen and became sensitized to OVA, as evidenced by their high IgE production and eosinophilic inflammation (B and C). (Adapted from reference (47).)

Additional reports support an essential role of Foxp3+ Treg cells derived from naïve Foxp3+ T cells for establishing tolerance in the respiratory mucosa.[47] In animal models, expansion of antigen-specific tolerance can be induced by transforming growth factor (TGF)-β and recent studies suggest that activated CD4+ Foxp3+ Treg cells that express TGF-β complexed to the latency-associated peptide (LAP) on their surface can generate *de novo* CD4+ Foxp3+ Treg cells in a cell-contact-dependent manner.[51] Tolerance has also been shown to extend to bystander antigens, suggesting a non antigen-specific component in the development of tolerance as well.[52]

These studies suggest that local regulation of T cell balance between effector T cells and "adaptive" regulatory T cells is critical for the development and chronicity of allergic diseases such as asthma. Moreover, it is likely that local DC regulate the T cell balance between these local effector T cells and "adaptive" Treg cells and that events that modify local or airway DC function will determine their ability to regulate T effector and

Treg cell function. Future studies are clearly needed to understand whether ambient PM or DEP regulate the balance of effector T cells and these "adaptive" peripheral regulatory T cells.

8.4 DC overview and subtypes

The immune response to a given antigen results from engagement of naïve T lymphocytes by an antigen-presenting cell (APC) in the context of T cell receptor and peptide-MHC (major histocompatibility) complex.[53] DC are heterogeneous and the subtype of DC as well as its activation state can determine the resulting Th1, Th2, Th17, Tf, Tr1 or Treg response.[54–56] DC can be of myeloid or lymphoid origin, although the origin does not determine the DC subtype. Human and mouse DC subtypes are defined on the basis of surface antigens, many of which are associated with pattern recognition and antigen presentation.

These subtypes respond differently to microbial products, produce different cytokines, and differ in their T cell response. DC subtypes have been described as follows:[54]

Pre-dendritic cells
plasmacytoid DC (pDC)
myeloid-derived DC (mDC)
Conventional DC (cDC)
Migratory DC
Lymphoid-tissue resident DC
Inflammatory DC

8.4.1 Pre-dendritic cells

Pre-DC include myeloid-derived DC, and in the presence of granulocyte-macrophage colony stimulating factor (GM-CSF; CSF2) both mouse and human pre-DC differentiate into $CD11c^+$ $MHCII^+$ DC, conventional migratory DC.[54, 55] Plasmacytoid DC (pDC) are pre-DC, which are found in the steady state in many tissues including blood, thymus, and lymphoid organs. In response to viruses, bacteria and certain toll-like receptor (TLR) agonists (TLR7, TLR8, TLR9), pDC show a characteristic type I interferon (IFN) response. In addition, pDC have specialized endosomal compartments for cross-presentation on MHC I. Migratory DC sample antigen in peripheral tissue and in the steady state, migrate to lymph nodes (LN) and undergo maturation where T cell presentation occurs; both migration and maturation is increased with a danger signal. Classic examples include Langerhans cells and dermal DC. Lymphoid-tissue resident DC are restricted to one lymphoid organ and collect and present foreign and self-antigens in the lymphoid organ. In the mouse, they include specialized subsets ($CD4^+CD8^-$, $CD4^-CD8^-$, $CD4^-CD8^+$). Inflammatory DC result from infection or inflammation and include pDC that have been exposed to viral or microbial stimuli and gained the capacity to produce TNF-α and inducible nitric-oxide synthase (iNOS).[(54)] Monocyte-derived DC (MDDC) are mDC generated by exposure of monocytes to granulocyte-macrophage colony stimulating factor (GM-CSF, CSF2) and IL-4 and used for *in vitro* studies of DC.[(56)] These cells are plastic and may represent inflammatory DC.

Signals derived from DC and their interactions with naïve T cells determine T cell fate as polarized effector T cells or Treg cells. Different DC populations can preferentially induce differentiation of naïve T cells into Th1, Th2, Th17, Tf, Tr1 or Treg cells.[(57)] The functional potential of DC is derived from the ontogeny of the DC as well as from additional factors that include microbial ligands for pattern recognition receptors, or environmental and endogenous stimuli.[(56)] In the presence of a microbial or tissue-derived signal, subtypes can mature and support multiple phenotypes.[(54, 57)] This flexibility is illustrated in studies in which mDC can be polarized as either Th1 or Th2 promoting cells depending on the microbial stimulus and the receptors that are activated.[(58)] Moreover, tissue derived factors from neighboring cells may induce, amplify or fine-tune a pathogen, particle, or allergen induced response and thus accelerate the maturation and polarization process. For example, adjuvant-derived signals administered with an innocuous antigen can regulate DC-T cell instruction.[(59, 60)] In addition, the presence of soluble factors such as PGE_2 or IL-10 during DC maturation results in DC that support Th2 polarization or Treg cell formation, whereas the presence of type I or II IFN results in DC that support Th-1 polarization.[(61–63)] One mechanism by which microbial and environmental stimuli effect myeloid DC-driven T cell polarization is by the induction of different Notch ligands on DC (64). Expression of Jagged on mDC is associated with the induction of Th2 differentiation, whereas Delta expression promotes Th1 differentiation.[(64, 65)] These data suggest that there is plasticity within the DC subtype and that during maturation these external signals regulate DC polarization. These signals can be derived from direct stimuli, or from the DC microenvironment.[(54, 66)]

8.5 DC in the lung

DC, abundant in animal and human lungs, are heterogeneous.[67–71] DC subsets in human lung digests include BDCA-1$^+$ and BDCA-3$^+$ mDC. These mDC are more abundant than pDC, and have been found throughout different anatomical locations in the lung.[72, 73] The different TLR expression on mDC and pDC in part regulates their different responses. Myeloid DC release TNF-α, IL1-β, IL-6 and IL-8 in response to specific TLR stimulation and induce robust T cell proliferation. In contrast, pDC express different TLR, release IFN-α in response to CpG oligonucleotides, but do not induce T cell proliferation.[74] The importance of lung DC in the induction and persistence of inflammation in asthma has been recognized in numerous studies using murine models.[75–84] However, some DC in the lung have opposing effects and reduce allergen induced airway hyperreactivity. Respiratory exposure to allergen, in contrast to intraperitoneal exposure, induces T cell tolerance and protection against the development of airway hyperreactivity.[85] Elegant studies in mice have shown that this process is mediated by the DC-dependent induction of Treg cells.[39, 86] In mice, pDC stimulate the induction of Treg cells[87, 88] and a subtype of pDC has been associated with the protection from antigen-induced asthma.[87] Most recently, adoptive transfer of a myeloid-derived regulatory DC has been shown to abolish antigen-specific IgE production and Th2 inflammation.[89] The abundance of DC in the lung and airway, and the presence of multiple subtypes and maturation states that can both promote inflammation and promote tolerance, suggest that regulation of DC recruitment and local activation state are important for expression of diseases such as asthma. We have proposed that ambient PM or DEP exert immunomodulatory effects by influencing DC trafficking and activation. Furthermore, since tissue-derived signals exert regulatory roles, and since airway epithelial cells are the first target for ambient pollutants, we have proposed that effects of PM or DEP are exerted via altering the DC microenvironment through epithelial cell-derived signals.

8.5.1 DC trafficking in the lung

DC are abundant in the nasal mucosa of the upper airway and in the conducting airways, where they exist as a meshwork in close proximity to airway epithelial cells.[90–97] These DC comprise both mDC and pDC although mDC predominate.[97] DC rapidly traffic through the airway ($t_{1/2} \leq 2$ days) and sample for antigen even in the absence of inflammation.[98, 99] Accumulation of airway DC, most likely derived from peripheral blood, is increased in animal models and humans after inhalation of a large variety of agents including infectious agents (bacteria, virus) and antigens.[97–103] After allergen inhalation in humans, there is a reduction in circulating mDC, but not pDC, suggesting that mDC are preferentially recruited to the airway.[104, 105] In contrast, recruitment of pDC may prevent reactions to harmless antigen.[87] The possibility therefore exists that ambient PM or DEP can exert airway effects via altering trafficking of DC subsets and that these effects are mediated by airway epithelial cells.

The chemokines and their cognate receptors that control DC trafficking to tissues such as the lung and airway differ in resting and inflamed states, and may control both numbers and composition of DC subtypes.[106] Trafficking of DC to the mucosa and subsequently to T cell areas is associated with the coordinated expression of specific chemokines and specific chemokine receptors on DC. Some immature mDC express CCR6, and respond to the CC chemokine MIP-3α/CCL20.[107, 108] Immature mDC or conventional DC also express CCR2, 1 and 5 and respond to MCP-1/CCL2, MCP-3/CCL7, MCP-4/CCL13, as well as MIP-1α/CCL3 and MIP-1β/CCL4 (109–111). Immature pDC express CCR2, 4, 5, 7 as well as CXCR3 and CXCR4 and respond to Mig/CXCL9, IP-10/CXCL10, I-TAC/CXCL11, as well as to SDF-1/CXCL12. Upon maturation, immature DC upregulate CCR7 and gain the ability to respond to MIP-3β/CCL19, SLC/CCL21 and migrate to lymphoid regions.[110]

The recruitment of DC precursors from the blood into inflamed peripheral tissues is regulated by multiple chemokines and both CCR2 and CCR6 and their respective ligands have been implicated in asthma models. CCR2 is important for recruitment of DC precursors into inflamed tissues.[112] CCR2 knockout mice exhibit defective DC activation[113] and the importance of CCR2 has been refined in studies of mice with both wild-type and knockout cells for select chemokine receptors. In these studies CCR2, but not CCR5 or CCR6, controlled DC recruitment into the lung after allergic airway inflammation.[114] However, CCR6 and its cognate ligand CCL20 is also associated with airway disease. Human lung DC express CCR6 and mRNA for CCL20 is expressed predominantly in inflamed mucosal tissues.[115] Human studies reveal an increase in epithelial associated DC, expression of CCR6 and an increase in CCL20 in airways of individuals with COPD, suggesting a role for CCR6 and its ligands in DC recruitment in this disease.[116] CCL20 is also upregulated in bronchoalveolar lavage fluid of asthmatics following endobronchial allergen provocation.[117] In an animal model of cockroach sensitization, antigen challenge induces CCL20 expression in the lung and CCR6 deficient mice have a reduced allergic pulmonary response.[118] Lung DC recruitment is attenuated in CCR6 knockout mice exposed to tobacco smoke.[119] A sequential role for CCR2 and CCR6 for recruitment of circulating DC to inflamed mucosal surfaces has been suggested.[120] Both CCR2 and CCR6 regulate immature mDC recruitment from the bloodstream in particulate antigen challenged mice.[121] These studies suggest that both CCR2 and CCR6 may play important, if different, roles in airway inflammation.

8.6 Ambient PM and DEP and DC trafficking

Ambient PM or DEP may exert effects on DC trafficking to lung tissue by altering epithelial cell expression of ligands for CCR2 or CCR6. We have demonstrated that primary culture human bronchial epithelial cells (HBEC) upregulate CCL20 mRNA and protein in response to pro-inflammatory cytokines (TNF-α and IL-1β) and Th2-type cytokines (IL-4 and IL-13).[122] We also demonstrated that size fractions of ambient PM upregulate CCL20 (122). Activation of mitogen activated protein kinase (MAPK) pathways ($MAPK^{erk1/2}$ and p38) was associated with and required for upregulation of CCL20. These studies were the first to show that human airway epithelial cells are a source of CCL20 in response to a broad spectrum of cytokines and ambient PM. The ability of alveolar epithelial cells to regulate DC trafficking via CCL20 has subsequently been demonstrated.[123] We have recently shown that physiologically relevant concentrations of DEP (1–10 $\mu g/cm^2$) upregulated both CCL20 and CCL2 release by human bronchial epithelial cells.[124] Moreover, exposure of immature mDC to DEP-treated bronchial epithelial cells in an *in vitro* system induced DC migration towards the epithelial cell layer. DC migration was reduced in the presence of anti-CCL20 or anti-CCL2.[124]

These data suggested that epithelial cell derived chemokines induced by DEP have potential to effect DC migration in the airway and that ambient PM or DEP can exert influences on local immune reactions in the airway, in part by enhancing the recruitment of DC in to the tissue. The question remains whether there is selective recruitment of different subsets by ambient PM or DEP-exposed airway epithelium and whether recruitment induced by ambient PM or DEP-exposed airway epithelial cells is associated with DC maturation and polarization. Finally, the question remains whether these findings can be corroborated in animal models of diesel or PM exposure.

8.7 DEP and bronchial epithelial cell induced DC maturation

The increased recruitment of DC to the airway in response to ambient PM or DEP-exposed airway epithelium suggests that these DC would be available to sample particles in the airway lumen and to respond to additional signals derived from a stimulated airway. Elegant studies of the gut show that DC penetrate gut epithelial monolayers and sample bacteria via their expression of tight junction proteins, which allows them to extend processes between epithelial cells without destroying the integrity of the monolayer.[125] Additional intravital two-photon imaging of the intestine shows that DC create trans-epithelial extensions constitutively. The extensions, however, increase in the presence of invasive or non-invasive bacteria and the increase is dependent on TLR signaling derived from the surrounding epithelium.[126] In the lung as well as in the gut, DC extend through the airway and constitutively sample lumen contents.[70] Studies in the rat lung have shown that a subset of airway mucosal DC constitutively extend processes through the airway lumen.[103]

In the murine lung, a CD103 (a_E)- b_7-integrin expressing DC population also express the tight junction proteins Claudin-1, Claudin-7, and ZO-2, suggesting that at least subtypes of airway DC have potential to traverse the lung epithelium in a manner analogous to that described for the gut.[127] These studies therefore suggest that airway mucosal DC would have the potential to directly sample inhaled particulate matter or DEP and that signals derived from this exposure might induce DC activation or maturation. This activation could potentially be induced via engagement of TLR, since TLR that recognize microbial molecules are widely expressed on DC[57] and TLR, including TLR-2 and -4 participate in DEP-and particle-induced induced inflammation in mice.[128–130]

Thus the possibility exists that DEP exert direct effects on DC maturation. Data supporting this process are described more fully in other chapters of this book; however, studies vary. Exposure to DEP has been shown to induce DC maturation of human monocyte-derived DC, but only in the presence of an adjuvant signal provided by lipopolysaccharide in some studies.[131] In others, urban ambient PM-treated human myeloid DC stimulated a Th2-type pattern of cytokine production in alloreactive naïve CD4+ T cells.[132, 133] These studies suggest a complexity in the response to DEP or ambient PM that may be due to differences in chemical components of the different particles as well as differences in the model.

We first tested whether DEP directly induced monocyte-derived DC maturation and used DEP derived from a 1.6-liter Volkswagen diesel engine

(40 kW).[134] Monocyte-derived DC (MDDC) were generated from human peripheral blood monocytes after treatment with CSF2 and low concentrations of IL-4 and were directly exposed to DEP (0.001–100 μg/ml, 48h). We failed to identify phenotypic DC maturation (CD80, CD83, CD86) or functional DC maturation measured by T cell proliferation in a mixed lymphocyte reaction (MLR) with alloreactive naïve CD4+ T cells.[134] These data suggested to us that local environment or tissue-derived signals might be needed for DEP-induced effects on DC. We therefore proposed that DEP act as an adjuvant and upregulate tissue-derived factors that modify DC maturation and polarization. Since the epithelium is the first target for DEP and ambient PM and is so closely and abundantly associated with DC, we proposed that epithelial cell derived factors from DEP-stimulated cells accelerated maturation and DC polarization.

To study epithelial cell-DC interactions, we used a co-culture system of MDDC and human airway epithelial cells (primary culture human bronchial epithelial cells, HBEC or 16HBE14o^{-} cells) to provide an *in vitro* model of the airway. We used flow cytometry to discriminate DC from epithelial cells using the expression of CD11c and CK18/19 and to examine the expression of maturation markers of DC. Using this system, we demonstrated that DEP-treated airway epithelial cells, but not resting airway epithelial cells, induced phenotypic maturation of DC.[134] To confirm that phenotypic maturation was functionally important, we also showed that DEP-treated bronchial epithelial cells induced functional DC maturation as measured by the ability of the flow-sorted DC to support T cell proliferation.[134]

To examine whether the effect of DEP-treated airway epithelial cells on DC maturation was due to direct cell contact or due to soluble mediators, we examined the effect of culture supernatants on DC function. Monoctye-derived DC exposed to supernatants derived from DEP-treated human bronchial epithelial cells but not from resting cells supported DC-dependent T cell proliferation.[134] These data suggested that DEP exert immumodulatory influences on DC-T cell function indirectly via activation of airway epithelial cells. Our subsequent studies clarify some of the mediators associated with this response.

8.8 Granulocyte-macrophage colony-stimulating factor (GM-CSF)

GM-CSF maintains the viability and functional maturation of DC.[53, 135, 136] The importance of bronchial epithelial cell-derived GM-CSF was first recognized for its ability to promote eosinophil activation and survival in asthma.[137] Subsequent studies using airway epithelial cell-restricted transgenic expression of GM-CSF show a critical role for the induction of sensitization to aerosolized OVA and also show that this sensitization is associated with an increase in mature DC in the airway.[138–142] A role for GM-CSF in diesel induced airway responses has been suggested with the use of murine models in which DEP induce airway hyperresponsiveness and the response is reduced in the presence of an antibody directed against GM-CSF.[143] Installation of DEP and antigen into murine airways upregulates GM-CSF as well as Th2-associated cytokines.[144]

DEP upregulate GM-CSF in a variety of airway epithelial cell models.[145–147] We have shown that New York City ambient PM, particularly the smallest particles, upregulate GM-CSF from primary and transformed human bronchial epithelial cells.[148] We and others have shown that DEP and ambient PM upregulation of epithelial cell GM-CSF is associated with phagocytosis of particles, and is induced by ROS and mitogen activated protein kinase pathways.[147–149] Recent studies demonstrate that ROS activate the NALP3 (Nacht Domain-, Leucine-Rich Repeat-, and PYD-Containing Protein 3) inflammasome[150] and it is intriguing to consider whether the inflammasome is involved in DEP-induced epithelial-cell activation.

In view of the evidence showing that DEP induce epithelial cell GM-CSF, the role for GM-CSF in animal models of DEP-induced airway disease, and the critical role of GM-CSF in DC function, it was logical to examine whether DEP-treated epithelial cells upregulate DC maturation via GM-CSF. To examine this question, we used our co-culture system of human MDDC and HBEC or 16HBE14o$^-$ cells.[134] Functional maturation of DC was measured by the ability of DC to support proliferation of alloreactive naïve CD4$^+$ T cells. Monocyte-derived DC exposed to DEP-treated epithelial cells, but not to resting epithelial cells, supported proliferation of alloreactive naïve CD4$^+$ T cells. The importance of GM-CSF for DC maturation induced by DEP-treated epithelial cells was demonstrated by the ability of anti-GM-CSF to abolish this effect if it was included in the co-culture. The epithelial source of GM-CSF was confirmed by studies using siRNA in which silencing of GM-CSF in 16HBE14o$^-$ cells inhibited the ability of DEP-treated epithelial cells to induce DC that supported T cell proliferation. These data demonstrate that epithelial cell-derived GM-CSF mediates phenotypic and functional DC maturation induced by DEP-treated human bronchial epithelial cells and begin to provide a mechanism by which DEP upregulate DC maturation with potential to promote Th2 responses.

8.9 Thymic stromal lymphopoietin (TSLP)

For DEP to participate in airway Th2 responses, DEP should have the potential to promote both DC maturation and DC polarization that supports Th2 cells. Thymic stromal lymphopoietin (TSLP), a member of the IL-7 family of cytokines,[151] induces maturation of mDC that support Th2 cell polarization[151] and promotes maintenance of the Th2 memory response.[152, 153] TSLP upregulates expression of MHC class II, CD80, CD83, but not IL-12 family members or type I interferons.[154] TSLP also upregulates mDC mRNA for chemokines that attract neutrophils and eosinophils, as well as thymus and activation regulated chemokine (TARC/CCL17), which attracts Th2 cells.[155] TSLP-treated mDC induce an inflammatory Th2 response that is associated with IL-5, IL-4, IL-13, and TNF-α but low IL-10.[151, 155, 156] Importantly, TLSP induces expression of the TNF superfamily protein OX40 ligand (OX40L), engagement of which signals the generation of Th2 inflammatory cells.[154] OX40L expression can also mediate inhibition of Treg suppressor function.[157] TSLP is expressed by human epithelial cells[151, 157] and is increased in asthmatic airways.[159, 160] The importance of TSLP in asthma is also supported by recent genetic studies showing that TSLP polymorphisms are associated with asthma in some populations.[161]

Little is known about the regulation of TSLP in airway cells. Recently, TNF-α, IL-4, IL-13, rhinovirus, and dsRNA acting via TLR3 have been described to upregulate TSLP in human bronchial epithelial cells.[162] We have recently shown that DEP upregulates TSLP mRNA and protein in primary culture human bronchial epithelial cells as well as in the 16HBE14o$^-$ transformed cell line (Figure 8.3A).[163] In these studies, the generation of ROS was associated with DEP-induction of TSLP transcription and DEP-induced TLSP mRNA was inhibited by N-acetyl cysteine (NAC). These data suggest that DEP upregulate epithelial cell TSLP in an oxidant-dependent manner.[163]

Since DEP upregulated epithelial cell-derived TSLP, we asked whether TSLP derived from DEP-treated human bronchial epithelial cells induced DC maturation and polarization resulting in T cell proliferation and Th2 polarization.[163] We demonstrated that human MDDC exposed to DEP-treated airway epithelial cells support proliferation of naïve T cells in an MLR. The presence of anti-TSLP antibody in the DC-epithelial cell co-culture reduced the ability of MDDC exposed to DEP-treated epithelial cells to support T cell proliferation (Figure 8.3B). The failure of TSLP-silenced 16HBE14o$^-$ cells treated with DEP to support DC maturation as measured by T cell proliferation confirmed the importance of epithelial cell-derived TSLP

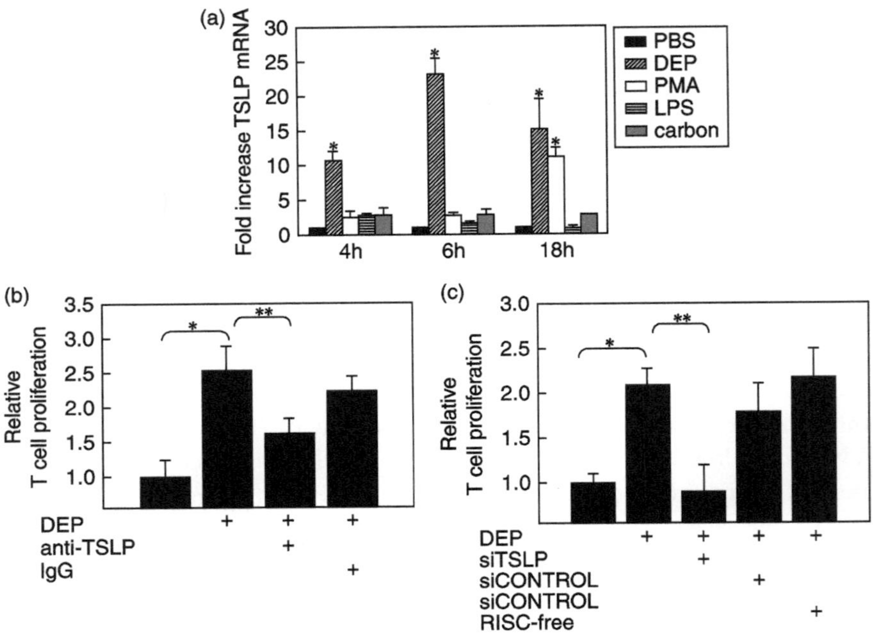

Figure 8.3 DEP upregulate TSLP in bronchial epithelial cells and promote DC maturation.

(a). Human bronchial epithelial cell (HBEC) TSLP mRNA was measured in response to DEP (3 μg/cm²), PMA (10 nM), LPS (1 μg/ml) or carbon (3 μg/cm²) (4–18h). RNA was isolated and quantified by realtime PCR, normalized to GAPDH and expressed as fold increase compared to unstimulated ($n = 3$, * = $p \leq 0.05$).

(b). TSLP derived from DEP-treated epithelial cells support DC maturation. Immature MDDC were exposed to resting or DEP (3 microg/cm²)-treated HBEC (48 h) in the absence or presence of anti-TSLP Ab. DC were FACS sorted, and T cell proliferation monitored by BrdU incorporation ($n = 3$, * DC derived from DEP-treated HBEC vs. resting, ** DC derived from DEP-treated HBEC compared to anti-TSLP $p < 0.05$).

(c). DEP-induced epithelial cell-derived TSLP supports DC maturation. Immature MDDC were exposed to resting, DEP-treated, or DEP-treated 16HBE14o⁻ cells pretreated with siTSLP or siCONTROLs. DC were FACS sorted, and their ability to support T cell proliferation monitored by BrdU incorporation ($n = 3$, * $p < 0.05$ DC derived from DEP-treated 16HBE14o⁻ cells vs. resting, ** $p < 0.05$ DC derived from DEP-treated 16HBE14o⁻ cells compared to siTSLP).

(Adapted from reference (163))

in this process (Fig. 8.3C). These data suggest that TSLP participates in the functional maturation of mDC exposed to DEP-treated HBEC.

The ability of DC to support T cell polarization depends on the ability of DC to express T helper polarizing cytokines (57). Dendritic cells activated by TSLP have been reported to express OX40L and Th2-attracting chemokines such as TARC/CCL17 but not Th1 cell polarizing cytokines such as IL-12 or interferon IFN-γ.[151, 155] We therefore examined whether DEP upregulated expression of OX40L and CCL17 in blood-derived mDC.[163] Direct exposure of DEP to mDC failed to change expression of OX40L, CCL17 or IL-12p35 mRNA consistent with the absence of Th2 polarization by DEP. As expected, exposure of mDC to human bronchial epithelial cells (16HBE14o$^-$) in the presence of cytokines known to induce Th2 responses (MF2) upregulated OX40L and TARC/CCL17 mRNA in contrast to cytokines known to induce Th1 responses (MF1) in FACS-sorted DC (Figure 8.4A). Exposure of mDC to DEP-treated 16HBE14o$^-$ cells significantly increased both CCL17 and OX40L mRNA in DC consistent with a Th2-priming pattern (Fig. 8.4A). The increased TARC/CCL17 and OX40L mRNA in DC induced by DEP-treated epithelial cells was due to TSLP as their expression was significantly reduced in the presence of anti-TSLP antibody.

We next confirmed that DEP-treated bronchial epithelial cells elicited DC with a functional ability to induce Th2 polarized T cells by the measurement of T cell IL-5/IFN-γ ratios. T cells were stimulated with blood-derived mDC exposed to bronchial epithelial cells (16HBE14o$^-$). T cell supernatants were isolated and IL-5 and IFN-γ measured by ELISA and expressed as the IL-5/IFN-γ ratio (Figure 8.4B). As expected, T cells exposed to mDC treated with MF1 showed a low IL-5/IFN-γ ratio. T cells exposed to mDC treated with MF2 expressed a high IL-5/IFN-γ ratio. T cells exposed to mDC cultured with resting epithelial cells (16HBE) had an elevated IL-5/IFN-γ ratio, suggesting that epithelial cells may provide a Th2 bias for DC. However, T cells exposed to mDC cultured with DEP-treated epithelial cells had a high IL-5/IFN-γ ratio that was greater than that seen for DC cultured with resting epithelial cells and similar to that seen in T cells exposed to DC cultured with MF2 and epithelial cells. TSLP was associated with the elevated IL-5/IFN-γ ratio since T cells exposed to mDC cultured with DEP-treated epithelial cells in the presence of anti-TSLP Ab had a significant decrease in the IL-5/IFN-γ ratio (Figure 8.4B). These studies suggest that DEP-treatment of epithelial cells induces functional Th2 polarization of DC and that TSLP is necessary for this response.[163]

In summary, disruption in the balance between effector and regulatory T cells in the airway may result in diseases such as asthma. This T cell balance is regulated by DC. Airway epithelial cells are the first target for ambient

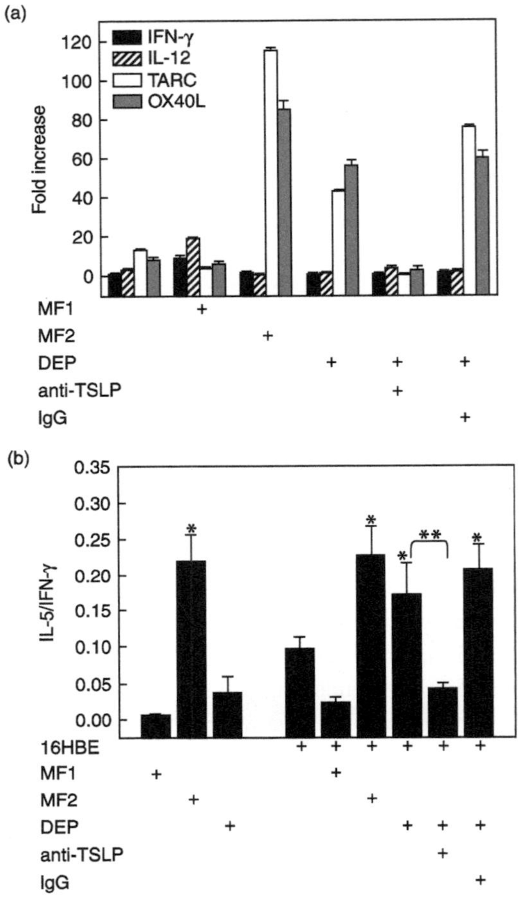

Figure 8.4 TSLP derived from DEP-treated epithelial cells supports DC expression of Th2 priming cytokines and DC-driven Th2 polarization.

(a). Immature mDC were exposed to epithelial cells (16HBE14o-) in the presence of defined cytokines that support Th1 (MF1) or Th2 (MF2) priming DC or with DEP (3 μg/cm2) +/– anti-TSLP Ab. mRNA from FACS-sorted DC was quantified for IFN-γ, IL-12p35, TARC and OX40L by realtime PCR (mean ± SE, n = 3).

(b). Immature mDC were exposed to MF1, MF2 or DEP in the absence or presence of 16HBE14o- cells and anti-TSLP Ab. DC were isolated and used as stimulator cells with allogeneic naïve T cells (1:10, 5 days). T cells were subsequently expanded (IL-2, 10 U/ml, 5 days), stimulated (PMA, 10 ng/ml and ionomycin, 1 mg/ml, 24 h) and cell-free supernatants analyzed for IFN-γ and IL-5 by ELISA. Data are expressed as ratio of IL-5/IFN-γ (n = 3, * $p < 0.05$ vs. resting epithelial cells, ** $p < 0.05$ DEP-treated epithelial cells vs. anti-TSLP Ab).

(Adapted from reference (163))

PM and DEP. DEP promote the release of chemokines, specifically CCL20 and CCL2, associated with DC recruitment. DEP also upregulate tissue-derived signals, including CSF2 and TSLP, that promote mDC maturation and Th2 polarization. Thus DEP may promote disruption of the airway T cell balance, and thus allergic asthma via the stimulation of epithelial cell-derived signals that regulate DC function.

References

1 Riedl MA. The effect of air pollution on asthma and allergy. *Curr Allergy Asthma Rep* 2008, 8: 139–146.

2 Janssen NA, Brunekreef B, van Vliet P, Aarts F, Meliefste K, Harssema H, Fischer P. The relationship between air pollution from heavy traffic and allergic sensitization, bronchial hyperresponsiveness, and respiratory symptoms in Dutch schoolchildren. *Environ Health Perspect* 2003, 111: 1512–1518.

3 Brugge D, Durant JL, Rioux C. Near-highway pollutants in motor vehicle exhaust: A review of epidemiologic evidence of cardiac and pulmonary health risks. *Environ Health* 2007, 6: 23.

4 Nordling E, Berglind N, Melen E, Emenius G, Hallberg J, Nyberg F, Pershagen G, Svartengren M, Wickman M, Bellander T. Traffic-related air pollution and childhood respiratory symptoms, function and allergies. *Epidemiology* 2008, 19: 401–408.

5 Morgenstern V, Zutavern A, Cyrys J, Brockow I, Koletzko S, Kramer U, Behrendt H, Herbarth O, von Berg A, Bauer CP, et al. Atopic diseases, allergic sensitization, and exposure to traffic-related air pollution in children. *Am J Respir Crit Care Med* 2008, 177: 1331–1337.

6 Li N, Hao M, Phalen RF, Hinds WC, Nel AE. Particulate air pollutants and asthma. A paradigm for the role of oxidative stress in PM-induced adverse health effects. *Clin Immunol* 2003, 109: 250–265.

7 Takenaka H, Zhang K, Diaz-Sanchez D, Tsien A, Saxon A. Enhanced human IgE production results from exposure to the aromatic hydrocarbons from diesel exhaust: Direct effects on B-cell IgE production. *J Allergy Clin Immunol* 1995, 95: 103–115.

8 Diaz-Sanchez D, Tsien A, Fleming J, Saxon A. Combined diesel exhaust particulate and ragweed allergen challenge markedly enhances human in vivo nasal ragweed-specific IgE and skews cytokine production to a T helper cell 2–type pattern. *J Immunol* 1997, 158: 2406–2413.

9 Fujieda S, Diaz-Sanchez D, Saxon A. Combined nasal challenge with diesel exhaust particles and allergen induces in vivo IgE isotype switching. *Am J Respir Cell Mol Biol* 1998, 19: 507–512.

10 Diaz-Sanchez D, Garcia MP, Wang M, Jyrala M, Saxon A. Nasal challenge with diesel exhaust particles can induce sensitization to a neoallergen in the human mucosa. *J Allergy Clin Immunol* 1999, 104: 1183–1188.

11 Mastrangelo G, Clonfero E, Pavanello S, Fedeli U, Fadda E, Turato A, Piccinni S, Montagnani R, Marcer G. Exposure to diesel exhaust enhances total IgE in

non-atopic dockers. *International archives of occupational and environmental health* 2003, 76: 63–68.
12 Manchester-Neesvig JB, Schauer JJ, Cass GR. The distribution of particle-phase organic compounds in the atmosphere and their use for source apportionment during the southern California children's health study. *J Air Waste Manag Assoc* 2003, 53: 1065–1079.
13 Polosa R, Salvi S, Di Maria GU. Allergic susceptibility associated with diesel exhaust particle exposure: clear as mud. *Arch Environ Health* 2002, 57: 188–193.
14 Schuetzle D, Lee FS, Prater TJ. The identification of polynuclear aromatic hydrocarbon (PAH) derivatives in mutagenic fractions of diesel particulate extracts. *Int J Environ Anal Chem* 1981, 9: 93–144.
15 Li N, Nel AE. The cellular impacts of diesel exhaust particles: Beyond inflammation and death. *Eur Respir J* 2006, 27: 667–668.
16 Oberdorster G, Utell MJ. Ultrafine particles in the urban air: To the respiratory tract–and beyond? *Environ Health Perspect* 2002, 110: A440–441.
17 Penttinen P, Timonen KL, Tiittanen P, Mirme A, Ruuskanen J, Pekkanen J. Ultrafine particles in urban air and respiratory health among adult asthmatics. *Eur Respir J* 2001, 17: 428–435.
18 Wichmann HE, Spix C, Tuch T, Wolke G, Peters A, Heinrich J, Kreyling WG, Heyder J. Daily mortality and fine and ultrafine particles in Erfurt, Germany part I: Role of particle number and particle mass. *Res Rep Health Eff Inst* 2000, 5–86; discussion 87–94.
19 McCreanor J, Cullinan P, Nieuwenhuijsen MJ, Stewart-Evans J, Malliarou E, Jarup L, Harrington R, Svartengren M, Han IK, Ohman-Strickland P, et al. Respiratory effects of exposure to diesel traffic in persons with asthma. *N Engl J Med* 2007, 357: 2348–2358.
20 Abe S, Takizawa H, Sugawara I, Kudoh S. Diesel exhaust (DE)-induced cytokine expression in human bronchial epithelial cells: A study with a new cell exposure system to freshly generated DE in vitro. *Am J Respir Cell Mol Biol* 2000, 22: 296–303.
21 Hiura TS, Kaszubowski MP, Li N, Nel AE. Chemicals in diesel exhaust particles generate reactive oxygen radicals and induce apoptosis in macrophages. *J Immunol* 1999, 163: 5582–5591.
22 Kumagai Y, Arimoto T, Shinyashiki M, Shimojo N, Nakai Y, Yoshikawa T, Sagai M. Generation of reactive oxygen species during interaction of diesel exhaust particle components with nadph-cytochrome p450 reductase and involvement of the bioactivation in the DNA damage. *Free Radical Biology & Medicine* 1997, 22: 479–487.
23 Li N, Venkatesan MI, Miguel A, Kaplan R, Gujuluva C, Alam J, Nel A. Induction of heme oxygenase-1 expression in macrophages by diesel exhaust particle chemicals and quinones via the antioxidant-responsive element. *J Immunol* 2000, 165: 3393–3401.
24 Li N, Kim S, Wang M, Froines J, Sioutas C, Nel A. Use of a stratified oxidative stress model to study the biological effects of ambient concentrated and diesel exhaust particulate matter. *Inhal Toxicol* 2002, 14: 459–486.
25 Lehmann I, Rehwagen M, Diez U, Seiffart A, Rolle-Kampczyk U, Richter M, Wetzig H, Borte M, Herbarth O. Enhanced in vivo IgE production and T cell

polarization toward the type 2 phenotype in association with indoor exposure to VOC: Results of the LARS study. *International Journal of Hygiene and Environmental Health* 2001, 204: 211–221.
26 Takano H, Yanagisawa R, Inoue K. Components of diesel exhaust particles diversely enhance a variety of respiratory diseases related to infection or allergy: Extracted organic chemicals and the residual particles after extraction differently affect respiratory diseases. *Journal of clinical Biochemistry and Nutrition* 2007, 40: 101–107.
27 Su DS, Serafino A, Muller JO, Jentoft RE, Schlogl R, Fiorito S. Cytotoxicity and inflammatory potential of soot particles of low-emission diesel engines. *Environ Sci Technol* 2008, 42: 1761–1765.
28 Woodfolk JA. T-cell responses to allergens. *J Allergy Clin Immunol* 2007, 119: 280–294; quiz 295–286.
29 Hammad H, Lambrecht BN. Dendritic cells and epithelial cells: Linking innate and adaptive immunity in asthma. *Nat Rev Immunol* 2008, 8: 193–204.
30 Akdis M. T cell tolerance to inhaled allergens: Mechanisms and therapeutic approaches. *Expert Opinion on Biological Therapy* 2008, 8: 769–777.
31 Curotto de Lafaille MA, Muriglan S, Sunshine MJ, Lei Y, Kutchukhidze N, Furtado GC, Wensky AK, Olivares-Villagomez D, Lafaille JJ. Hyper immunoglobulin E response in mice with monoclonal populations of B and T lymphocytes. *J Exp Med* 2001, 194: 1349–1359.
32 Curotto de Lafaille MA, Lafaille JJ. The role of regulatory T cells in allergy. *Springer Semin Immunopathol* 2004, 25: 295–310.
33 Curotto de Lafaille MA, Lino AC, Kutchukhidze N, Lafaille JJ. CD25- T cells generate cd25+foxp3+ regulatory T cells by peripheral expansion. *J Immunol* 2004, 173: 7259–7268.
34 Ling EM, Smith T, Nguyen XD, Pridgeon C, Dallman M, Arbery J, Carr VA, Robinson DS. Relation of CD4+CD25+ regulatory T-cell suppression of allergen-driven T-cell activation to atopic status and expression of allergic disease. *Lancet* 2004, 363: 608–615.
35 Akdis M, Verhagen J, Taylor A, Karamloo F, Karagiannidis C, Crameri R, Thunberg S, Deniz G, Valenta R, Fiebig H, et al. Immune responses in healthy and allergic individuals are characterized by a fine balance between allergen-specific T regulatory 1 and T helper 2 cells. *J Exp Med* 2004, 199: 1567–1575.
36 Mamessier E, Nieves A, Lorec AM, Dupuy P, Pinot D, Pinet C, Vervloet D, Magnan A. T-cell activation during exacerbations: A longitudinal study in refractory asthma. *Allergy* 2008, 63: 1202–1210.
37 Akbari O, DeKruyff RH, Umetsu DT. Pulmonary dendritic cells producing IL-10 mediate tolerance induced by respiratory exposure to antigen. *Nat Immunol* 2001, 2: 725–731.
38 Umetsu DT, McIntire JJ, Akbari O, Macaubas C, DeKruyff RH. Asthma: An epidemic of dysregulated immunity. *Nat Immunol* 2002, 3: 715–720.
39 Akbari O, Freeman GJ, Meyer EH, Greenfield EA, Chang TT, Sharpe AH, Berry G, DeKruyff RH, Umetsu DT. Antigen-specific regulatory T cells develop via the icos–icos–ligand pathway and inhibit allergen-induced airway hyperreactivity. *Nat Med* 2002, 8: 1024–1032.
40 Fontenot JD, Gavin MA, Rudensky AY. Foxp3 programs the development and function of CD4+CD25+ regulatory T cells. *Nat Immunol* 2003, 4: 330–336.

41 Hori S, Nomura T, Sakaguchi S. Control of regulatory T cell development by the transcription factor foxp3. *Science* 2003, 299: 1057–1061.
42 Khattri R, Cox T, Yasayko SA, Ramsdell F. An essential role for scurfin in CD4+CD25+ T regulatory cells. *Nat Immunol* 2003, 4: 337–342.
43 Shevach EM, DiPaolo RA, Andersson J, Zhao DM, Stephens GL, Thornton AM. The lifestyle of naturally occurring CD4+ CD25+ foxp3+ regulatory T cells. *Immunol Rev* 2006, 212: 60–73.
44 Apostolou I, von Boehmer H. In vivo instruction of suppressor commitment in naive T cells. *J Exp Med* 2004, 199: 1401–1408.
45 Cobbold SP, Castejon R, Adams E, Zelenika D, Graca L, Humm S, Waldmann H. Induction of foxp3+ regulatory T cells in the periphery of T cell receptor transgenic mice tolerized to transplants. *J Immunol* 2004, 172: 6003–6010.
46 Mucida D, Kutchukhidze N, Erazo A, Russo M, Lafaille JJ, Curotto de Lafaille MA. Oral tolerance in the absence of naturally occurring Tregs. *J Clin Invest* 2005, 115: 1923–1933.
47 Curotto de Lafaille MA, Kutchukhidze N, Shen S, Ding Y, Yee H, Lafaille JJ. Adaptive foxp3+ regulatory T cell-dependent and -independent control of allergic inflammation. *Immunity* 2008, 29: 114–126.
48 Ruprecht CR, Gattorno M, Ferlito F, Gregorio A, Martini A, Lanzavecchia A, Sallusto F. Coexpression of CD25 and CD27 identifies foxp3+ regulatory T cells in inflamed synovia. *J Exp Med* 2005, 201: 1793–1803.
49 Saruta M, Yu QT, Fleshner PR, Mantel PY, Schmidt-Weber CB, Banham AH, Papadakis KA. Characterization of foxp3+CD4+ regulatory T cells in Crohn's disease. *Clin Immunol* 2007, 125: 281–290.
50 Sasaki M, Ikeda H, Sawada S, Sato Y, Nakanuma Y. Naturally-occurring regulatory T cells are increased in inflamed portal tracts with cholangiopathy in primary biliary cirrhosis. *Journal of Clinical Pathology* 2007, 60: 1102–1107.
51 Andersson J, Tran DQ, Pesu M, Davidson TS, Ramsey H, O'Shea JJ, Shevach EM. Cd4+ foxp3+ regulatory T cells confer infectious tolerance in aTGF-beta-dependent manner. *J Exp Med* 2008, 205: 1975–1981.
52 Van Hove CL, Maes T, Joos GF, Tournoy KG. Prolonged inhaled allergen exposure can induce persistent tolerance. *Am J Respir Cell Mol Biol* 2007, 36: 573–584.
53 Banchereau J, Steinman RM. Dendritic cells and the control of immunity. *Nature* 1998, 392: 245–252.
54 Shortman K, Naik SH. Steady-state and inflammatory dendritic-cell development. *Nat Rev Immunol* 2007, 7: 19–30.
55 Naik SH. Demystifying the development of dendritic cell subtypes, a little. *Immunology and Cell Biology* 2008, 86: 439–452.
56 Steinman RM. Dendritic cells in vivo: A key target for a new vaccine science. *Immunity* 2008, 29: 319–324.
57 Kapsenberg ML. Dendritic-cell control of pathogen-driven T-cell polarization. *Nat Rev Immunol* 2003, 3: 984–993.
58 de Jong EC, Vieira PL, Kalinski P, Schuitemaker JH, Tanaka Y, Wierenga EA, Yazdanbakhsh M, Kapsenberg ML. Microbial compounds selectively induce TH1 cell-promoting or Th2 cell-promoting dendritic cells in vitro with diverse th cell-polarizing signals. *J Immunol* 2002, 168: 1704–1709.

59 Eisenbarth SC, Piggott DA, Huleatt JW, Visintin I, Herrick CA, Bottomly K. Lipopolysaccharide-enhanced, Toll-like receptor 4-dependent T helper cell type 2 responses to inhaled antigen. *J Exp Med* 2002, 196: 1645–1651.
60 Brimnes MK, Bonifaz L, Steinman RM, Moran TM. Influenza virus-induced dendritic cell maturation is associated with the induction of strong T cell immunity to a coadministered, normally nonimmunogenic protein. *J Exp Med* 2003, 198: 133–144.
61 Muthuswamy R, Urban J, Lee JJ, Reinhart TA, Bartlett D, Kalinski P. Ability of mature dendritic cells to interact with regulatory T cells is imprinted during maturation. *Cancer Res* 2008, 68: 5972–5978.
62 Sato K, Yamashita N, Baba M, Matsuyama T. Modified myeloid dendritic cells act as regulatory dendritic cells to induce anergic and regulatory T cells. *Blood* 2003, 101: 3581–3589.
63 Kalinski P, Hilkens CM, Wierenga EA, Kapsenberg ML. T-cell priming by type-1 and type-2 polarized dendritic cells: The concept of a third signal. *Immunol Today* 1999, 20: 561–567.
64 Amsen D, Blander JM, Lee GR, Tanigaki K, Honjo T, Flavell RA. Instruction of distinct CD4 T helper cell fates by different notch ligands on antigen-presenting cells. *Cell* 2004, 117: 515–526.
65 Liotta F, Frosali F, Querci V, Mantei A, Fili L, Maggi L, Mazzinghi B, Angeli R, Ronconi E, Santarlasci V, et al. Human immature myeloid dendritic cells trigger a Th2-polarizing program via jagged–1/notch interaction. *J Allergy Clin Immunol* 2008, 121: 1000–1005 e1008.
66 Kapsenberg ML, Kalinski P. The concept of type 1 and type 2 antigen-presenting cells. *Immunol Lett* 1999, 69: 5–6.
67 Xia WJ, Schneeberger EE, McCarthy K, Kradin RL. Accessory cells of the lung. Ii. Ia+ pulmonary dendritic cells display cell surface antigen heterogeneity. *Am J Respir Cell Mol Biol* 1991, 5: 276–283.
68 Gong JL, McCarthy KM, Telford J, Tamatani T, Miyasaka M, Schneeberger EE. Intraepithelial airway dendritic cells: A distinct subset of pulmonary dendritic cells obtained by microdissection. *J Exp Med* 1992, 175: 797–807.
69 van Haarst JM, Hoogsteden HC, de Wit HJ, Verhoeven GT, Havenith CE, Drexhage HA. Dendritic cells and their precursors isolated from human bronchoalveolar lavage: Immunocytologic and functional properties. *Am J Respir Cell Mol Biol* 1994, 11: 344–350.
70 Sertl K, Takemura T, Tschachler E, Ferrans VJ, Kaliner MA, Shevach EM. Dendritic cells with antigen-presenting capability reside in airway epithelium, lung parenchyma, and visceral pleura. *J Exp Med* 1986, 163: 436–451.
71 Cochand L, Isler P, Songeon F, Nicod LP. Human lung dendritic cells have an immature phenotype with efficient mannose receptors. *Am J Respir Cell Mol Biol* 1999, 21: 547–554.
72 Demedts IK, Brusselle GG, Vermaelen KY, Pauwels RA. Identification and characterization of human pulmonary dendritic cells. *Am J Respir Cell Mol Biol* 2005, 32: 177–184.
73 Masten BJ, Olson GK, Tarleton CA, Rund C, Schuyler M, Mehran R, Archibeque T, Lipscomb MF. Characterization of myeloid and plasmacytoid dendritic cells in human lung. *J Immunol* 2006, 177: 7784–7793.

74 Demedts IK, Bracke KR, Maes T, Joos GF, Brusselle GG. Different roles for human lung dendritic cell subsets in pulmonary immune defense mechanisms. *Am J Respir Cell Mol Biol* 2006.
75 Moller GM, Overbeek SE, Van Helden-Meeuwsen CG, Van Haarst JM, Prens EP, Mulder PG, Postma DS, Hoogsteden HC. Increased numbers of dendritic cells in the bronchial mucosa of atopic asthmatic patients: Downregulation by inhaled corticosteroids. *Clin Exp Allergy* 1996, 26: 517–524.
76 Bocchino V, Bertorelli G, Zhuo X, Grima P, Di Comite V, Damia R, Chetta A, Del Donno M, Foresi A, Casalini A, et al. Short-term treatment with a low dose of inhaled fluticasone propionate decreases the number of CD1a+ dendritic cells in asthmatic airways. *Pulm Pharmacol Ther* 1997, 10: 253–259.
77 Lambrecht BN, Carro-Muino I, Vermaelen K, Pauwels RA. Allergen-induced changes in bone-marrow progenitor and airway dendritic cells in sensitized rats. *Am J Respir Cell Mol Biol* 1999, 20: 1165–1174.
78 Hammad H, Lambrecht BN, Pochard P, Gosset P, Marquillies P, Tonnel AB, Pestel J. Monocyte-derived dendritic cells induce a house dust mite-specific Th2 allergic inflammation in the lung of humanized scid mice: Involvement of CCR7. *J Immunol* 2002, 169: 1524–1534.
79 Graffi SJ, Dekan G, Stingl G, Epstein MM. Systemic administration of antigen-pulsed dendritic cells induces experimental allergic asthma in mice upon aerosol antigen rechallenge. *Clin Immunol* 2002, 103: 176–184.
80 Lambrecht BN, Peleman RA, Bullock GR, Pauwels RA. Sensitization to inhaled antigen by intratracheal instillation of dendritic cells. *Clin Exp Allergy* 2000, 30: 214–224.
81 Julia V, Hessel EM, Malherbe L, Glaichenhaus N, O'Garra A, Coffman RL. A restricted subset of dendritic cells captures airborne antigens and remains able to activate specific T cells long after antigen exposure. *Immunity* 2002, 16: 271–283.
82 Lambrecht BN, Salomon B, Klatzmann D, Pauwels RA. Dendritic cells are required for the development of chronic eosinophilic airway inflammation in response to inhaled antigen in sensitized mice. *J Immunol* 1998, 160: 4090–4097.
83 Lambrecht BN, Hammad H. Taking our breath away: Dendritic cells in the pathogenesis of asthma. *Nat Rev Immunol* 2003, 3: 994–1003.
84 van Rijt LS, Jung S, Kleinjan A, Vos N, Willart M, Duez C, Hoogsteden HC, Lambrecht BN. In vivo depletion of lung CD11c+ dendritic cells during allergen challenge abrogates the characteristic features of asthma. *J Exp Med* 2005, 201: 981–991.
85 McMenamin C, Schon-Hegrad M, Oliver J, Girn B, Holt PG. Regulation of IgE responses to inhaled antigens: Cellular mechanisms underlying allergic sensitization versus tolerance induction. *Int Arch Allergy Appl Immunol* 1991, 94: 78–82.
86 Ostroukhova M, Seguin-Devaux C, Oriss TB, Dixon-McCarthy B, Yang L, Ameredes BT, Corcoran TE, Ray A. Tolerance induced by inhaled antigen involves CD4(+) T cells expressing membrane-bound TGF-beta and FOXP3. *J Clin Invest* 2004, 114: 28–38.
87 de Heer HJ, Hammad H, Soullie T, Hijdra D, Vos N, Willart MA, Hoogsteden HC, Lambrecht BN. Essential role of lung plasmacytoid dendritic cells in preventing asthmatic reactions to harmless inhaled antigen. *J Exp Med* 2004, 200: 89–98.

88 Ito T, Yang M, Wang YH, Lande R, Gregorio J, Perng OA, Qin XF, Liu YJ, Gilliet M. Plasmacytoid dendritic cells prime IL-10-producing T regulatory cells by inducible costimulator ligand. *J Exp Med* 2007, 204: 105–115.
89 Fujita S, Yamashita N, Ishii Y, Sato Y, Sato K, Eizumi K, Fukaya T, Nozawa R, Takamoto Y, Yamashita N, et al. Regulatory dendritic cells protect against allergic airway inflammation in a murine asthmatic model. *J Allergy Clin Immunol* 2008, 121: 95–104 e107.
90 Holt PG, Schon-Hegrad MA, Oliver J, Holt BJ, McMenamin PG. A contiguous network of dendritic antigen-presenting cells within the respiratory epithelium. *Int Arch Allergy Appl Immunol* 1990, 91: 155–159.
91 Holt PG, Schon-Hegrad MA, McMenamin PG. Dendritic cells in the respiratory tract. *Int Rev Immunol* 1990, 6: 139–149.
92 Casolaro MA, Bernaudin JF, Saltini C, Ferrans VJ, Crystal RG. Accumulation of Langerhans' cells on the epithelial surface of the lower respiratory tract in normal subjects in association with cigarette smoking. *Am Rev Respir Dis* 1988, 137: 406–411.
93 Soler P, Moreau A, Basset F, Hance AJ. Cigarette smoking-induced changes in the number and differentiated state of pulmonary dendritic cells/Langerhans cells. *Am Rev Respir Dis* 1989, 139: 1112–1117.
94 Mellman I, Steinman RM. Dendritic cells: Specialized and regulated antigen processing machines. *Cell* 2001, 106: 255–258.
95 Mahnke K, Schmitt E, Bonifaz L, Enk AH, Jonuleit H. Immature, but not inactive: The tolerogenic function of immature dendritic cells. *Immunology and cell biology* 2002, 80: 477–483.
96 Lambrecht BN. Allergen uptake and presentation by dendritic cells. *Curr Opin Allergy Clin Immunol* 2001, 1: 51–59.
97 Jahnsen FL, Moloney ED, Hogan T, Upham JW, Burke CM, Holt PG. Rapid dendritic cell recruitment to the bronchial mucosa of patients with atopic asthma in response to local allergen challenge. *Thorax* 2001, 56: 823–826.
98 McWilliam AS, Nelson D, Thomas JA, Holt PG. Rapid dendritic cell recruitment is a hallmark of the acute inflammatory response at mucosal surfaces. *J Exp Med* 1994, 179: 1331–1336.
99 Vermaelen KY, Carro-Muino I, Lambrecht BN, Pauwels RA. Specific migratory dendritic cells rapidly transport antigen from the airways to the thoracic lymph nodes. *J Exp Med* 2001, 193: 51–60.
100 Holt PG, Stumbles PA. Characterization of dendritic cell populations in the respiratory tract. *J Aerosol Med* 2000, 13: 361–367.
101 McWilliam AS, Napoli S, Marsh AM, Pemper FL, Nelson DJ, Pimm CL, Stumbles PA, Wells TN, Holt PG. Dendritic cells are recruited into the airway epithelium during the inflammatory response to a broad spectrum of stimuli. *J Exp Med* 1996, 184: 2429–2432.
102 Tager AM, Luster AD, Leary CP, Sakamoto H, Zhao LH, Preffer F, Kradin RL. Accessory cells with immunophenotypic and functional features of monocyte-derived dendritic cells are recruited to the lung during pulmonary inflammation. *J Leukoc Biol* 1999, 66: 901–908.
103 Jahnsen FL, Strickland DH, Thomas JA, Tobagus IT, Napoli S, Zosky GR, Turner DJ, Sly PD, Stumbles PA, Holt PG. Accelerated antigen sampling and

transport by airway mucosal dendritic cells following inhalation of a bacterial stimulus. *J Immunol* 2006, 177: 5861–5867.
104 Upham JW, Denburg JA, O'Byrne PM. Rapid response of circulating myeloid dendritic cells to inhaled allergen in asthmatic subjects. *Clin Exp Allergy* 2002, 32: 818–823.
105 Farrell E, O'Connor TM, Duong M, Watson RM, Strinich T, Gauvreau GM, O'Byrne PM. Circulating myeloid and plasmacytoid dendritic cells after allergen inhalation in asthmatic subjects. *Allergy* 2007, 62: 1139–1145.
106 Alvarez D, Vollmann EH, von Andrian UH. Mechanisms and consequences of dendritic cell migration. *Immunity* 2008, 29: 325–342.
107 Greaves DR, Wang W, Dairaghi DJ, Dieu MC, Saint-Vis B, Franz-Bacon K, Rossi D, Caux C, McClanahan T, Gordon S, et al. CCR6, a CC chemokine receptor that interacts with macrophage inflammatory protein 3alpha and is highly expressed in human dendritic cells. *J Exp Med* 1997, 186: 837–844.
108 Kucharzik T, Hudson JT, 3rd, Waikel RL, Martin WD, Williams IR. Ccr6 expression distinguishes mouse myeloid and lymphoid dendritic cell subsets: Demonstration using a CCR6 egfp knock-in mouse. *Eur J Immunol* 2002, 32: 104–112.
109 Schutyser E, Struyf S, Van Damme J. The CC chemokine CCL20 and its receptor CCR6. *Cytokine Growth Factor Rev* 2003, 14: 409–426.
110 Caux C, Vanbervliet B, Massacrier C, Ait-Yahia S, Vaure C, Chemin K, Dieu N, Mc, Vicari A. Regulation of dendritic cell recruitment by chemokines. *Transplantation* 2002, 73: S7–11.
111 Lukacs-Kornek V, Engel D, Tacke F, Kurts C. The role of chemokines and their receptors in dendritic cell biology. *Front Biosci* 2008, 13: 2238–2252.
112 Geissmann F, Jung S, Littman DR. Blood monocytes consist of two principal subsets with distinct migratory properties. *Immunity* 2003, 19: 71–82.
113 Chiu BC, Freeman CM, Stolberg VR, Hu JS, Zeibecoglou K, Lu B, Gerard C, Charo IF, Lira SA, Chensue SW. Impaired lung dendritic cell activation in CCR2 knockout mice. *The American Journal of Pathology* 2004, 165: 1199–1209.
114 Robays LJ, Maes T, Lebecque S, Lira SA, Kuziel WA, Brusselle GG, Joos GF, Vermaelen KV. Chemokine receptor CCR2 but not CCR5 or CCR6 mediates the increase in pulmonary dendritic cells during allergic airway inflammation. *J Immunol* 2007, 178: 5305–5311.
115 Power CA, Church DJ, Meyer A, Alouani S, Proudfoot AE, Clark-Lewis I, Sozzani S, Mantovani A, Wells TN. Cloning and characterization of a specific receptor for the novel CC chemokine MIP–3alpha from lung dendritic cells. *J Exp Med* 1997, 186: 825–835.
116 Demedts IK, Bracke KR, Van Pottelberge G, Testelmans D, Verleden GM, Vermassen FE, Joos GF, Brusselle GG. Accumulation of dendritic cells and increased CCL20 levels in the airways of patients with chronic obstructive pulmonary disease. *Am J Respir Crit Care Med* 2007, 175: 998–1005.
117 Francis JN, Sabroe I, Lloyd CM, Durham SR, Till SJ. Elevated CCR6+ CD4+ T lymphocytes in tissue compared with blood and induction of CCL20 during the asthmatic late response. *Clin Exp Immunol* 2008, 152: 440–447.
118 Lukacs NW, Prosser DM, Wiekowski M, Lira SA, Cook DN. Requirement for the chemokine receptor CCR6 in allergic pulmonary inflammation. *J Exp Med* 2001, 194: 551–555.

119 Bracke KR, D'Hulst A I, Maes T, Moerloose KB, Demedts IK, Lebecque S, Joos GF, Brusselle GG. Cigarette smoke-induced pulmonary inflammation and emphysema are attenuated in CCR6-deficient mice. *J Immunol* 2006, 177: 4350–4359.

120 Vanbervliet B, Homey B, Durand I, Massacrier C, Ait-Yahia S, de Bouteiller O, Vicari A, Caux C. Sequential involvement of CCR2 and CCR6 ligands for immature dendritic cell recruitment: Possible role at inflamed epithelial surfaces. *Eur J Immunol* 2002, 32: 231–242.

121 Osterholzer JJ, Ames T, Polak T, Sonstein J, Moore BB, Chensue SW, Toews GB, Curtis JL. CCR2 and CCR6, but not endothelial selectins, mediate the accumulation of immature dendritic cells within the lungs of mice in response to particulate antigen. *J Immunol* 2005, 175: 874–883.

122 Reibman J, Hsu Y, Chen LC, Bleck B, Gordon T. Airway epithelial cells release MIP-3alpha/CCL20 in response to cytokines and ambient particulate matter. *Am J Respir Cell Mol Biol* 2003, 28: 648–654.

123 Thorley AJ, Goldstraw P, Young A, Tetley TD. Primary human alveolar type II epithelial cell CCL20 (macrophage inflammatory protein-3alpha)-induced dendritic cell migration. *Am J Respir Cell Mol Biol* 2005, 32: 262–267.

124 Bleck B, Tse D, Ahmed R, Liu M, Reibman J. Diesel exhaust particle-treated human bronchial epithelial cells release chemokines associated with mDC and pDC recruitment. *American Journal of Respiratory and Critical Care Medicine* 2008, 177: A349.

125 Rescigno M, Urbano M, Valzasina B, Francolini M, Rotta G, Bonasio R, Granucci F, Kraehenbuhl JP, Ricciardi-Castagnoli P. Dendritic cells express tight junction proteins and penetrate gut epithelial monolayers to sample bacteria. *Nat Immunol* 2001, 2: 361–367.

126 Chieppa M, Rescigno M, Huang AY, Germain RN. Dynamic imaging of dendritic cell extension into the small bowel lumen in response to epithelial cell TLR engagement. *J Exp Med* 2006, 203: 2841–2852.

127 Sung SS, Fu SM, Rose CE, Jr., Gaskin F, Ju ST, Beaty SR. A major lung CD103 (alphae)-beta7 integrin-positive epithelial dendritic cell population expressing langerin and tight junction proteins. *J Immunol* 2006, 176: 2161–2172.

128 Inoue K, Takano H, Yanagisawa R, Hirano S, Ichinose T, Shimada A, Yoshikawa T. The role of Toll-like receptor 4 in airway inflammation induced by diesel exhaust particles. *Archives of Toxicology* 2006, 80: 275–279.

129 Hollingsworth JW, 2nd, Cook DN, Brass DM, Walker JK, Morgan DL, Foster WM, Schwartz DA. The role of Toll-like receptor 4 in environmental airway injury in mice. *Am J Respir Crit Care Med* 2004, 170: 126–132.

130 Becker S, Fenton MJ, Soukup JM. Involvement of microbial components and Toll-like receptors 2 and 4 in cytokine responses to air pollution particles. *Am J Respir Cell Mol Biol* 2002, 27: 611–618.

131 Verstraelen S, Van Den Heuvel R, Nelissen I, Witters H, Verheyen G, Schoeters G. Flow cytometric characterisation of antigen presenting dendritic cells after in vitro exposure to diesel exhaust particles. *Toxicol In Vitro* 2005, 19: 903–907.

132 Porter M, Karp M, Killedar S, Bauer SM, Guo J, Williams D, Breysse P, Georas SN, Williams MA. Diesel-enriched particulate matter functionally activates human dendritic cells. *Am J Respir Cell Mol Biol* 2007, 37: 706–719.

133 Williams MA, Porter M, Horton M, Guo J, Roman J, Williams D, Breysse P, Georas SN. Ambient particulate matter directs nonclassic dendritic cell activation and a mixed TH1/TH2-like cytokine response by naive CD4+ T cells. *J Allergy Clin Immunol* 2007, 119: 488–497.
134 Bleck B, Tse DB, Jaspers I, Curotto de Lafaille MA, Reibman J. Diesel exhaust particle-exposed human bronchial epithelial cells induce dendritic cell maturation. *J Immunol* 2006, 176: 7431–7437.
135 Witmer-Pack MD, Olivier W, Valinsky J, Schuler G, Steinman RM. Granulocyte/macrophage colony-stimulating factor is essential for the viability and function of cultured murine epidermal Langerhans cells. *J Exp Med* 1987, 166: 1484–1498.
136 Sallusto F, Lanzavecchia A. Efficient presentation of soluble antigen by cultured human dendritic cells is maintained by granulocyte/macrophage colony-stimulating factor plus interleukin 4 and downregulated by tumor necrosis factor alpha. *J Exp Med* 1994, 179: 1109–1118.
137 Soloperto M, Mattoso VL, Fasoli A, Mattoli S. A bronchial epithelial cell-derived factor in asthma that promotes eosinophil activation and survival as GM-CSF. *Am J Physiol* 1991, 260: L530–538.
138 Lei XF, Ohkawara Y, Stampfli MR, Gauldie J, Croitoru K, Jordana M, Xing Z. Compartmentalized transgene expression of granulocyte-macrophage colony-stimulating factor (GM-CSF) in mouse lung enhances allergic airways inflammation. *Clin Exp Immunol* 1998, 113: 157–165.
139 Stampfli MR, Wiley RE, Neigh GS, Gajewska BU, Lei XF, Snider DP, Xing Z, Jordana M. GM-CSF transgene expression in the airway allows aerosolized ovalbumin to induce allergic sensitization in mice. *J Clin Invest* 1998, 102: 1704–1714.
140 Wang J, Snider DP, Hewlett BR, Lukacs NW, Gauldie J, Liang H, Xing Z. Transgenic expression of granulocyte-macrophage colony-stimulating factor induces the differentiation and activation of a novel dendritic cell population in the lung. *Blood* 2000, 95: 2337–2345.
141 Cates EC, Gajewska BU, Goncharova S, Alvarez D, Fattouh R, Coyle AJ, Gutierrez-Ramos JC, Jordana M. Effect of GM-CSF on immune, inflammatory, and clinical responses to ragweed in a novel mouse model of mucosal sensitization. *J Allergy Clin Immunol* 2003, 111: 1076–1086.
142 Swirski FK, Sajic D, Robbins CS, Gajewska BU, Jordana M, Stampfli MR. Chronic exposure to innocuous antigen in sensitized mice leads to suppressed airway eosinophilia that is reversed by granulocyte macrophage colony-stimulating factor. *J Immunol* 2002, 169: 3499–3506.
143 Ohta K, Yamashita N, Tajima M, Miyasaka T, Nakano J, Nakajima M, Ishii A, Horiuchi T, Mano K, Miyamoto T. Diesel exhaust particulate induces airway hyperresponsiveness in a murine model: Essential role of GM-CSF. *J Allergy Clin Immunol* 1999, 104: 1024–1030.
144 Takano H, Yoshikawa T, Ichinose T, Miyabara Y, Imaoka K, Sagai M. Diesel exhaust particles enhance antigen-induced airway inflammation and local cytokine expression in mice. *Am J Respir Crit Care Med* 1997, 156: 36–42.
145 Devalia JL, Bayram H, Rusznak C, Calderon M, Sapsford RJ, Abdelaziz MA, Wang J, Davies RJ. Mechanisms of pollution-induced airway disease: In vitro studies in the upper and lower airways. *Allergy* 1997, 52: 45–51.

146 Ohtoshi T, Takizawa H, Okazaki H, Kawasaki S, Takeuchi N, Ohta K, Ito K. Diesel exhaust particles stimulate human airway epithelial cells to produce cytokines relevant to airway inflammation in vitro. *J Allergy Clin Immunol* 1998, 101: 778–785.
147 Boland S, Baeza-Squiban A, Fournier T, Houcine O, Gendron MC, Chevrier M, Jouvenot G, Coste A, Aubier M, Marano F. Diesel exhaust particles are taken up by human airway epithelial cells in vitro and alter cytokine production. *Am J Physiol* 1999, 276: L604–613.
148 Reibman J, Hsu Y, Chen LC, Kumar A, Su WC, Choy W, Talbot A, Gordon T. Size fractions of ambient particulate matter induce granulocyte macrophage colony-stimulating factor in human bronchial epithelial cells by mitogen-activated protein kinase pathways. *Am J Respir Cell Mol Biol* 2002, 27: 455–462.
149 Boland S, Bonvallot V, Fournier T, Baeza-Squiban A, Aubier M, Marano F. Mechanisms of GM-CSF increase by diesel exhaust particles in human airway epithelial cells. *Am J Physiol Lung Cell Mol Physiol* 2000, 278: L25–32.
150 Petrilli V, Dostert C, Muruve DA, Tschopp J. The inflammasome: A danger sensing complex triggering innate immunity. *Curr Opin Immunol* 2007, 19: 615–622.
151 Liu YJ, Soumelis V, Watanabe N, Ito T, Wang YH, Malefyt Rde W, Omori M, Zhou B, Ziegler SF. TSLP: An epithelial cell cytokine that regulates T cell differentiation by conditioning dendritic cell maturation. *Annu Rev Immunol* 2007, 25: 193–219.
152 Wang YH, Ito T, Wang YH, Homey B, Watanabe N, Martin R, Barnes CJ, McIntyre BW, Gilliet M, Kumar R, et al. Maintenance and polarization of human Th2 central memory T cells by thymic stromal lymphopoietin-activated dendritic cells. *Immunity* 2006, 24: 827–838.
153 Angkasekwinai P, Park H, Wang YH, Wang YH, Chang SH, Corry DB, Liu YJ, Zhu Z, Dong C. Interleukin 25 promotes the initiation of proallergic type 2 responses. *J Exp Med* 2007, 204: 1509–1517.
154 Liu YJ. Thymic stromal lymphopoietin and OX40 ligand pathway in the initiation of dendritic cell-mediated allergic inflammation. *J Allergy Clin Immunol* 2007, 120: 238–244.
155 Ito T, Wang YH, Duramad O, Hori T, Delespesse GJ, Watanabe N, Qin FX, Yao Z, Cao W, Liu YJ. TSLP-activated dendritic cells induce an inflammatory T helper type 2 cell response through OX40 ligand. *J Exp Med* 2005, 202: 1213–1223.
156 Liu YJ. Thymic stromal lymphopoietin: Master switch for allergic inflammation. *J Exp Med* 2006, 203: 269–273.
157 Valzasina B, Guiducci C, Dislich H, Killeen N, Weinberg AD, Colombo MP. Triggering of OX40 (CD134) on CD4(+)CD25+ T cells blocks their inhibitory activity: A novel regulatory role for OX40 and its comparison with GITR. *Blood* 2005, 105: 2845–2851.
158 Soumelis V, Reche PA, Kanzler H, Yuan W, Edward G, Homey B, Gilliet M, Ho S, Antonenko S, Lauerma A, et al. Human epithelial cells trigger dendritic cell mediated allergic inflammation by producing TSLP. *Nat Immunol* 2002, 3: 673–680.
159 Ying S, O'Connor B, Ratoff J, Meng Q, Mallett K, Cousins D, Robinson D, Zhang G, Zhao J, Lee TH, et al. Thymic stromal lymphopoietin expression is

increased in asthmatic airways and correlates with expression of Th2-attracting chemokines and disease severity. *J Immunol* 2005, 174: 8183–8190.
160 Ying S, O'Connor B, Ratoff J, Meng Q, Fang C, Cousins D, Zhang G, Gu S, Gao Z, Shamji B, et al. Expression and cellular provenance of thymic stromal lymphopoietin and chemokines in patients with severe asthma and chronic obstructive pulmonary disease. *J Immunol* 2008, 181: 2790–2798.
161 Hunninghake GM, Lasky-Su J, Soto-Quiros ME, Avila L, Liang C, Lake SL, Hudson TJ, Spesny M, Fournier E, Sylvia JS, et al. Sex-stratified linkage analysis identifies a female-specific locus for IgE to cockroach in Costa Ricans. *Am J Respir Crit Care Med* 2008, 177: 830–836.
162 Kato A, Favoreto S, Jr., Avila PC, Schleimer RP. TLR3- and TH2 cytokine-dependent production of thymic stromal lymphopoietin in human airway epithelial cells. *J Immunol* 2007, 179: 1080–1087.
163 Bleck B, Tse DB, Curotto de Lafaille MA, Zhang F, Reibman J. Diesel exhaust particle-exposed human bronchial epithelial cells induce dendritic cell maturation and polarization via thymic stromal lymphopoietin. *J Clin Immunol* 2008, 28: 147–156.

9

Role of macrophages in adverse pulmonary effects of particulate pollutants

Raymond Pieters

Abstract. Macrophages constitute a very diverse type of leukocytes of great importance in innate immunity and modulation of adaptive immune responses, including allergic responses. Lung or alveolar macrophages are known to engulf airborne particulates and retain these phagocytosed particles for a considerable time period. In addition other substances (e.g. chemicals attached to particles) may affect alveolar macrophages. The role of macrophages in pollutant-induced lung effects is complex as they may have opposite immunomodulating capacities. Stimulation of allergic responses may occur by extensive formation or release of proinflammatrory cytokines by macrophages that are stressed because they cannot destroy inert particles. On the other hand the down-regulating function of macrophages may be affected. In this chapter, the effects of particulate pollutants will be discussed from the point of view of the macrophage.

Keywords: macrophages, allergic inflammation, innate immunity, allergic asthma, diesel exhaust particulate matter, pulmonary inflammation, oxidative stress, reactive oxygen species, reactive nitrogen species, scavenger receptors, toll-like receptors, endocytosis, phagocytosis, antioxidant defense, viral infections, disease exacerbations

9.1 Introduction

The respiratory tract, in particular the huge gas-exchanging surface of the lungs, is continuously exposed to undesired substances in the air. These substances include microbes and microbial components, but also many different airborne chemical substances, including particles.

Results from epidemiological studies have demonstrated a link between increases of airway allergy and exposure to particulate matter, such as diesel exhaust particles (DEP), and have fueled concerns about the influence of air pollution on human health. Subsequent animal studies confirmed that particulates may indeed be responsible for triggering or inducing allergic airway responses.[1, 2, 3] Notably, particles were found to stimulate the release of adjuvant signals from innate cells of the immune system that subsequently caused activation of adaptive immune responses, including T and B cells. Based on in vivo and in vitro studies it has been suggested that macrophages play an important role in the particulate matter-mediated stimulation of adaptive immune responses.

The present chapter should be considered a brief summary of recently gathered and reviewed[4, 5] research in order to identify important caveats of knowledge in the view of human risk assessment of particulate air pollutants.

9.2 Macrophages as immunomodulating cells

More than a century after Metchnitkoff's discovery in 1883 that they are experts in phagocytosis, macrophages are regarded as one of the major innate effector cells of the immune system.[6, 7] It is now clear that macrophages are also producers of, for instance, various cytokines and chemokines, but in addition are very well capable of antigen presentation. As such, macrophages have a very important function in first-line defense and in translating the recognition of various potentially dangerous molecules to the adaptive immune system. Macrophages are found abundantly at sites where organisms come in contact with the environment, such as the skin, where they are called Langerhans cells. Conceivably, in an organ like the lungs that is continuously exposed to microbes and environmental pollutants macrophages are also abundantly present. With respect to airborne pollutants, e.g. particulates or occupational chemicals, alveolar macrophages are among the first cells that will encounter and respond to these pollutants. In the case of particulates the response consists of activation (for instance production of proinflammatory cytokines), phagocytosis and production of reactive species, such as reactive oxygen species[8] and reactive nitrogen species (RNS).

By their specific properties, macrophages can modulate responses of other innate immune cells, dendritic cells (DC) and lymphocytes, scavenge pathogens and kill these pathogens directly by ROS and RNS. Alveolar cells cooperate with other pulmonary cells, in particular epithelial cells and dendritic cells. All these cells have been demonstrated to be involved in responses to airborne particulates, but because of their unique scavenging ability macrophages may be considered the main target cells of particulates. Chemical pollutants may target any of the cells mentioned, but the main focus of this chapter will be on particulates, because of their link with macrophages.

9.3 Ubiquitous role of macrophages in immune homeostasis

Macrophages are mostly regarded as phagocytes that engulf larger microbes and all kinds of particulate matter, but they also influence the function of other innate cells as well as adaptive cells.[7] Phagocytosis triggers production of proinflammatory cytokines and chemokines and ROS/RNS. As a result of cytokine production, other cells may be attracted and inflammatory responses may ensue, whereas ROS/RNS help to kill and destroy microbes. These products of respiratory burst are also involved in antigen processing and presentation. Although macrophages are less effective as antigen presenting cells than professional antigen presenting DC, they express the whole machinery (including MHC class II and costimulatory molecules such as CD80 and CD86) required to sensitize T lymphocytes.

Macrophages express many different receptors to recognize foreign substances. These include so-called macrophage scavenger receptors (e.g. the SR called MARCO or macrophage receptor with collagenous structure), Fc and complement receptors (binding receptors for antibodies or complement that help to recognize opsonized substances), and a whole range of additional receptors that belong to a group of receptors collectively called pattern recognition receptors (PRRs). Well-known PRRs are toll-like receptors (TLRs), NOD-like receptors (NLRs), and carbohydrate receptors (e.g. DC-SIGN). Moreover, macrophages have a battery of receptors for optimal functioning such as integrins, cytokine receptors and receptors to cross-talk with neural cells.

Macrophages may occur in different appearances, be stimulated in a number of different ways, and also have different effects on other immune cells. Depending on growth factors released from the cellular environment type 1 or type 2 macrophages, analogous to Th1 and Th2 cells may evolve, which are designated Mφ-1 and Mφ-2, respectively.[9, 10] Such different macrophage subsets have been described for the human situation, but also in mice different subsets of macrophages may occur (e.g. C57BL1 mice may have predominantly Mφ-1 macrophages, whereas macrophages of BALB/c mice are predominantly Mφ-2).[11] The growth factors involved (GM-CSF for Mφ-1 cells, and CSF for Mφ-2 for instance) may originate from surrounding tissue cells, but also in a sort of reverse activation signal from Th1 cells (for Mφ-1 cells) and from Th2 cells (for Mφ-2 cells).

These two extreme types of macrophages have contrasting effects on the adaptive immune response. Mφ-1 cells produce IL-23 and IL-12 (leading to production of IFN-γ by Th1 cells, cytotoxic T lymphocytes and NK cells) and are proinflammatory, whereas Mφ-2 cells produce IL10 and are expected to dampen immune responses, in particular Th1 responses. In addition, Mφ-2 cells may be involved in processes such as wound healing, scavenging debris and angiogenesis. Although Mφ-1 and Mφ-2 cells may counteract each other in a similar way to that in which Th1 and Th2 cells would,[12] in reality their interaction may lead to much more complicated responses. For instance, at incidences when allergic inflammation is ongoing the addition of IFN-γ to counteract Th2 cells may result in a more pronounced allergic reaction. Much has to be learned about the diverse population of macrophages, but for now it should be realized that macrophages cannot be regarded as a homogenous cell population. Rather, macrophages are from a family of cells with a central but varying role in immune homeostasis or are cells that may have opposite functions under different environmental circumstances. How functional alterations within this population relate to particulate-induced immune effects in the lungs has become increasingly clear over the past decade.

9.4 Particulate matter and macrophages

After administration via the respiratory tract (of mice), particulate matter such as diesel exhaust particles (DEP) or carbon black particles (CBP) is mostly found cell-free in the lung fluid (broncho-alveolar lavage fluid or BALF) or in macrophages. Even long after initial exposure (up to 21 days) particulates can be found in macrophages isolated by lung flushing. Conceivably, macrophages are regarded as one of the prime target cell of particulates in the lungs.

A recent review has compared 27 studies on effects of particulate matter on monocytes or macrophages.[5] Cells or cell lines that have been used are freshly isolated alveolar macrophages (AM), Human Peripheral Blood Mononuclear Cells (HPBMNC), J774.4, RAW264.7, THP-1 and U937. The comparative study by Mitschik et al.[5] focused on inflammatory cytokines, in the case of macrophages primarily TNF-α and IL-6, MIP1α and IL1α. All kinds of particles, including DEP, TiO2 and concentrated ambient air, have been tested in this way in concentrations ranging from

1 mg/μL for 24 hrs to 500 mg/μL for 2, 8 or 24 hrs and in all cases increases in the formation of these cytokines/chemokines were observed. Most incubations were performed with concentrations of 50 and 100 μg/mL, at durations of 9 to 24 hrs, but the lowest concentration that showed effects (on cytokine mRNA) was 5 to 10 μg/mL.

9.4.1 Particles and oxidative stress in macrophages

The underlying mechanism by which particles stimulate macrophages to produce proinflammatory mediators may involve similar processes to those triggered by other substances, including microbes. Many particles, however, cannot be degraded (easily) by macrophages, so they may keep on triggering the same (oxidative) processes for a long time.

It is well known that oxidative stress signals trigger activation processes in macrophages (and other leukocytes), leading to release of proinflammatory mediators (e.g. cytokines, chemokines) and upregulation of adhesion molecules. Indeed, particles have been shown to stimulate the formation of ROS and to trigger various signaling pathways in various cell types, including macrophages [13] and epithelial cells. [14] Conceivably, the consequence of ROS on macrophages depends on the amount of ROS formed and hence also on the concentration or dose of particles. Li et al. [4] have recently reviewed the possible outcomes of ROS-induction in relation to particle (DEP) exposure and have suggested a three-tier model to categorize the cellular responses in relation to the amount of ROS induced. At low ROS level protective effects are mediated by the transcription factor Nrf2 that elicits antioxidant defense mechanisms. These antioxidant mechanisms include well-known phase 2 enzymes such as HO-1, GST, catalase and SOD. Once this protective Tier 1 is overwhelmed by ROS, MAPK, NF-κB and AP-1 pathways will become active, which results in formation of proinflammatory mediators and increase of costimulatory molecules (on macrophage and dendritic cells, DCs). At an even higher dose of particles and ROS induction, severe cell stress with severe mitochondrial damage and death (apoptosis of necrosis) may occur. Particles may elicit oxidative stress simply because they contain redox-cycling chemicals, including transition metals (e.g. Fe, Co, Cr), polycyclic aromatic hydrocarbons (PAH) or quinones.

Beck-Speier et al. [15] have described a crucial role for arachidonic acid (AA)-related lipid mediators in the elemental carbon (EC)-induced oxidative stress. In this process both cPLA2, responsible for hydrolysis of membrane phospholipids and providing AA, and NADPH oxidase, involved in generation of ROS, appeared decisive since blocking either one of these enzymes with specific blocking agents prevented respiratory burst. Via the metabolization of AA, which serves as substrate for 5-lipoxygenase (5-LO) and cyclooxygenase (COX), a number of immunomodulating and activating mediators can be produced, including LTB4 and PGE2. In addition, as a result of ROS, isoprostanes may be formed that trigger further oxidative stress. Together these studies link early effects on membranes and membrane-related enzymes with release of proinflammatory and immunodulating signals.

For instance, Beck-Speier et al. [15] also showed that Printex 90, Printex G and DEP, which have low to weak oxidative potential compared to EC, only stimulated AA and PGE2/XTB2 (and not 8-isoprostane and LTB4 as did EC). In addition, in contrast to freshly suspended EC, aged EC (suspended for 24 hrs) caused mild oxidative stress and did not activate LTB4, whereas both fresh and aged EC were capable of inducing the formation of AA and PGE2/XTB2. EC had the strongest oxidative potential and this may suggest that optimum formation of lipid mediators is dependent on this potential. But the other particles, showing weak oxidative potential, also induced some formation of lipid mediators. Based on these studies the surface area of the particles, rather than their oxidative potential, appeared the main predictive factor for the cellular oxidative stress response (15). Apparently, a number of particle properties may be involved in the extent of macrophage activation. Which of these properties (e.g. size, surface, oxidative potential) are most important for adverse airways effect in humans is not yet fully understood and remains an important research topic for the future, in particular for the assessment of health risks of certain particles.

9.4.2 Receptors involved in particle uptake by macrophages

A receptor that has been shown to be involved in uptake of particles by macrophages is the scavenger receptor (SR) with collagenous structure MARCO (macrophage receptor with collagenous structure). MARCO has been demonstrated to mediate ingestion of unopsonized environmental particles such as TiO_2, Fe_2O_3, latex beads [16, 17, 18] and silica. [19] Whether binding and/or uptake of nanosize particles is mediated by SR-mediated processes is not completely clear. In a recent paper, [20] it has been demonstrated that (fluorescent) polystyrene particles as small as 20 nm are associated by MARCO-transfected COS-7 cells, but not by vector-only transfected COS-7 cells. The binding could not be completely inhibited by the MARCO ligand polyG, which is suggestive of a specific binding or binding to other unknown molecules. Larger particles (200 nm and 1 μm) were taken up by the MARCO+COS-7 cells, but to some extent also by COS-7 cells transfected with an empty vector. Despite the fact that the 20 nm particles were able to associate to the MARCO+COS-7 cells they were not internalized (although they formed small agglomerates). Contrarily, Geiser et al.[21] have demonstrated that ultrafine TiO2 (0.078 m) can be taken up by (porcine) lung macrophages in an endocytosis- and actin-independent manner. Obviously, depending on specific characteristics (e.g. size) particles may be taken up by macrophages in any of the different ways: by phagocytosis, pinocytosis or patocytosis (i.e. via specific membrane channels).[22, 21]

Other receptors involved in effects induced by particles are TLRs, in particular concerning ambient PM, or ultrafine engineered particles. In the case of ambient particles adhered TLR ligands such as LPS (lipopolysaccharide from Gram-negative bacteria, binding to TLR4) or LTA (Lipoteichoic Acid from Gram-positive bacteria, binding to TLR2) may stimulate responses induced by particles.[23] On the other hand particles may affect synthesis of TLR, thereby interfering with innate immune responses.[24]

Engineered nanosize particles may interfere with all kind of receptors on macrophages, including TLRs, mannose receptors, Fc receptors, complement receptors and scavenger receptors. The binding specificity clearly depends on the nature (e.g. attached sugar moieties), and effort can be made to minimize the binding (for instance by modification with PEG). Depending on the binding characteristics different nanoparticles may influence different functions.[25]

9.5 Link between particle-induced macrophage activation, respiratory allergy and lung infections

In vivo studies have shown that particles (e.g. DEP, CBP) elicit allergic responses to bystander antigens (OVA or pollen for instance).[1, 3, 26, 27] This effect is caused by a so-called adjuvant effect of particles, involving release of pro-inflammatory cytokines and induction of Th2-driven immune responses. Several studies have also demonstrated that exposure to particles, in particular DEP, decreases clearance of bacteria such as *Listeria monocytogenes*.[28] Still other studies have shown that exposure to DEP can enhance the susceptibility to viral infections, such as influenza virus[29] and respiratory syncytial virus (RSV).[8] The decreased clearance of bacteria may be due to the effect of DEP on macrophages, whereas the increased susceptibility to viruses is most probably the result of decreased function of epithelial cells, which are the main target cells of virus infections. In vitro studies with DEP-treated epithelial cells have revealed that oxidative stress interfered with protective innate mechanisms, possibly production of surfactant proteins, resulting in increased virus attachment and entrance.[29]

After having engulfed DEP, alveolar macrophages produce more ROS, HO-1 and IL-10 but less TNF-α, IL1-β, IL-12.[28, 30, 31] T cells which normally occur after Listeria infection are less well developed and able to produce IL-2 and IFN-γ.[32] The effect of DEP appeared to result to a great extent from the adhered organic compounds, since washed-DEP and CPB were less effective in modulating macrophage function, and organic extracts of DEP were as effective as DEP as such.

As mentioned, at extremes macrophages display Mφ-1 or Mφ-2 phenotypes. Although these subsets or phenotypic appearances of macrophages have not been studied extensively in relation to the lungs their distinctive function may help to explain to why particles inhibit bacterial clearance on one hand and stimulate allergic responses on the other. Both in mice and rats such Mφ-1 or Mφ-2 have been found and studied. Alveolar macrophages (AM) isolated from Brown Norway rats, which have been used in models of asthma, produce all kind of cytokines including IL-12, IL-10 and IL-13 and increased levels of NO.[33] AM isolated from asthma-resistant Sprague-Dawley rats produce high amounts of TNF-α, but lower amounts of all other cytokines, particularly of type-2 cytokines. Also in different mouse strains opposite macrophage subsets have been found. The phagocytosis capacity of Mφ-1 or Mφ-2 bronchoalveolar macrophages isolated from respectively C57BL/6 mice or BALB/c mice in resting conditions is very different.[34] Under normal resting conditions, the capacity to phagocytose unopsonized particles (carboxylate-modified fluorescent latex beads of 2 μm), expression of MARCO and production NO-species was higher in C57BL/6-derived alveolar Mφ-1 macrophages than in BALB/c-derived alveolar Mφ-2 macrophages. Under stressful conditions (i.e. macrophages were isolated from mice that had undergone severe exercise) the functional capacity of Mφ-2 cell changed remarkably. Stressed Mφ-2 macrophages (isolated from BALB/c mice that had undergone severe exercise) showed increased MARCO expression and phagocytic activity, similar to Mφ-1 macrophages. The high macrophage activity of the Mφ-1-type of macrophages is possibly involved in the high protection of C57BL/6 mice to tuberculosis infection, whereas the high production of NO-related suppressors by Mφ-1 macrophages may to some extent inhibit further immune activation (of phagocytosis and activation of acquired immunity) and inhibit in particular Th1-mediated immune responses.

These differences in macrophage phenotypes may be involved in the DEP-mediated decreased defense against bacteria (Listeria, see above) and the concurrent increase of allergic responses. Although no research data are available, the apparently contradicting effect of DEP is due to a misbalance of various subsets of macrophages. Briefly, Mφ-1 cells, which are efficient in phagocytosis, that have taken up particles will produce high amounts of nitric compounds. As a result further phagocytosis as well as production of type-1 cytokines (in particular IL-12, which is an IFN-γ stimulating cytokine) will be inhibited. This will provide room for Mφ-2 macrophages that under stress conditions become more efficient phagocytotic cells. Mφ-2 cells can thus be activated as well (due to a stressful situation of particle exposure) and start to produce PGE2 and IL-10, thus promoting allergic responses.[35] Although the mechanism described may be important, other studies (not related to particles) have shown that viral infections stimulate the formation of IFN-γ and TNF-α, thereby contributing to the exacerbation of asthma.[36] Possibly, the unique effect of inert particles or extracts, and the timing of various exposures (particles versus bacteria or viruses) determine the sequence of effects and the final outcome.

The role of macrophages in particulate matter-induced respiratory effects has to be considered in the context of the presence of other pulmonary cells, including epithelial cells (which are also target of viruses), fibroblasts, neurons and other immune cells including mast cells and DC. DC, which are closely related to macrophages, are likely to be involved in translating signals released from macrophages to the adaptive immune response cells, i.e. T and B lymphocytes. Recently, it has been shown that carbon black particles particularly activate myeloid or conventional DC (mDC or cDC) and not plasmacytoid DC (pDC).[37] This is of relevance in view of the idea that pDC may have an immunoregulatory role in the lungs, in contrast to mDC that may have a stimulating role.

All of the cells mentioned, although some of these are less equipped with phagocytic machinery than macrophages, may respond quite similarly to interaction and uptake of particles: i.e. all these cells may respond to particles with increased production of ROS and RNS and various inflammatory mediators. Conceivably, it is very likely that of the various pulmonary cells more than a single one is involved in the final respiratory effects of particle exposure, but also that the macrophage, because of its unique properties, is indeed one of the most important ones involved.

9.6 Future perspectives

Over the last decade a lot of information has been gathered on the role of macrophages in adverse respiratory effects by particulate matter. However, a number of key questions remain to be resolved. For societal reasons, studies that aim at determining which of the particle characteristics is most crucial in modulation of macrophage activity seem extremely relevant. This knowledge, i.e. direct linking of particle characteristics with possible health effects, would facilitate effective risk assessment and management of health effects.

Mechanistic knowledge of cellular effects of particles on macrophages (and other cells) is already extensive. But the exact pathophysiological role of these cellular effects in combination with the different phenotypes of macrophages that occur in the lungs is not known. Since different phenotypes of macrophages may have a diverse capacity to clear particles and to modulate acquired immune responses further, elucidation of the exact role of macrophages in the context of other pulmonary cells is clearly warranted.

References

1 Nilsen, A., Hagemann, R., and Eide, I. 1997. The adjuvant activity of diesel exhaust particles and carbon black on systemic IgE production to ovalbumin in mice after intranasal instillation. *Toxicology* 124: 225–232.

2 Li, N., Hao, M., Phalen, R.F., Hinds, W.C., and Nel, A.E. 2003. Particulate air pollutants and asthma. A paradigm for the role of oxidative stress in PM-induced adverse health effects. *Clin. Immunol.* 109: 250–265.

3 van Zijverden, M., de Haar, C., van Beelen, A., van Loveren, H., Penninks, A., and Pieters, R. 2001. Coadministration of antigen and particles optimally stimulates the immune response in an intranasal administration model in mice. *Toxicol. Appl. Pharmacol.* 177: 174–178.

4 Li, N., Xia, T., and Nel, A.E. 2008. The role of oxidative stress in ambient particulate matter-induced lung diseases and its implications in the toxicity of engineered nanoparticles. *Free Radic. Biol. Med.* 44: 1689–1699.

5 Mitschik, S., Schierl, R., Nowak, D., and Jorres, R.A. 2008. Effects of particulate matter on cytokine production in vitro: a comparative analysis of published studies. *Inhal. Toxicol.* 20: 399–414.

6 Tauber, A.I., 1990. Metchnikoff, the modern immunologist. *J. Leukoc. Biol.* 47: 561–567.

7 Gwinn, M.R., Vallyathan, V. 2006. Respiratory burst: role in signal transduction in alveolar macrophages. *J. Toxicol. Environ. Health B Crit. Rev.* 9: 27–38.

8 Harrod, K.S., Jaramillo, R.J., Rosenberger, C.L., Wang, S.Z., Berger, J.A., McDonald JD, Reed MD. 2003. Increased susceptibility to RSV infection by exposure to inhaled diesel engine emissions. *Am. J. Respir. Cell. Mol. Biol.* 28: 451–463.

9 Verreck, F.A.W., de Boer, T., Langenberg, D.M., Hoeve, M.A., Kramer, M., Vaisberg, E., Kastelein, R., Kolk, A., de Waal Malefyt, R., and Ottenhof, T.H.M. 2004. Human IL-23-producing type 1 macrophages promote but IL-10-

producing type 2 macrophages subvert immunity to (myco)bacteria. *Proc. Natl. Acad. Sci. USA* 101: 4560–4565.

10 Verreck, F.A.W., de Boer, T., Langenberg, D.M., van der Zanden, L., and Ottenhoff, T.H. 2006. Phenotypic and functional profiling of human proinflammatory type-1 and anti-inflammatory type-2 macrophages in response to microbial antigens and IFN-gamma- and CD40L-mediated costimulation. *J. Leukoc. Biol.* 79: 285–293.

11 Mills, C.D., Kincaid, K., Alt, J.M., Heilman, M.J., and Hill, A.M. 2000. M-1/M-2 macrophages and the Th1/Th2 paradigm. *J. Immunol.* 164: 6166–6173.

12 Tang, C., Inman, M.D., van Rooijen, N., Yang, P., Shen, H., Matsumoto, K., and Byrne P.M.O. 2001. Th type 1-stimulating activity of lung macrophages inhibits Th2-mediated allergic airway inflammation by an IFN-gamma-dependent mechanism. *J. Immunol.* 166: 1471–1481.

13 Li, N., Venkatesan, M.I., Miguel, A., Kaplan, R., Gujuluva, C., Alam, J., and Nel A.E. 2000. Induction of heme oxygenase-1 expression in macrophages by diesel exhaust particle chemicals and quinones via the antioxidant-responsive element. *J. Immunol.* 165: 3393–3401.

14 Li, N., Wang, M., Oberley, T.D., Sempf, J.M., and Nel, A.E. 2002. Comparison of the pro-oxidative and proinflammatory effects of organic diesel exhaust particle chemicals in bronchial epithelial cells and macrophages. *J. Immunol.* 169: 4531–4541.

15 Beck-Speier, I., Dayal, N., Karg, E., Maier, K.L., Schumann, G., Schulz, H., Semmler, M., Takenaka, S., Stettmaier K., Bors, W., Ghio, A., Samet, J.M., and Heyder, J. 2005. Oxidative stress and lipid mediators induced in alveolar macrophages by ultrafine particles. *Free Radic. Biol. Med.* 38: 1080–1092.

16 Kobzik, L. 1995. Lung macrophage uptake of unopsonized environmental particulates. Role of scavenger-type receptors. *J. Immunol.* 155: 367–374.

17 Palecanda A, Paulauskis J, Al-Mutairi E, Imrich A, Qin G, Suzuki, H., Kodama, T., Truggvason, K., Koziel, H., and Kobzik, L. 1999. Role of the scavenger receptor MARCO in alveolar macrophage binding of unopsonized environmental particles *J. Exp. Med.* 189: 1497–1506.

18 Arredouani, M.S., Palecanda, A., Koziel, H., Huang, Y.C., Imrich, A., Sulahian, T.H., Ning, Y.Y., Yang, Z., Pikkarainen, T., Sankala, M., Vargas, S.O., Takeya, M., Truggvason, K., and Kobzik, L. 2005. MARCO is the major binding receptor for unopsonized particles and bacteria on human alveolar macrophages. *J. Immunol,* 175: 6058–6064.

19 Hamilton, R.F., Jr., Thakur, S.A., Holian, A. 2008. Silica binding and toxicity in alveolar macrophages. *Free Radic. Biol. Med.* 44: 1246–1258.

20 Kanno, S., Furuyama, A., Hirano, S. 2007. A murine scavenger receptor MARCO recognizes polystyrene nanoparticles. *Toxicol. Sci.* 97: 398–406.

21 Geiser, M., Rothen-Rutishauser, B., Kapp, N., Schurch, S., Kreyling, W., Schulz, H., Semmler, M., Im Hof, V., Heyder, J., and Gehr, P. 2005. Ultrafine particles cross cellular membranes by nonphagocytic mechanisms in lungs and in cultured cells. *Environ. Health Perspect.* 113: 1555–1560.

22 Kruth, H.S., Chang, J., Ifrim, I., Zhag, W.Y., 1999. Characterization of patocytosis: endocytosis into macrophage surface-connected compartments. *Eur. J. Cell. Biol.* 78: 91–99.

23 Mundandhara, S.D., Becker, S., and Madden, M.C. 2006. Effects of diesel exhaust particles on human alveolar macrophage ability to secrete inflammatory mediators in response to lipopolysaccharide. *Toxicol. In Vitro* 20: 614–624.
24 Becker, S., Mundandhara, S., Devlin, R.B., and Madden, M. 2005. Regulation of cytokine production in human alveolar macrophages and airway epithelial cells in response to ambient air pollution particles: further mechanistic studies. *Toxicol. Appl. Pharmacol.* 207: 269–275.
25 Dobrovolskaia, M.A., and McNeil S.E. 2007. Immunological properties of engineered nanomaterials. *Nat. Nanotechnol.* 2: 469–478.
26 Whitekus, M.J., Li, N., Zhang, M., Wang, M., Horwitz, M.A., Nelson, S.K., Horwitz, L.D., Brechun, N., Diaz-Sanchez, D., and Nel, A.E. 2002. Thiol antioxidants inhibit the adjuvant effects of aerosolized diesel exhaust particles in a murine model for ovalbumin sensitization *J. Immunol.* 168: 2560–2567.
27 de Haar, C., Hassing, I., Bol, M., Bleumink, R., and Pieters, R. 2006. Ultrafine but not fine particulate matter causes airway inflammation and allergic airway sensitization to co-administered antigen in mice. *Clin. Exp. Allergy* 36: 1469–1479.
28 Yin XJ, Dong CC, Ma JY, Antonini JM, Roberts JR, Barger, M.W., and Ma, J.K.H. 2005. Sustained effect of inhaled diesel exhaust particles on T-lymphocyte-mediated immune responses against Listeria monocytogenes. *Toxicol. Sci.* 88: 73–81.
29 Jaspers, I., Ciencewicki, J.M., Zhang, W., Brighton, L.E., Carson, J.L., Beck, M.A., and Madden, M.C. 2005. Diesel exhaust enhances influenza virus infections in respiratory epithelial cells. *Toxicol. Sci.* 85: 990–1002.
30 Yin, X.J., Ma, J.Y., Antonini, J.M., Castranova, V., and Ma, J.K. 2004. Roles of reactive oxygen species and heme oxygenase-1 in modulation of alveolar macrophage-mediated pulmonary immune responses to Listeria monocytogenes by diesel exhaust particles. *Toxicol. Sci.* 82: 143–153.
31 Nilsen, A.M., Hagemann, R., Eikas, H., Egeberg, K., Norkov, T., and Sundan, A. 2003. Reduction of IL-12 p40 production in activated monocytes after exposure to diesel exhaust particles. *Int. Arch. Allergy Immunol.* 131: 201–208.
32 Yin, X.J., Dong, C.C., Ma, J.Y., Roberts, J.R., Antonini, J.M., and Ma, J.K. 2007. Suppression of phagocytic and bactericidal functions of rat alveolar macrophages by the organic component of diesel exhaust particles. *J. Toxicol. Environ. Health A* 70: 820–828.
33 Sirois, J., Bissonnette, E.Y. 2001. Alveolar macrophages of allergic resistant and susceptible strains of rats show distinct cytokine profiles. *Clin. Exp. Immunol.* 126: 9–15.
34 Su, S.H., Chen, H., and Jen, C.J. 2001. C57BL/6 and BALB/c bronchoalveolar macrophages respond differently to exercise. *J. Immunol.*, 167: 5084–5091.
35 Kapsenberg, M.L. 2003. Dendritic-cell control of pathogen-driven T-cell polarization. *Nat. Rev. Immunol.* 3: 984–993.
36 Dery, R.E., and Bissonnette, E.Y. 1999. IFN-gamma potentiates the release of TNF-alpha and MIP-1alpha by alveolar macrophages during allergic reactions. *Am. J. Respir. Cell. Mol. Biol.* 20: 407–412.
37 de Haar, C., Kool, M., Hassing, I., Bol, M., Lambrecht, B.N., Pieters, R. 2008. Lung dendritic cells are stimulated by ultrafine particles and play a key role in particle adjuvant activity. *J. Allergy Clin. Immunol.* 121: 1246–1254.

10

Particulate air pollution and vulnerability to respiratory infections in children

Jonathan Grigg

Abstract. Children are especially vulnerable to particulate matter (PM) air pollution since their respiratory rate is higher and defences against oxidative stress may be impaired. Increased vulnerability to bacterial pneumonia due to exposure to high levels of PM from the burning of biomass fuels is one of the most important global environmental threats to children's health. Children in the developed world are exposed to lower levels of PM – predominantly from fossil fuel combustion and environmental tobacco smoke. In this population, the association between exposure and vulnerability to bacterial and viral respiratory infection remains poorly defined. The mechanism whereby PM increases vulnerability of respiratory cells to infection is also unclear, but chronic oxidative stress is likely to be involved.

Keywords: air pollution, pediatric health, smog, particulate matter, airway inflammation, airway macrophages, ultrafine particulate matter, development, oxidative stress, genetic susceptibility, gene polymorphisms, respiratory infections, respiratory syncytial virus, biomass particulate matter, environmental tobacco smoke

10.1 Introduction

Some of the first evidence that particulate matter (PM) air pollution increases vulnerability of children to respiratory infections is provided by Logan's classic report of the London air pollution incident of 1952.[1] The pollution incident lasted from Friday December 5th to early in the morning of Tuesday December 9th and during this period, deaths of infants aged 1 to 12 months more than doubled, and deaths in children rose by a third.

Subgroup analysis, albeit relatively crude, found that most of these pediatric deaths were from either "bronchitis" or "pneumonia" – both conditions associated with primary infections of the lower respiratory tract (Table 10.1).[1]

Since the London smog event was associated with a dramatic increase in several air pollutants, including carbonaceous particulate matter (PM), sulphur dioxide and nitrogen dioxide, PM may not have been the major toxic agent. However, recently Hunt et al. (2) studied autopsy lung specimens from individuals who died shortly after the smog event, which were stored at the Royal London Hospital, Whitechapel. Microanalysis of this lung tissue revealed that the common feature of the exogenous PM in all lung compartments was aggregates of fine carbonaceous material (unit size ≤0.1 μm) associated with a variety of fine (generally ≤1.0 μm) inorganic particles; a finding that was interpreted as being consistent with the hypothesis that carbonaceous PM – especially those containing metals – was the important toxic agent for The London Smog Event of 1952. One of the 18 subjects was a child aged six months who died of "bronchitis" (in retrospect probably bacterial pneumonia). In this case, no "quantifiable" amounts of exogenous PM were found in this child's lung tissue.[2]

There is, however, no doubt that inhaled carbonaceous PM reach pediatric lower airway cells – even under conditions of relatively low exposure. For example, in a study based in a medium-sized UK city, we sampled airway macrophages (AM) from children with no respiratory symptoms undergoing elective surgery. Cells were sampled using a blindly wedged suction catheter, and the resulting fluid was centrifuged and the cell pellet fixed for electron microscopy. Next, 100 nm thick sections of AM were examined to locate particles. We detected PM in AM in all children – the percentage of particle-containing AM ranged from 1 percent to 16 percent per child (Figure 10.1). Furthermore, all particles in AM were ultrafine (<0.1 μm diameter) (Figure 10.1), and microanalysis was consistent with a carbonaceous core.[3] Lower airway cells in children living in London in 1952 must therefore have been exposed to high levels of carbonaceous PM aggregates. The apparent

Table 10.1 Deaths from bronchitis and pneumonia in infants for the London Administrative County during December 1952 (1). Deaths during the air pollution incident are given in the December 13th column.

	Dec 6th	Dec 13th	Dec 20th
Bronchitis under 1 years	2	6	1
Pneumonia under 1 years	5	9	7

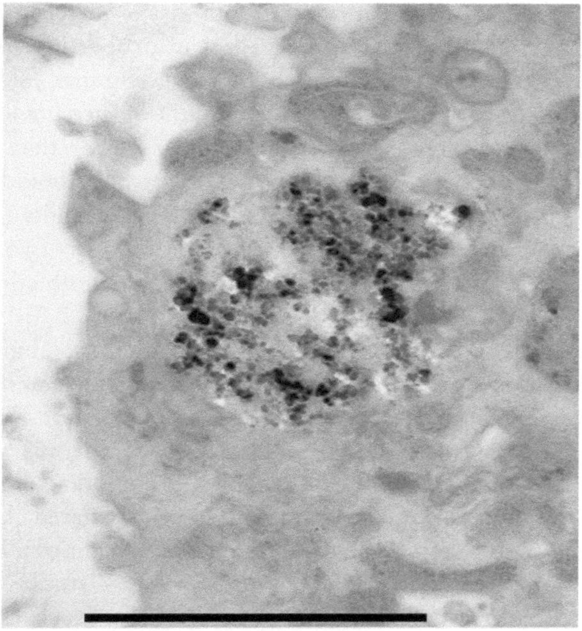

Figure 10.1 Electron micrograph of an airway macrophage removed from a healthy three-month-old boy undergoing elective surgery using bronchoalveolar lavage. Aggregates of carbonaceous nanoparticles, compatible with inhaled fossil fuel PM, are present in the phagolysosome. Bar represents 1000 nm.

paucity of PM in the six-month-old child in the study of Hunt et al.[(2)] may still therefore represent much higher levels than we observed under modern-day exposure conditions.

The aim of this chapter is to assess the recent evidence that particulate air pollution is an important vulnerability factor for childhood infections. This chapter will review why lung physiology, immaturity in airway cell function, and lung growth, may result in increased vulnerability of children to PM-associated health effects, and then consider the strength of the epidemiological evidence for the association between particulate air pollution and pediatric lung infections.

10.2 Developmental vulnerability

From birth to eight years of age, the lung grows by developing new alveoli and capillaries. Subsequently lung growth is via expansion of these structures. Since the surface area of the air–tissue interface of the lung ($3m^2$ at birth, $75m^2$ in adulthood) increases in proportion to the rest of the body, exposure of lower airway cells to pollutants, including PM, is approximately the same from birth to adulthood *per breath*. However, the metabolic rate of children is proportionally higher than adults, and in order to match oxygen consumption with carbon dioxide excretion, children need to take more breaths *per minute* than adults (Table 10.2). Thus for the same concentration of particles, the airways of young children will be exposed to more particles (and gases) per minute compared with adults.

Many studies (reviewed in Chapter 5) suggest that the ability of PM to induce an oxidative stress in airway cells modulates their toxicity and the resulting adverse health effects. Although there is concern that children's airway cells are more vulnerable to oxidative stress, there is a remarkable paucity of data on developmental changes in pulmonary antioxidant enzymes (AOEs) and enzyme induction, and age-associated changes in the concentrations of the key alveolar epithelial lining antioxidants such as glutathione and ascorbate. In one of the very few studies in humans, Asikainen et al.[4] measured the mRNA and activity levels of superoxide dismutases (SOD), catalyse (CAT), and glutathione peroxidase (GPx) in adult, neonatal (35 to 42 week gestation), and fetal (15 to 19 week gestation) lung tissue samples. Although large individual variations in mRNA and activity were found, SOD and CAT mRNA tended to be lower in fetusus and neonates, and GPx mRNA was similar to adult levels.

Confusingly, AOE activity did not mirror mRNA expression: SOD activity was not impaired, CAT activity was reduced, and GPx activity tended to be higher in neonates compared with adults. Overall, these data do not convincingly show that cells from young children are more vulnerable to oxidative stress – but there is a lack of robust data. Recent data, currently published only in abstract, does, however, provide preliminary evidence for developmental changes in cellular responses to PM. Lin et al.[5] performed

Table 10.2 Normal range for respiratory rate

Age	Breaths per minute
Birth to 1 year	30 to 60
1 to 3 years	24 to 40
3 to 6 years	22 to 34
6 to 12 years	18 to 30
12 to 18 years	12 to 16

Source: www.health.state.ny.us/nysdoh/ems/pdf/assmttools.pdf

diesel exhaust particle (DEP) exposures of 0 to 300 μg/m^3 to 20 adults and 15 children aged 10 to 15 years. At highest exposure, children had increased nasal passage cellular inflammation, and decreased mRNA expression of the antioxidant gene glutathione S-transferase pi (GSTP1) compared with adults.

A major difference between children and adults is that children's lungs are growing. Reduced lung growth, from whatever cause, is a non-specific risk factor for increased respiratory symptoms associated with a range of respiratory diseases. For example, infants with lower lung function in the first weeks of life are at increased risk of developing symptoms of RSV-bronchiolitis.(6) Although there are no data from children, in a prospective longitudinal study of over 13,000 adults, reduced lung function was found to be consistently related to both pneumonia-related mortality and hospitalization.(7) There is, however, good evidence that PM exposure impairs children's lung function growth. In the seminal 12 Community Southern California study, Gauderman et al.(8) measured lung function growth in 1,759 school-age children between the ages of 10 and 18 years. Over an eight-year period, reduced lung growth was associated with both $PM_{2.5}$ and black carbon. Furthermore, the proportion of 18-year-olds with clinically significantly low lung function was 4.9 times higher in communities with the highest levels of exposure to $PM_{2.5}$. Additional support for these data was provided by our study of the association between lung function in normal children and the amount of inhaled carbonaceous material in lower AM. Using image analysis we quantified the median area of AM carbon from 100 cells per child (n=64). For each increase of 1.0 μm^2 in carbon content we found a reduction of 17 percent (95 percent CI, 5.6 to 28.4) in forced expiratory volume in one second (the maximum volume of breath that can be forcibly expelled in one second), and a reduction of 34.7 percent (95 percent CI; 11.3 to 58.1) in the forced expiratory flow between 25 and 75 percent of the forced vital capacity (a marker of smaller airway function).(9) In summary, there are several reasons why children may be more vulnerable to the PM-induced vulnerability to infection. These include increased minute deposition of PM in the lower airway, attenuated antioxidant defenses, and impaired lung growth.

10.3 Respiratory infections in children

Infection-associated respiratory diseases in children include bacterial pneumonia, viral-bronchiolitis, and viral-triggered wheeze. Pneumonia is due to infection-triggered inflammation of the lung tissue. In children, the major causative pathogens for pneumonia change with age. In neonates less than three weeks of age, pneumonia is often caused by acquisition of bacteria from the mother around the time of birth. Common organisms include *Escherichia coli*, Group B streptococci, and *Listeria monocytogenes*. In preschool children, respiratory viruses (adenovirus, influenza virus, parainfluenza virus 1 to 3, and respiratory syncytial virus) are the most frequent cause of clinical pneumonia. In children who are more unwell with high fever and lethargy, bacterial pneumonia caused by *Streptococcus pneumoniae* is common. The signs of bacterial pneumonia are localized inspiratory crackles over the area of the infected lung, and in some cases, reduced breath sounds resulting from accumulation of pus in the pleural space (empyema). In the teenage years, *Mycoplasma pneumoniae* increasingly becomes an important etiologic agent. Bronchiolitis is a seasonal condition, predominately seen in infants less than 12 months of age, and is caused by direct respiratory viral infection of the smaller airways (bronchioles). Respiratory syncytial virus (RSV) is the commonest cause of bronchiolitis and the terms "bronchiolitis and "RSV-bronchiolitis" are often used interchangeably by pediatricians. Bronchiolitis is characterized by generalized fine inspiratory crackles throughout the whole lung, an increased respiratory rate, and a moist "bubbly" cough.[(10)] Some children require admission to hospital because of poor feeding and need for supplemental oxygen. Bronchiolitis is not a relapsing condition since, in general, subsequent RSV infections cause only viral colds. In most children these viral colds are clinically trivial. However, in preschool children respiratory viruses, including RSV, can trigger attacks of wheeze (called "preschool viral-wheeze"). These attacks are clinically distinct from bronchiolitis since widespread crackles in the chest are infrequent and bilateral wheeze (a whistling sound on expiration) predominates.

Viral colds also trigger wheeze attacks in older children with allergic asthma. Children with preschool viral-wheeze tend to wheeze for a few days every time they get a viral cold, but do not wheeze between colds.[(11)] In contrast, children with asthma tend to have daily wheeze and cough, with superimposed viral-triggered wheezing "attacks".[(12)] The wide overlap in pathogens and symptoms between respiratory diseases in children presents a major problem when interpreting epidemiological studies into the association between PM exposure and vulnerability to respiratory infection, especially in children under six years of age. On one hand, RSV may cause either bronchiolitis, or vial pneumonia, or viral-wheeze. On the other hand, high fever with raised respiratory rate may occur in infants with either RSV bronchiolitis, or RSV pneumonia, or bacterial pneumonia.

10.4 Bacterial pneumonia in the developing world

The most plausible data for an association between PM and vulnerability to infection is provided by epidemiological studies in the developing world. Indeed, over the last decade, indoor air pollution from the burning of biomass fuels is now considered one of the most important threats to children's health, predominantly via an increased vulnerability to bacterial pneumonia.[13, 14] Since *Streptococcus pneumoniae* is the major cause of mortality from pneumonia in children in the developed world,[15] any environmental factor that increases vulnerability to *Streptococcus pneumoniae* will have a major impact. In a recent meta-analysis Dherani et al.[16] assessed whether risk of pneumonia is determined by aetiological agent and pneumonia severity in children less than five years of age exposed to emissions from solid fuels. Twenty-five studies were identified as meeting the meta-analysis criteria. The analysis suggested that the risk of pneumonia in young children is increased by exposure to unprocessed solid fuels by a factor of 1.78 (95 percent CI; 1.45 to 2.18).

This robust finding supports the World Health Organization's (WHO) statement that indoor air pollution is the eighth most important risk factor – responsible for 2.7 percent of the global burden of disease. The WHO estimates that: i) indoor smoke is responsible for an estimated 3.7 percent of the global disease burden, making it the most lethal killer after malnutrition, unsafe sex and lack of safe water and sanitation; and ii) acute lower respiratory infections represent the single most important cause of air pollution-related death in children under five years. The odds ratios (OR) from the meta-analysis of Dherani et al.[16] further support the WHO's view that exposure to indoor air pollution more than doubles the risk of pneumonia and is thus responsible for more than 900,000 of the two million annual deaths from pneumonia.[17]

A major limitation of the epidemiological data used by the WHO in estimating PM-induced health effects is that identification of causative pathogens is difficult in the developing world. Studies to date therefore cannot identify whether the effect of biomass smoke on respiratory infection in children is via increased susceptibility to viral infection, bacterial infection, or a combination of both. The independent effect of the biomass PM is difficult to assess in these developing world studies. However, PM remains the most plausible pollutant, since indoor air levels of PM in the developing world often exceed 1000 $\mu g/m^3$[14] – an order of magnitude greater than inhalable PM levels in the developed world.[18] High PM levels in air and near to huts in the developing world certainly result in increased exposure of lower airway lung cells to PM. For example, in a study in Gondar (Ethiopia) we sampled airway macrophages (AM) from mothers and children using sputum induction. Examination of the cells under light microscopy showed very high levels of phagocytosed carbon from both children and mothers living in biomass-burning huts (Figure 10.2).[19]

In the developing world "indoor" smoke is not the only source of biomass PM exposure. Indeed in Asia, biomass contributes to both "indoor" and outdoor "background" PM. For example, Gutafsson et al.,[20] using radiocarbon measurements of winter monsoon aerosols from western India and the Indian Ocean, determined that biomass combustion (from residential cooking and agricultural burning) produced 75 percent of the bulk carbonaceous aerosols. Levels of carbonaceous PM are not only higher in the developing world, but also the particles themselves may be more toxic on a mass for mass basis than those generated from fossil fuels.

For example, we assessed the pro-oxidative activity of PM derived from the burning of biomass fuel dung cake by examining their capacity to deplete antioxidants from a model human respiratory tract lining fluid.[21] For comparison, the observed oxidative activity was compared with that of

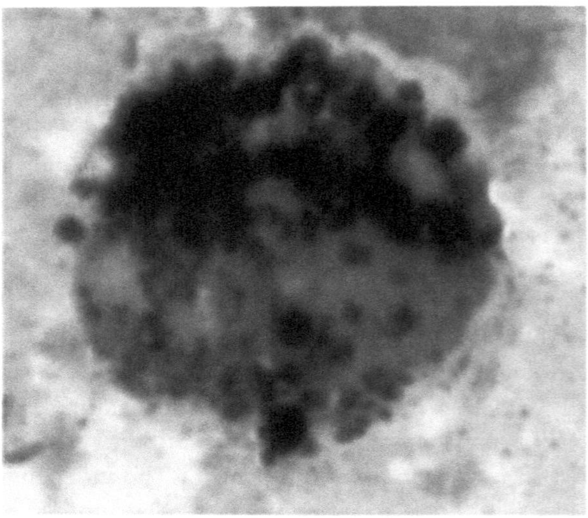

Figure 10.2 Airway macrophage from a healthy Ethiopian child chronically exposed to biomass smoke from an open cooking stove. Airway macrophages were sampled using induced sputum, smeared onto a microscope slide, stained with Diff-Quik, and imaged under oil immersion and light microscopy (x1000). The extensive back material represents inhaled carbon.

PM derived from vehicular sources. Incubation of the dung cake particle PM in the human respiratory tract lining fluid for four hours resulted in a mean loss of ascorbate, which was attenuated by co-incubation with a metal chelator (Figure 10.3).[21] In this model, reduced glutathione was also depleted by dung cake PM. Since dung cake PM had a significantly increased capacity to deplete ascorbate compared to diesel or gasoline particles (Figure 10.3),[21] children in the developing world are not only exposed to much higher levels of PM, but PM may be more toxic as a result of increased adsorbed metals.

As discussed above, biomass smoke contains not only inhalable particles of carbon, but compounds such as carbon monoxide and nitrogen oxides.[22, 23] Thus studies using PM and pathogens in animal and *in vitro* models are required in order to establish biological plausibility for the adverse effects of PM. To date, few animal studies have modeled the interaction between carbonaceous PM and infections that are relevant to children. Some supportive data is provided by Hatch et al.,[24] who instilled a range of particles into the lungs of mice (at a dose of 100 μg), then infected animals with aerosolised Group C *Streptococcus* sp (24). In this model, a single dose of carbonaceous particles significantly increases mortality from streptococcal infection, with detrimental effects seen with carbonaceous particles from ambient air (90 percent increase in mortality), and particles of pure carbon (39 percent increase).[24]

10.5 Bacterial pneumonia in the developed world

A recent case-crossover study of daily numbers of hospital admissions in five Australian and New Zealand cities[25] suggests that levels of PM found in developed world cities may also increase vulnerability to pneumonia. This study found that, in children of one to four years of age with doctor-diagnosed "pneumonia or bronchitis", there was a 2.4 percent (95 percent CI; 0.1 to 4.7) increase in admissions for an interquartile increase in $PM_{2.5}$ averaged over the current and previous day – an association that was not confounded by temperature. The study's limitations are: (a) "bronchitis" is a relatively imprecise diagnosis – usually meaning increased mucus production in the larger airways after viral infection; and (b) no distinction was made between bacterial and viral pneumonia.

Despite this, it provides the first convincing evidence that relatively low concentrations of fossil-fuel derived PM increase vulnerability to pneumonia – especially in young children. Exposure to environmental tobacco smoke (ETS) is also a potential source of PM exposure in children.

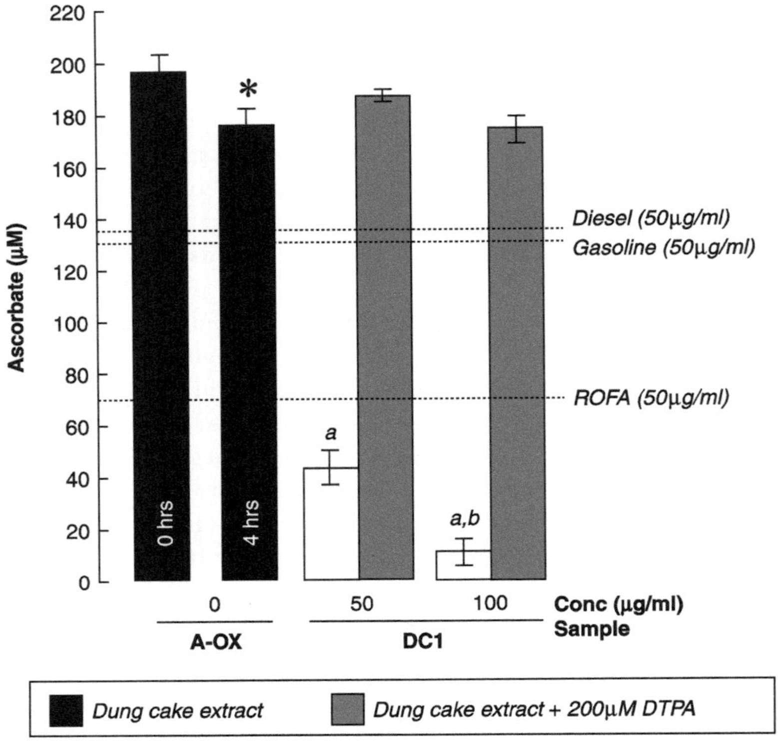

Figure 10.3 Ascorbate acid (AA) remaining in synthetic respiratory tract lining fluid following a four-hour incubation with dung cake (DC) particle samples at 50 and 100 µg/ml (white bars). The impact of co-incubation with the transition metal chelator DTPA (200mM) is illustrated by the grey bars. Pre (0hr) and post (4hr) AA concentrations in the particle-free controls are illustrated with black bars. The losses observed with 50mg/ml doses of fresh diesel and gasoline PM2.5, as well as residual oil fly ask (ROFA) are also illustrated. Data represent the mean (SD) of three separate experiments: "a" indicates that AA concentrations after the four-hour incubation were significantly lower ($P<0.05$) than the four-hour particle-free control values; "b" illustrates that the losses observed at 100 mg/ml are significantly greater than those seen at the lower 50 µg/ml concentration. The "*" illustrates a significant loss of AA in the particle free control over the four-hour incubation period.

For example, in a French study (of adults) using personal sampling, exposure to $PM_{2.5}$ in the home was primarily influenced by exposure to ETS. [26] Recently, Suzuki et al., in a cross-sectional survey of 24,781 Vietnamese children under five years of age, found that ETS exposure was independently associated with hospitalizations for pneumonia (adjusted odds ratio 1.55; 95 percent CI 1.25 to 1.92). From these data, the authors estimated that 28.7 percent of childhood pneumonia in Vietnam is attributable to ETS.[27]

Increased capacity of respiratory cells to support pneumococcal adhesion and colonization is one putative mechanism for increased vulnerability to pneumonia due to ETS-exposed children. Support for this is provided by a cross-sectional surveillance study of 208 Israeli children less than 60 months of age. In this study, carriage rate was significantly increased (76 percent) in ETS exposed children, compared with non-ETS-exposed children (60 percent). Although there are no data on the PM component of ETS, Ozlu et al.[28] reported that *S. pneumoniae* adherence to the buccal mucosa of rats was significantly increased in animals chronically exposed to cigarette smoke. Whether the PM component of ETS *per se* is responsible for these effects is unclear. It is, however, tempting to speculate that PM is the common factor underlying increased vulnerability infection associated with both exposure to biomass smoke and ETS.

10.6 Bronchiolitis

Few studies have addressed the effect of PM on infant bronchiolitis. Ségala et al. obtained two series of Paris hospital admission data for bronchiolitis in children under three years of age. In the period from 1997 to 2001 there were 50,857 emergency hospital consultations and 16,588 hospitalizations. After adjustment for holidays and metrological variables, a case-crossover model showed that PM_{10} was associated with both consultations and hospitalizations. For a lag of 0 to 4 days, each 10 $\mu g/m^3$ increase in PM_{10} was associated with odds ratio of 1.06 (1.04 to 1.08) for consultations and 1.06 (1.03 to 1.10) for admissions.[29]

A different perspective is provided by Karr et al.,[30] who used birth-hospital-discharge records of 18,596 infants born between 1995 and 2000 in the South Coast Air Basin of California. Cases with a hospital discharge for bronchiolitis in infancy were matched to ten age- and gestational-age-matched controls. Exposures in the month prior to hospitalization and mean lifetime exposure were estimated from data derived from the California Air Resources Board. In conditional logistic regression, both previous month and lifetime $PM_{2.5}$ exposures were associated with increased risk of bronchiolitis (adjusted OR for both exposure durations 1.09 (1.04 to 1.14) per $10\mu/m^3$. These studies suggest that there may be both chronic and acute effects of PM on vulnerability to RSV bronchiolitis.

There are animal studies to provide biologic plausibility for these epidemiological associations. Harrod et al.[31] exposed relatively RSV-resistant mice to diesel exhaust emissions (DEP; 30 or 1000 μg/m^3, six hours a day for six days), then infected animals with RSV. Histologically, both lung inflammation and airway epithelial remodelling to RSV were augmented by prior exposure to DEP. Although this model does not replicate the clinical syndrome of RSV bronchiolitis, it does suggest that DEP-exposed lungs may be more vulnerable to the first RSV infection. Lambert et al.[32] instilled 40 μg of ultrafine carbon black (i.e. aggregates of 14 nm pure carbon particles) into the lungs of mice, followed by infection with RSV. Although particle exposure did not enhance the replication of RSV in lung tissue, carbon black-exposed animals had more pulmonary neutrophils, and higher levels of lung tumor necrosis factor.

10.7 Interactions between viruses and bacteria

An important observation in the RSV study of Harrod et al. (31), described above, is that secondary bacterial pneumonia was only seen in animals exposed to both carbon and RSV. Delayed clearance of bacteria has also been reported after Influenza A infection,[33] but to date no study has explored the interaction between exposure to PM and this clinically important virus. In mice, RSV infection delays pulmonary clearance of *Pneumococcus, Staphylococcus aureus* and *Pseudomonas* for up to seven days.[34] It is therefore possible that the association between PM exposure and acute bacterial pneumonia is, in part, mediated via a PM-associated increase in vulnerability to *viral* infection. Indeed, Sigaud et al.[35] hypothesised that lungs that have recently been exposed to a respiratory virus would be "primed" by upregulation of interferon-gamma (IFN-γ). To model this, mice were first exposed to aerosolized IFN-γ, then concentrated ambient particles (CAPs), and finally pneumococcal infection. Overall clearance of bacteria from the lung was impaired in animals exposed to CAPs, an effect that was dramatically enhanced in IFN-γ "primed" animals.

10.8 Conclusions

The extent to which PM increases vulnerability to bacterial and viral respiratory infection and the underlying biological mechanism for this interaction are relevant and important questions. Epidemiological data to date strongly suggest that children are especially vulnerable to the adverse effect of PM – with potentially hundreds of thousands of excess deaths from bacterial pneumonia attributable to exposure to carbonaceous PM from biomass fuels. The extent to which relatively low levels of PM from both fossil fuels and ETS increases vulnerability to common respiratory infections in the developed world remains unclear, but may be one of the most important "reversible" environmental factors.

References

1 Logan WP. Mortality in the London fog incident, 1952. *Lancet* 1953, 1: 336–8.
2 Hunt A, Abraham JL, Judson B, Berry CL. Toxicologic and epidemiologic clues from the characterization of the 1952 London smog fine particulate matter in archival autopsy lung tissues. *Environ Health Perspect* 2003, 111: 1209–14.
3 Bunn HJ, Dinsdale D, Smith T, Grigg J. Ultrafine particles in alveolar macrophages from normal children. *Thorax* 2001, 56: 932–4.
4 Asikainen TM, Raivio KO, Saksela M, Kinnula VL. Expression and developmental profile of antioxidant enzymes in human lung and liver. *Am J Respir Cell Mol Biol* 1998, 19: 942–9.
5 Lin EM, Zhang L, Diaz-Sanchez D. Children demonstrate diminished antioxidant defences against diesel exhaust particles. *J Allergy Clin Immunol* 2007, 119: S236.
6 Young S, O'Keeffe PT, Arnott J, Landau LI. Lung function, airway responsiveness, and respiratory symptoms before and after bronchiolitis. *Arch Dis Child* 1995, 72: 16–24.
7 Lange P, Vestbo J, Nyboe J. Risk factors for death and hospitalization from pneumonia. A prospective study of a general population. *Eur Respir J* 1995, 8: 1 694–8.
8 Gauderman WJ, Avol E, Gilliland F, et al. The effect of air pollution on lung development from 10 to 18 years of age. *N Engl J Med* 2004, 351: 1057–67.
9 Kulkarni N, Pierse N, Rushton L, Grigg J. Carbon in airway macrophages and lung function in children. *N Engl J Med* 2006, 355: 21–30.
10 Stafler P. Dexamethasone for bronchiolitis. *N Engl J Med* 2007, 357: 1659–60; author reply 60.
11 Grigg J, Silverman M. Wheezing disorders in young children: one disease or several phenotypes? *Eur Respir Mon* 2006, 37: 6.
12 Johnston SL, Pattemore PK, Sanderson G, et al. Community study of role of viral infections in exacerbations of asthma in 9–11 year old children. *Bmj* 1995, 310: 1225–9.
13 Smith KR, Samet JM, Romieu I, Bruce N. Indoor air pollution in developing countries and acute lower respiratory infections in children. *Thorax* 2000, 55: 518–32.
14 Bruce N, Perez-Padilla R, Albalak R. Indoor air pollution in developing countries: a major environmental and public health challenge. *Bull World Health Organ* 2000, 78: 1078–92.
15 Scott JA. The preventable burden of pneumococcal disease in the developing world. *Vaccine* 2007, 25: 2398–405.

16 Dherani M, Pope D, Mascarenhas M, Smith KR, Weber M, Bruce N. Indoor air pollution from unprocessed solid fuel use and pneumonia risk in children aged under five years: a systematic review and meta-analysis. *Bull World Health Organ* 2008, 86: 390–8C.
17 World Health Organization. Indoor air pollution and health. 2005. (Accessed 9/1/2009, at http://www.who.int/mediacentre/factsheets/fs292/en/index.html.)
18 Air Quality, Expert Group. *Particulate Matter in the United Kingdom*. London: Defra Publications, 2005: 6–15.
19 Kulkarni NS, Prudon B, Panditi SL, Abebe Y, Grigg J. Carbon loading of alveolar macrophages in adults and children exposed to biomass smoke particles. *Sci Total Environ* 2005, 345: 23–30.
20 Gustafsson O, Krusa M, Zencak Z, et al. Brown clouds over South Asia: biomass or fossil fuel combustion? *Science* 2009, 323: 495–8.
21 Mudway IS, Duggan ST, Venkataraman C, Habib G, Kelly FJ, Grigg J. Combustion of dried animal dung as biofuel results in the generation of highly redox active fine particulates. *Part Fibre Toxicol* 2005, 2: 6.
22 Seagrave J, McDonald JD, Reed MD, Seilkop SK, Mauderly JL. Responses to subchronic inhalation of low concentrations of diesel exhaust and hardwood smoke measured in rat bronchoalveolar lavage fluid. *Inhal Toxicol* 2005, 17: 657–70.
23 Kocbach A, Johansen BV, Schwarze PE, Namork E. Analytical electron microscopy of combustion particles: a comparison of vehicle exhaust and residential wood smoke. *Sci Total Environ* 2005, 346: 231–43.
24 Hatch GE, Boykin E, Graham JA, et al. Inhalable particles and pulmonary host defense: in vivo and in vitro effects of ambient air and combustion particles. *Environ Res* 1985, 36: 67–80.
25 Barnett AG, Williams GM, Schwartz J, et al. Air pollution and child respiratory health: a case-crossover study in Australia and New Zealand. *Am J Respir Crit Care Med* 2005, 171: 1272–8.
26 Mosqueron L, Momas I, Le Moullec Y. Personal exposure of Paris office workers to nitrogen dioxide and fine particles. *Occup Environ Med* 2002, 59: 550–5.
27 Suzuki M, Thiem VD, Yanai H, et al. Environmental tobacco smoking exposure is associated with an increased risk of hospitalized pneumonia among children under 5 years old in Vietnam. *Thorax* 2009.
28 Ozlu T, Celik I, Oztuna F, Bulbul Y, Ozsu S. Streptococcus pneumoniae adherence in rats under different degrees and durations of cigarette smoke. *Respiration* 2008, 75: 339–44.
29 Segala C, Poizeau D, Mesbah M, Willems S, Maidenberg M. Winter air pollution and infant bronchiolitis in Paris. *Environ Res* 2008, 106: 96–100.
30 Karr C, Lumley T, Schreuder A, et al. Effects of subchronic and chronic exposure to ambient air pollutants on infant bronchiolitis. *Am J Epidemiol* 2007, 165: 553–60.
31 Harrod KS, Jaramillo RJ, Rosenberger CL, et al. Increased susceptibility to RSV infection by exposure to inhaled diesel engine emissions. *Am J Respir Cell Mol Biol* 2003, 28: 451–63.
32 Lambert AL, Trasti FS, Mangum JB, Everitt JI. Effect of preexposure to ultrafine carbon black on respiratory syncytial virus infection in mice. *Toxicol Sci* 2003, 72: 331–8.

33 LeVine AM, Koeningsknecht V, Stark JM. Decreased pulmonary clearance of S. pneumoniae following influenza A infection in mice. *J Virol Methods* 2001, 94: 173–86.
34 Stark JM, Stark MA, Colasurdo GN, LeVine AM. Decreased bacterial clearance from the lungs of mice following primary respiratory syncytial virus infection. *J Med Virol* 2006, 78: 829–38.
35 Sigaud S, Goldsmith CA, Zhou H, et al. Air pollution particles diminish bacterial clearance in the primed lungs of mice. *Toxicol Appl Pharmacol* 2007, 223: 1–9.

11

The intersection of respiratory syncytial virus infection, innate immunity and allergic lung disease

Michael H. Chi, Martin L. Moore and R. Stokes Peebles, Jr

Abstract. Respiratory syncytial virus (RSV) infection is the leading cause of bronchiolitis, pneumonia, and respiratory failure in infants younger than one year of age and is becoming more prevalently associated with serious illness and morbidity in elderly patients. A better understanding of the innate immune response to RSV infection may lead to developing effective therapy. The main objective of this chapter is to discuss the interplay between RSV infection, the environment, and the host innate immune response. Alterations in the host innate immune response as a result of allergic inflammation, ozone exposure, and ambient particulate matter may determine disease severity from RSV infection. In turn, RSV infection may modify host immunity to environmental stimuli. The impact of RSV infection on host innate immunity with comparison between the allergic asthmatic host and non-allergic, non-asthmatic host will be highlighted. Effects of RSV on inflammatory responses in the airway will also be discussed. Defining the factors that modulate the host innate immune response to RSV infection will shed light on the pathogenesis of this virus and provide insights into the development of treatment and prevention strategies.

Keywords: respiratory syncytial virus (RSV), pulmonary immunity, lung infections, innate immunity, asthma, chronic obstructive pulmonary disease (COPD), ambient particulate matter, ozone, pattern recognition receptors, toll-like receptor pathway, diesel engine emissions, airway hyperreactivity (AHR), airway inflammation, inflammatory cytokines, inflammatory chemokines

11.1 Introduction

In the United States, RSV is the most frequent cause of bronchiolitis, mechanical ventilation, and respiratory failure in infants. More than half of infants less than 12 months of age are infected with RSV, while almost all children have been infected with RSV by two years of age.[1] It is estimated that RSV-induced bronchiolitis causes more than 100,000 infant hospitalizations per year in the US.[2] RSV-induced illness is also becoming a prevalent cause of hospitalization in the elderly, chronic asthmatics, and those with chronic obstructive pulmonary disease (COPD).[3] There are currently no effective vaccines or post-infection treatments available for RSV. It is necessary to understand the mechanisms by which RSV infection causes illness in order to develop effective vaccines or treatments.

One important characteristic of RSV infection is that it results in little protective immunity; this often results in recurrent infections.[4] RSV's lack of immunogenicity could possibly be dependent on the complex mechanisms of the host innate immunity. Therefore, understanding how RSV interacts with the innate immune system could potentially lead to vaccines or treatments.

RSV infection has also been shown to alter allergic responses and has been postulated to result in chronic asthma. Exposure to ambient particulate matter and pollution affects RSV disease severity, while the timing of infection and allergen sensitization affects allergic response severity during later allergen challenges. Having a firm grasp on these relationships will help determine risk factors to predict augmented RSV-induced illness.

This chapter will discuss the interplay between RSV infection and host innate immunity. It will also focus on RSV infection with respect to allergic disease. The main topics to be discussed are pollution, ambient particulate matter and ozone, innate immunity gene polymorphisms, surfactant proteins (SPs), toll-like receptors (TLRs), interferon-α (IFN-α), dendritic cells (DCs), natural killer (NK) cells, and timing of infection and allergic sensitization and challenge. Results from experiments and studies in the human model will be included for sections when possible, but the amount of information is limited, due to the difficulties of exploring RSV pathogenesis in humans. Results from experimental *in vitro* and mouse models of RSV infection, as well as clinical studies will be included.

11.2 Pollution, ambient particulate matter, and ozone

Symptoms of RSV infection are affected by the environment. One important determinant of disease severity caused by RSV infection is exposure to contaminants in the air, such as pollution. A study was performed of children under the age of three years admitted to the emergency department for bronchiolitis during the RSV season (5). Particulate matter 10 (PM_{10}), black smoke (BS), sulfur dioxide (SO_2), and nitrogen dioxide (NO_2) were positively correlated with hospitalization for bronchiolitis using the generalized additive and case-crossover statistical models.[5] This study suggests that air pollution, including PM_{10}, BS, SO_2, and NO_2, plays a role in acute severe RSV bronchiolitis.

In a separate study, severe bronchiolitis was positively correlated to cigarette smoke.[6] Infants under 12 months old with severe bronchiolitis who tested positive for RSV were included in a cohort study to correlate RSV-induced bronchiolitis and environmental factors.[6] This study showed that postnatal cigarette smoke exposure altered lung function in RSV-infected infants while home allergen levels had no effect.[6] More specifically, this alteration of lung function caused by smoke exposure resulted in significantly decreased O_2 saturation.[6] These findings suggest that exposure to smoke may exacerbate RSV-induced illness in infants.

Pollution in the form of diesel engine emissions (DEE) showed similar effects to postnatal cigarette smoke. Mice exposed to DEE for six hours a day for seven days prior to RSV infection had exacerbated pulmonary inflammation compared to RSV infected mice not exposed to DEE.[7] The number of inflammatory cells in the bronchoalveolar lavage (BAL) fluid was also increased in mice exposed to DEE prior to RSV infection, while histology revealed inflammation linked to the exposure with DEE.[7] These findings suggest that pollution is a key factor in determining RSV-induced disease severity.

In addition to outdoor air pollution, contaminants of indoor air affect RSV disease. Two common biologically active indoor air contaminants are bacterial lipopolysaccharides (LPS) and house dust mite allergen (*Der p* I). Airway epithelial cells inoculated with LPS four hours before or at the same time as RSV infection exhibited a dose-dependent decrease in viral infectious yield (8). A decrease in the expression of IL-8 occurred when the cells were inoculated with LPS at the same time as RSV infection.[8] In a parallel experiment, airway epithelial cells were inoculated with *Der p* I at the same time as RSV infection.[8] These cells exhibited contrasting results from the LPS experiment; there was an increase in RSV replication as well as IL-8 production.[8] These results suggest that common indoor air contaminants play a role in the innate immune response to RSV and can modify RSV disease severity.

Along with pollution, ambient particulate matter exhibits effects on RSV pathogenesis. Mice infected with RSV and exposed to carbon black (CB) particles three days post-infection had elevated neutrophil and lymphocyte counts in the lung as well as enhanced RSV-induced airway hyperreactivity

(AHR) compared to control mice that were RSV-infected and exposed to saline.[9] Different results were found in an *in vitro* study using guinea pig alveolar macrophages. When ambient particulate matter was added to RSV-infected guinea pig alveolar macrophages, it diminished RSV replication and proinflammatory cytokine production.[10] Furthermore, the results were found to be independent of the relative timing of RSV infection and exposure to particulate matter.[10] These two reports using different models highlight the complex interactions of RSV, the environment, and innate immunity. Exposure to ambient particulate matter in the setting of RSV infection may lead to macrophage activation, resulting in decreased viral replication yet enhanced immunopathology.

Along with pollution and particulate matter, ozone is another common air contaminant. In an *in* vitro study, ozone exposure of human alveolar macrophages prior to RSV infection had no effect on RSV replication or cytokine production compared to normal air.[11] These findings support the hypothesis that ozone does not play a role in RSV infection. Further studies in animal models, however, may reveal a role for ozone in RSV pathogenesis.

11.3 Innate immunity gene polymorphisms

Current known risk factors for severe RSV disease include premature birth and underlying lung diseases such as bronchopulonary dysplasia. These risk factors, however, cannot fully account for the differential disease severity seen with RSV infection. In a genetic association study of 470 children, it was recently shown that single-nucleotide polymorphisms (SNPs) are associated with RSV bronchiolitis.[12] Out of 384 SNPs analyzed, the four with the strongest association to RSV bronchiolitis were found in the vitamin D receptor (VDR), JUN, interferon-α5 (IFNA5), and nitric oxide synthase 2 (NOS2) innate immune genes.[12] VDR and JUN both participate in signal transduction for innate immunity.[13, 14] IFNA5 plays a role in the interferon pathway of innate immunity, while NOS2A is involved in the proinflammatory and airway mucosal responses. These results suggest that genetic polymorphisms could be risk factors for severe RSV disease. They also suggest that innate immune responses play key roles in RSV-induced illness.

Cytokines also play an important role in innate and adaptive immunity by activating and recruiting immune cells. Some cytokines that have important roles in innate immunity include TNF-α, TGF-β1, IL-10, IL-6, and IFN-γ. In genetic association studies of infants or adults, polymorphisms in many of these cytokine genes were shown to mediate RSV disease severity in terms of clinical outcomes such as lower respiratory illness severity, blood O_2 saturation, length of hospital stay, RSV-specific serum IgG titers, and nasal cytokine protein levels.[15, 16] More specifically, IFN-γ, IL-6, IL-10, and TGF-β1 were associated with more severe RSV disease in infants.[15] In adults, IFN-γ, TNF-α, and IL-6 were associated with severe RSV disease.[16] Like VDR, JUN, IFNA5, and NOS2 gene polymorphisms, these cytokine gene polymorphisms have the potential to be used to distinguish patients at risk for severe RSV disease.

A chemokine that is important in the innate immune response to RSV is regulated on activation, normal T cell expressed and secreted (RANTES). RANTES, also known as CCL5, can be produced by epithelial cells, fibroblasts, and platelets, and it attracts T cells, monocytes, basophils, eosinophils, NK cells, DCs, and mast cells.[17, 18] A study of 106 children hospitalized with RSV-induced bronchiolitis showed that a certain RANTES promoter genotype, which consists of a combination of two specific nucleotide polymorphisms, is associated with severe RSV infection.[19] A previous study showed that RSV induced RANTES expression *in vitro*, suggesting that RANTES plays a key role in RSV pathogenesis.[20] Therefore, increased RANTES expression due to the specific promoter genotype could possibly explain the increased RSV disease severity. This hypothesis is supported by other investigators. In a supporting study, mice infected with RSV showed an increase in the level of RANTES in the lungs.[21] RANTES also increased the allergen-induced inflammatory response after RSV infection.[21]

TLR-4 is a signaling receptor that is activated by bacterial LPS. It is also activated by the RSV fusion (F) protein.[22] A study of 105 RSV positive infants and children revealed that two SNPs (Asp299Gly and Thr399Ile) were associated with symptomatic RSV disease.[23] An *in vitro* study using epithelial cells and peripheral blood mononuclear cells (PBMCs) showed that the same two SNPs caused a decrease in NF-κB, IFNs, IL-8, IL-10, IL-12p35, IL-18, and CCL8.[24] These studies, along with many others, suggest that these two TLR4 polymorphisms together play a role in RSV disease and may be risk factors for RSV disease severity.[25, 26] Furthermore, as TLR4 mediates innate immune activation by LPS and RSV F, polymorphisms in TLR4 may modulate complex interactions between exposures to LPS and RSV.

11.4 Surfactant proteins

SP-A and SP-D are produced by Type II alveolar epithelial cells, are located on mucosal surfaces, are critical for lung homeostasis and maintenance of surface tensions, and recognize and bind bacterial, fungal, and viral pathogens. This enhances the opsonization and killing of these pathogens by phagocytic cells. SP-A deficient mice exhibited more severe pulmonary infiltration of inflammatory cells and slightly increased viral load after RSV infection compared to control mice.[27] SP-A deficiency also increased the levels of pro-inflammatory cytokines such as TNF-α and IL-6, suggesting that SP-A somehow limits the production of cytokines during viral infection.[27] A modified enzyme-linked immunosorbent assay (ELISA) showed that SP-A binds to the F glycoprotein of RSV, while a neutralization assay showed that the binding of SP-A to RSV F neutralizes the virus.[28] These results strongly suggest that SP-A is an important innate immune component against RSV infection. In another experiment, control and SP-D -/- mice were infected with RSV.[29] In this study, increased viral titers were found in the SP-D deficient mice compared to control mice, which could be attributed to SP-D-enhanced phagocytosis of RSV by alveolar macrophages and/or neutrophils.[29] SP-D deficient mice were also found to have more severe lung inflammation (29). These data show that both SP-A and SP-D play important roles in innate anti-viral defense in the lung.

11.5 Toll-like receptors

TLRs are critical components of the innate immune response. TLRs in DC membranes sense proteins or lipids from viruses and bacteria, while TLRs in endosomal membranes detect viral and bacterial nucleic acids. While TLR3 may not play a role in RSV clearance, it has been shown to play a role in limiting RSV-induced disease.[30] TLR3 deficient mice infected with RSV exhibited increased mucus in the airways compared to RSV infected wild-type mice.[30] TLR3-deficient mice infected with RSV also exhibited increased IL-5 and IL-13 production over wild-type controls. In a separate study, human epithelial kidney (HEK) 293 cells were transfected with a TLR3-expressing or control plasmid.[31] These cells were infected with RSV and found to differentially express the chemokines CXCL8 and CCL5 (31). In cells expressing TLR3, there was an increase in induction of both chemokines compared to cells transfected with the control plasmid (31). Taken together, these data imply that TLR3 has an important role in RSV infection by limiting mucus production and inducing chemokines such as CXCL8 and CCL5.

In addition to TLR3, TLR4 also plays a key role in the innate immune response via LPS signaling.[32] TLR4 has also been recently shown to mediate the innate immune response to RSV F.[22] In one experiment,

TLR4-deficient mice infected with RSV exhibited higher titers of virus than control mice infected with RSV.[22] In a similar experiment using TLR4-deficient and control mice, the TLR4-deficient mice showed a decrease in virus clearance.[33] TLR4-deficient mice also showed reduced NK cell and $CD14^+$ cell trafficking, deficient NK cell function, and reduced interleukin-12 expression.[33] These results suggest that TLR4 plays a critical role in the innate immune response to RSV.

The role of TLR4 in the innate immune response to RSV is further established in an experiment on blood samples of infants infected with RSV and healthy controls (34). In this study, flow cytometry analysis revealed that only $CD14^+$ monocytes expressed TLR4 in both groups of infants and there was significantly greater expression of TLR4 in RSV infected infants compared to healthy controls.[34] An *in vitro* study using lung epithelial cells (A549) confirmed that TLR4 expression *in vitro* increases with RSV infection.[35] This study also showed that RSV infection led to increased LPS binding to A549 cells.[35] It is hypothesized that the increase in TLR4 expression due to RSV infection leads to the increased LPS binding to epithelial cells, suggesting that RSV infection causes lung inflammatory responses through TLR4 signaling.[35]

11.6 Interferon-α

IFN-α is an antiviral cytokine of the type I IFN innate immune response of most cell types. IFN-α exhibits anti-viral activity via the induction of protective genes that inhibit viral replication and impede viral dissemination. In a recent study, whole blood samples were taken from adults with allergic asthma and healthy controls.[36] These samples were incubated with RSV or Newcastle Disease Virus (NDV, an avian paramyxovirus known to induce high levels of IFN-α *in vitro*) for five hours and tested for IFN-α2 expression.[36] The study showed that IFN-α2 response to RSV or NDV infection was reduced in the allergic asthmatic adult compared to healthy controls, suggesting a modified innate immune response to RSV in allergic asthmatic hosts.[36]

Similar results of decreased IFN-α in response to NDV infection were found in allergic asthmatic children.[37] Blood samples were taken from healthy children, children with nonallergic asthma, children with allergic asthma, and children with allergic rhinitis.[37] Whole blood cultures and PBMCs from the blood cultures were incubated with NDV for 20 hours, after which IFN-α levels were measured.[37] In allergic asthmatic children, IFN-α was significantly reduced in both the whole blood and PBMC cultures when incubated with NDV compared to nonallergic asthmatic children. These findings suggest that a decrease in IFN-α levels could possibly be used as a marker of allergic asthma.

11.7 Dendritic cells

DCs rapidly produce cytokines in response to antigens. They also act as antigen presenting cells (APCs), linking the innate immune system to the adaptive immune system. Experiments have been performed investigating the role of conventional DCs (cDCs), myeloid DCs (mDCs), and plasmacytoid DCs (pDCs) in the mouse model of RSV infection. In one experiment, mice were infected with RSV and their lungs and lung-draining lymph nodes were analyzed using flow cytometry at different times post-infection.[38] The number of cDCs and pDCs both increased in the lungs and lung-draining lymph nodes of RSV infected mice.[38] To further elucidate the effect of pDCs on RSV-induced disease, pDCs were ablated from mice using a depleting antibody.[38] These mice showed greater AHR as seen by histology.[38] These results suggest that pDCs play a protective role in RSV infection.

RSV also alters DC phenotype and function. In another study, inoculated mouse bone marrow derived pDCs or mDCs were exposed to RSV and the expression of maturation markers CD40, CD80, and CD86 after 48 hours of inoculation was investigated.[39] The expression of these maturation markers by mDCs was enhanced by RSV exposure, while there was no effect of RSV on pDC maturation.[39] mDCs were then stimulated with both RSV and ovalbumin (OVA) to study the induction of OVA-specific T cells.[39] These RSV- and OVA-stimulated mDCs were able to induce proliferation of OVA-specific T cells.[39] pDCs stimulated with both RSV and OVA were unable to induce proliferation of OVA-specific T cells.[39] These results suggest that mDCs may function as a link between RSV infection and allergic inflammation at the interface of innate and adaptive immunity.

DCs link innate to adaptive immunity by several mechanisms, one of which is TLR activation by MyD88 adapter protein signaling.[40] To examine the contribution of MyD88 signaling in RSV pathogenesis, MyD88 deficient mice were infected with RSV and cDC counts and mucus expression were examined.[40] MyD88-deficient mice had reduced numbers of cDCs in their lungs and also had increased mucus expression compared to control mice.[40] MyD88-deficient mouse bone marrow-derived DCs were infected with RSV and shown to produce less *delta-like4* and IL-12 than wild-type bone marrow-derived DCs.[40] This suggests that MyD88 plays an important role in regulating DC development of Th1 immune responses during RSV infection.[40] More research needs to be done to fully understand the complex connections between DCs and adaptive immunity.

DC production of Type I IFN has also been investigated in the context of RSV infection. Mouse DCs were infected with influenza A virus or RSV.[41] Production of type I IFNs was increased by influenza A virus and RSV infection *in vitro*, but only influenza A virus infection increased production of type I IFNs *in vivo* in a mouse model.[41] Reduced type I IFN responses *in vivo* may contribute to weak immunogenicity elicited by RSV in humans compared to influenza viruses. Another group, however, found that human DCs elicited type I IFN production via pDCs when triggered by RSV infection.[42] These conflicting results using two different DC lines emphasizes the fact that more research is necessary in order to elucidate the complex interaction between RSV infection, DCs, and type I IFN production.

11.8 Natural killer cells

NK cells are recruited locally and act as part of innate immunity during viral infection by secreting IFN-γ and direct cytolytic killing of infected cells. They are also involved in antibody-dependent cell-mediated cytotoxicity. One study examined the PBMCs of infants 1 to 21 months old who were hospitalized for RSV infection.[43] Compared to controls, infants infected with RSV had increased numbers of NK cells.[43] In another experiment, mice were infected with RSV, BAL fluid was collected at certain time points post-infection, and NK cell cytotoxicity assays were performed on the BAL samples.[44] This study showed that mice infected with RSV exhibited higher NK cell cytotoxicity.[44] This upregulation of NK cells and increase in NK cell cytotoxicity suggests that NK cells have a role in the innate immune response to RSV infection.

11.9 Timing

The age of initial infection with RSV is a factor that regulates inflammatory airway disease.[45] Seven-day-old mice were infected with RSV then sensitized and challenged with OVA as adults.[45] The mice infected with RSV as neonates exhibited chronic AHR and reduced airway function as adults.[45] TNF-α was elevated in the BAL fluid soon after RSV infection. Combined with the earlier mentioned results, it suggests that early RSV infection is able to alter the pulmonary function in adults, possibly through a mechanism involving TNF-α.

The relative timing of RSV infection and allergen sensitization is also an important factor that can lead to inflammatory airway disease.[46] Our group studied mice that were either infected with RSV then allergically sensitized to OVA, or allergically sensitized to OVA before infection with RSV.[46] Allergen-induced AHR decreased when mice were infected with RSV before being sensitized to OVA, but AHR increased when mice were sensitized to OVA before being infected with RSV.[46] RSV infection before OVA sensitization also reduced RSV-induced weight loss, allergen-induced lung eosinophilia, and lung IL-13 production, which strongly implies that the relative timing of RSV infection and allergen sensitization is important in determining the severity of future RSV-induced disease.[46] These findings also support the hypothesis that hosts with prior allergic disease exhibit more severe RSV-associated airway dysfunction compared to RSV infected non-allergic hosts. It also supports the possibility that allergen sensitization is a risk factor for severe RSV disease.

To further explore the importance of relative timing between RSV infection and allergen sensitization, mice were sensitized to OVA and infected with RSV shortly before or during allergic challenge.[47] These mice exhibited an increase in IL-4, IL-5, and IL-13 expression as well as goblet cell hyperplasia.[47] In another experiment, mice were infected with RSV during OVA sensitization.[48] These mice exhibited allergen-induced AHR, but no increase in IL-4, IL-5, or IL-13 expression.[48] These results further support the implication that the sequence of RSV infection and allergen sensitization is critical in determining RSV-induced disease severity.

11.10 Future directions

An exciting recent development in the field of RSV pathogenesis is the recognition that the phenotypic response to viral infection is at least in part regulated by the strain of RSV used in the infection model. In collaboration with Dr Nick Lukacs at the University of Michigan, our groups found that the line19 strain of RSV induced lung IL-13, mucus, and airway responsiveness in BALB/c mice, whereas laboratory RSV A2 strain did not.[49] We are currently engaged in examining the ability of RSV clinical isolates to also induce variable IL-13 and mucus responses in mice. Thus, RSV pathogenesis is a complex interaction of host genetics, viral genetics, and environmental factors. One important aspect of this work will be determining the interaction of the viral proteins and the host innate immune response in regulating the differential airway disease phenotypes. These studies will be important for vaccine strategy development.

11.11 Conclusions

RSV infection is the leading cause of bronchiolitis, pneumonia, and respiratory failure in infants in the US. RSV infection is also becoming more frequently recognized as a significant cause of morbidity in elderly patients. Understanding the innate immune response to RSV infection, especially in the allergic or asthmatic host, is therefore critical to developing an effective therapy. Research has shown that Type I IFN response in the allergic or asthmatic human host is different from that of the normal human host. Innate immunity gene polymorphisms and pollution have also been show to play a role in causing more severe RSV disease in humans.

Because of obvious difficulties in experimentally infecting humans, much more is known about the relationship between RSV and innate immunity in rodent models and *in vitro*. SPs, DCs, TLRs, and NK cells all act as an innate defense against RSV infection and disease. Similarly to in the human model, ambient particulate matter and pollution both augmented disease severity. RSV disease severity was also dependent on the relative timing of infection, allergen sensitization, and allergen challenge. These mouse model and *in vitro* studies suggest that innate immunity in humans plays a huge role during RSV infection, and that there is a significant and complex interaction between RSV infection and allergies.

Acknowledgements

This work was supported by NIH HL 069949, AI054660, AI 070672, HL 090664, and GM 15431. MLL was supported by T32 GM07569 and T32 HL069765.

References

1 Glezen, W.P., Taber, L.H., Frank, A.L., and Kasel, J.A. 1986. Risk of primary infection and reinfection with respiratory syncytial virus. *Am. J. Dis. Child.* 140: 543–554.

2 Openshaw, P.J., Dean, G.S., and Culley, F.J. 2003. Links between respiratory syncytial virus bronchiolitis and childhood asthma: clinical and research approaches. *Pediatr. Infect. Dis. J.* 22: S58–S4.
3 Falsey, A.R. 2007. Respiratory syncytial virus infection in adults. *Semin. Respir. Crit. Care Med.* 28: 171–81.
4 Power, U.F. 2008. Respiratory syncytial virus (RSV) vaccines–two steps back for one leap forward *J. Clin. Virol.* 41: 38–44.
5 Segala, C., Poizeau, D., Mesbah M., Willems S., and Maidenberg, M. 2008. Winter air pollution and infant bronchiolitis in Paris. *Environ. Res.* 106: 96–100.
6 Bradley, J.P., Bacharier L.B., Bonfiglio, J., Schechtman, K.B., Strunk, R., Storch, G., and Castro, M. 2005. Severity of respiratory syncytial virus bronchiolitis is affected by cigarette smoke exposure and atopy. *Pediatrics* 115: e7–14.
7 Harrod, K.S., Jaramillo, R.J., Rosenberger, C.L., Wang, S.Z., Berger, J.A., McDonald, J.D., and Reed, M.D.. 2003. Increased susceptibility to RSV infection by exposure to inhaled diesel engine emissions. *Am. J. Respir. Cell Mol. Biol.* 28: 451–463.
8 Foster, S., Bedford, K.J., Gould, M.E., Coward, W.R., and Hewitt, C.R. 2003. Respiratory syncytial virus infection and virus-induced inflammation are modified by contaminants of indoor air. *Immunology* 108: 109–115.
9 Lambert, A.L., Mangum, J.B., DeLorme, M.P., and Everitt, J.I. 2003. Ultrafine carbon black particles enhance respiratory syncytial virus-induced airway reactivity, pulmonary inflammation, and chemokine expression. *Toxicol. Sci.* 72: 339–346.
10 Kaan, P.M. and Hegele, R.G. 2003. Interaction between respiratory syncytial virus and particulate matter in guinea pig alveolar macrophages. *Am. J. Respir. Cell Mol. Biol.* 28: 697–704.
11 Soukup, J., Koren, H.S., and Becker, S. 1993. Ozone effect on respiratory syncytial virus infectivity and cytokine production by human alveolar macrophages. *Environ. Res.* 60: 178–186.
12 Janssen, R., Bont, L., Siezen, C.L., Hodemaekers, H.M., Ermers, M.J., Doornbos, G., van 't, S.R., Wijmenga, C., Goeman, J.J., Kimpen, J.L., van Houwelingen, H. C., Kimman, T.G., and Hoebee, B.. 2007. Genetic susceptibility to respiratory syncytial virus bronchiolitis is predominantly associated with innate immune genes. *J. Infect. Dis.* 196: 826–834.
13 Cutolo, M. and Otsa, K. 2008. Review: vitamin D, immunity and lupus. *Lupus* 17: 6–10.
14 Dong, C., Davis, R.J., and Flavell, R.A.. 2001. Signaling by the JNK group of MAP kinases. c-jun N-terminal Kinase. *J. Clin. Immunol* 21: 253–257.
15 Gentile, D.A., Doyle, W.J., Zeevi, A., Howe-Adams, J., Kapadia, S., Trecki, J., and Skoner, D.P. 2003. Cytokine gene polymorphisms moderate illness severity in infants with respiratory syncytial virus infection. *Hum. Immunol.* 64: 338–344.
16 Gentile, D.A., Doyle, W.J., Zeevi, A., Piltcher, O., and Skoner, D.P. 2003. Cytokine gene polymorphisms moderate responses to respiratory syncytial virus in adults. *Hum. Immunol.* 64: 93–98.
17 Appay, V. and Rowland-Jones, S.L. 2001. RANTES: a versatile and controversial chemokine. *Trends Immunol.* 22: 83–87.
18 Schall, T.J. 1991. Biology of the RANTES/SIS cytokine family. *Cytokine* 3: 165–183.

19 Amanatidou, V., Sourvinos, G., Apostolakis, S., Neonaki, P., Tsilimigaki, A., Krambovitis, E., and Spandidos, D.A. 2008. RANTES promoter gene polymorphisms and susceptibility to severe respiratory syncytial virus-induced bronchiolitis. *Pediatr. Infect. Dis. J.* 27: 38–42.
20 Miller, A.L., Bowlin, T.L., and Lukacs, N.W. 2004. Respiratory syncytial virus-induced chemokine production: linking viral replication to chemokine production in vitro and in vivo. *J. Infect. Dis.* 189: 1419–1430.
21 John, A.E., Berlin, A.A., and Lukacs, N.W. 2003. Respiratory syncytial virus-induced CCL5/RANTES contributes to exacerbation of allergic airway inflammation. *Eur. J. Immunol.* 33: 1677–1685.
22 Kurt-Jones, E.A., Popova, L., Kwinn, L., Haynes, L.M., Jones, L.P., Tripp, R.A., Walsh, E.E., Freeman, M.W., Golenbock, D.T., Anderson, L.J., and Finberg, R.W. 2000. Pattern recognition receptors TLR4 and CD14 mediate response to respiratory syncytial virus. *Nat. Immunol.* 1: 398–401.
23 Awomoyi, A.A., Rallabhandi, P., Pollin, T.I., Lorenz, E., Sztein, M.B., Boukhvalova, M.S., Hemming, V.G., Blanco, J.C., and Vogel, S.N., 2007. Association of TLR4 polymorphisms with symptomatic respiratory syncytial virus infection in high-risk infants and young children. *J. Immunol.* 179: 3171–3177.
24 Tulic, M.K., Hurrelbrink, R.J., Prele, C.M., Laing, I.A., Upham, J.W., Le Souef, P., Sly, P.D., and Holt, P.G., 2007. TLR4 polymorphisms mediate impaired responses to respiratory syncytial virus and lipopolysaccharide. *J. Immunol.* 179: 132–140.
25 Mandelberg, A., Tal, G., Naugolny, L., Cesar, K., Oron, A., Houri, S., Gilad, E., and Somekh, E., 2006. Lipopolysaccharide hyporesponsiveness as a risk factor for intensive care unit hospitalization in infants with respiratory syncitial virus bronchiolitis. *Clin. Exp. Immunol.* 144: 48–52.
26 Tal, G., Mandelberg, A., Dalal, I., Cesar, K., Somekh, E., Tal, A., Oron, A., Itskovich, S., Ballin, A., Houri, S., Beigelman, A., Lider, O., Rechavi, G., and Amariglio, N. 2004. *J. Infect. Dis.* 189: 2057–2063.
27 LeVine, A.M., Gwozdz, J., Stark, J., Bruno, M., Whitsett, J., and Korfhagen, T. 1999. Association between common Toll-like receptor 4 mutations and severe respiratory syncytial virus disease. *J. Clin. Invest.* 103: 1015.
28 Ghildyal, R., Hartley, C., Varrasso, A., Meanger, J., Voelker, D.R., Anders, E.M., and Mills, J. 1999. Surfactant protein A binds to the fusion glycoprotein of respiratory syncytial virus and neutralizes virion infectivity. *J. Infect. Dis.* 180: 2009–2013.
29 LeVine, A.M., Elliott, J., Whitsett, J.A., Srikiatkhachorn, A., Crouch, E., DeSilva, N., and Korfhagen, T. 2004. Surfactant protein-d enhances phagocytosis and pulmonary clearance of respiratory syncytial virus. *Am. J. Respir. Cell Mol. Biol.* 31: 193–199.
30 Rudd, B.D., Smit, J.J., Flavell, R.A., Alexopoulou, L., Schaller, M.A., Gruber, A., Berlin, A.A., and Lukacs, N.W. 2006. Deletion of TLR3 alters the pulmonary immune environment and mucus production during respiratory syncytial virus infection. *J. Immunol.* 176: 1937–1942.
31 Rudd, B.D., Burstein, E., Duckett, C.S., Li, X., and Lukacs, N.W. 2005. Differential role for TLR3 in respiratory syncytial virus-induced chemokine expression. *J. Virol.* 79: 3350–3357.

32 Chow, J.C., Young, D.W., Golenbock, D.T., Christ, W.J., and Gusovsky, F. 1999. Toll-like receptor-4 mediates lipopolysaccharide-induced signal transduction. *J. Biol. Chem.* 274: 10689–10692.

33 Haynes, L.M., Moore, D.D., Kurt-Jones, E.A., Finberg, R.W., Anderson, L.J., and Tripp, R.A. 2001. Involvement of toll-like receptor 4 in innate immunity to respiratory syncytial virus. *J. Virol.* 75: 10730–10737.

34 Gagro, A., Tominac, M., Krsulovic-Hresic, V., Bace, A., Matic, M., Drazenovic, V., Mlinaric-Galinovic, G., Kosor, E., Gotovac, K., Bolanca, I., Batinica, S., and Rabatic, S.. 2004. Increased Toll-like receptor 4 expression in infants with respiratory syncytial virus bronchiolitis. *Clin. Exp. Immunol.* 135: 267–272.

35 Monick, M.M., Yarovinsky, T.O., Powers, L.S., Butler, N.S., Carter, A.B., Gudmundsson, G., and Hunninghake, G.W. 2003. Respiratory syncytial virus up-regulates TLR4 and sensitizes airway epithelial cells to endotoxin. *J. Biol. Chem.* 278: 53035–53044.

36 Gehlhar, K., Bilitewski, C., Reinitz-Rademacher, K., Rohde, G., and Bufe, A. Impaired virus-induced interferon-alpha2 release in adult asthmatic patients. 2006. *Clin. Exp. Allergy* 36: 331–337.

37 Bufe, A., Gehlhar, K., Grage-Griebenow, E., and Ernst, M. 2002. Atopic phenotype in children is associated with decreased virus-induced interferon-alpha release. *Int. Arch. Allergy Immunol.* 127: 82–88.

38 Smit, J.J., Rudd, B.D., and Lukacs, N.W. 2006. Plasmacytoid dendritic cells inhibit pulmonary immunopathology and promote clearance of respiratory syncytial virus. *J. Exp. Med.* 203: 1153–1159

39 Boogaard, I., van Oosten, M., van Rijt, L.S., Muskens, F., Kimman, T.G., Lambrecht, B.N., and Buisman, A.M. 2007. Respiratory syncytial virus differentially activates murine myeloid and plasmacytoid dendritic cells. *Immunology* 122: 65–72.

40 Rudd, B.D., Schaller, M.A., Smit, J.J., Kunkel, S.L., Neupane, R., Kelley, L., Berlin, A.A., and Lukacs, N.W. 2007. MyD88-mediated instructive signals in dendritic cells regulate pulmonary immune responses during respiratory virus infection *J. Immunol.* 178: 5820–5827.

41 Jewell, N.A., Vaghefi, N., Mertz, S.E., Akter, P., Peebles Jr., R.S., Bakaletz, L.O., Durbin, R.K., Flano, E, and Durbin, J.E. 2007. Differential type I interferon induction by respiratory syncytial virus and influenza a virus in vivo. *J. Virol.* 81: 9790–9800.

42 Guerrero-Plata, A., Casola, A., Suarez, G., Yu, X., Spetch, L., Peeples, M.E., and Garofalo, R.P. 2006. Differential response of dendritic cells to human metapneumovirus and respiratory syncytial virus. *Am. J. Respir. Cell Mol. Biol.* 34: 320–329.

43 Tripp, R.A., Moore, D., Barskey, A., Jones, L., Moscatiello, C., Keyserling, H., and Anderson, L.J. 2002. Peripheral blood mononuclear cells from infants hospitalized because of respiratory syncytial virus infection express T helper-1 and T helper-2 cytokines and CC chemokine messenger RNA *J. Infect. Dis.* 185: 1388–1394.

44 Hussell, T. and Openshaw, P.J. 1998. Intracellular IFN-gamma expression in natural killer cells precedes lung CD8+ T cell recruitment during respiratory syncytial virus infection. *J. Gen. Virol.* 79: 2593–2601.

45 You, D., Becnel, D., Wang, K., Ripple, M., Daly, M., and Cormier, S.A. 2006. Exposure of neonates to respiratory syncytial virus is critical in determining subsequent airway response in adults. *Respir. Res.* 7: 107.
46 Peebles, R.S., Jr., Hashimoto, K., Collins, R.D., Jarzecka, K., Furlong, J., Mitchell, D.B., Sheller, J.R., and Graham, B.S. 2001. Immune interaction between respiratory syncytial virus infection and allergen sensitization critically depends on timing of challenges. *J. Infect. Dis.* 184: 1374–1379.
47 Barends, M., van Oosten, M., De Rond, C.G., Dormans, J.A., Osterhaus, A.D., Neijens, H.J., and Kimman, T.G. 2004. Timing of infection and prior immunization with respiratory syncytial virus (RSV) in RSV-enhanced allergic inflammation. *J. Infect. Dis.* 189: 1866–1872.
48 Peebles Jr., R.S., Sheller, J.R., Collins, R.D., Jarzecka, A.K., Mitchell, D.B., Parker, R.A., and Graham, B.S. 2001. Respiratory syncytial virus infection does not increase allergen-induced type 2 cytokine production, yet increases airway hyperresponsiveness in mice. *J. Med. Virol.* 63: 178–188.
49 Lukacs, N.W., Moore, M.L., Rudd, B.D., Berlin, A.A., Collins, R.D., Olson, S.J., Ho, S.B., and Peebles Jr, R.S. 2006. Differential immune responses and pulmonary pathophysiology are induced by two different strains of respiratory syncytial virus. *Am. J. Pathol.* 169: 977–986.

12

Interactions between allergens and dendritic cells: pattern recognition receptors and their function in the pathogenesis of allergic respiratory diseases

Stephanie T. Yerkovich and John W. Upham

Abstract. Allergic diseases are characterized by excessive and inappropriate responses to allergens leading to a Th2 skewed immune environment. While the exact mechanisms involved are not completely understood, Th2 polarization is likely to involve both dendritic cell (DC) and T cell dependent factors. Furthermore, allergens themselves are now no longer viewed as inert proteins, but have their own biological properties that can skew immune responses. Such "intrinsic properties" of allergens may influence DC function, and this subsequently has profound effects on allergic inflammation. This chapter will focus on common aeroallergens such as house dust mite (HDM) and pollens, and the mechanisms by which these allergens alter DC cytokine, prostaglandin, and chemokine synthesis and the expression of costimulatory molecules. Some of the effects of allergens on DC differ between atopic and healthy subjects, while other DC responses are similar in both groups. This chapter will also discuss how HDM and pollen allergens activate DC, and the mounting evidence to suggest that pathogen recognition receptors, in particular the C-type lectins, play an important role in the dysregulated allergic immune response. While most of the population is exposed to common aeroallergens, only a proportion will develop allergic disease and our understanding of allergen-DC-T cell interactions and mechanisms involved in this process is increasing. In the future this should allow for more targeted therapies to reduce the impact of allergic disease.

Keywords: allergic lung disease, allergic inflammation, allergens, house-dust mite antigen, allergic asthma, aeroallergens, innate immunity, dendritic cells, allergic T helper cells, T regulatory cells (Tregs), co-stimulation, immune tolerance, pattern-recognition receptors, toll-like receptors, C-type lectins, phagocytosis, endocytosis, antigen processing and presentation, immunomodulation

12.1 Introduction

The incidence of allergic disease has rapidly increased over the last few decades in Westernized countries and unfortunately this trend is not abating. The impact of allergic disease is wide ranging, being responsible for high levels of morbidity, and, in some instances, severe asthma and anaphylaxis may even be fatal. The impact on society is also great with increased health costs and lost productivity. To date the only treatment for allergic disease has been to attempt to reduce the symptoms once established. It has therefore become imperative to gain a better understanding of the mechanisms leading to the development of allergic disease so in future medical science may provide more targeted therapies and ultimately prevent its development.

Allergic diseases encompass a spectrum of disorders characterized by the development of an overactive immune response to an otherwise harmless allergen, resulting in a Th2 polarized cytokine response to the allergen and the production of an IgE antibody response. Allergic diseases are manifested in a number of different ways. For example, contact allergies result in a rash at the site of contact, while ingestion of some food allergens, such as the widely publicized peanut allergy, results in systemic affects with life-threatening anaphylaxis. The focus of this chapter will be on those allergic diseases affecting the respiratory system, especially rhino-sinusitis and asthma. Allergic respiratory disease is triggered by the inhalation of a number of both indoor and outdoor airborne allergens, the more important and widely studied being house dust mite (HDM), cat, moulds, fungi and grass pollens.

12.2 Allergic respiratory diseases: the key instigators and cellular players

12.2.1 The instigators: aeroallergens

Allergens by definition are any substance that can cause an allergic reaction and accordingly allergenic components have been found in a wide range of different plant and animal species. In most temperate climates of the world, HDM are a major source of many of the allergens in house dust. A large number of individuals show positive reactivity to this allergen and mite allergens sensitize and induce rhinitis and allergic asthma in a large proportion of those with allergic disease. There are several mite species with *Dermatophagoides pteronyssinus* and *Dermatophagoides farinae* the most prevalent in the Western world.[1] Historically, allergens have been classified as a "major allergen" if greater than 50 percent of the population allergic to that species show IgE binding, and there is considerable evidence to suggest that Der p 1 and Der p 2 are the major allergens of *D pteronyssinus* due to their high IgE binding capacity and high concentration of these 2 allergens in HDM extracts.[2] Similar considerations apply to Der f 1 and Der f 2. While Der p 1 and Der p 2 are classified as major allergens, a number of other HDM allergens have been described and indeed there are now over 20 different HDM allergens listed by the International Union of Immunological Societies nomenclature, with the capacity to bind IgE varying between these allergens.[3, 4] In terms of the ability of these allergens to individually induce an allergic T cell response there have been limited studies, but it does appear that while Der p 1 can induce both high Th2 cytokine and IgE levels, other minor allergens are also capable of inducing a T cell cytokine response, even in the absence of detectable IgE antibody responses.[5] Therefore while HDM has many different allergenic components, the majority, if not all, of these contribute to allergic response elicited by HDM and hence many studies investigating the *in vitro* response to HDM tend to use a whole HDM extract that contains a mix of major and several minor allergens. While only the HDM allergen is described in detail here, a similar classification system exists for most other allergens.

It is also interesting to note that the major HDM allergen Der p 1 is a cysteine protease, belonging to the same family as papain and cathepsin L, and similarly to these enzymes it shows a broad range of specificity. This is of particular interest as enzymatically active Der p 1 is more allergenic in a mouse model of airway inflammation compared to the inactive form.[6] Similarly, the enzymatic properties of Der p 1[7, 8] and especially the protease activity of allergens[9] are important for many of the responses elicited. A number of allergens from different sources have been reported to have protease activity and the full implication of this in the allergic response will be discussed in more detail in section 12.3.2. In conclusion, airborne allergens come from a number of different sources such as dust mites, domestic pets, moulds and fungi and pollens of grasses and other plant species and all are capable of eliciting an allergic immune response. The classification of allergens has progressed to allow the identification and characterization of many different allergens, yet our understanding of how these allergens promote allergic disease and the mechanisms involved is still incomplete.

12.2.2 The players: overview

Allergic manifestations involve multiple cell types including antigen presenting cells (APC), such as dendritic cells (DC), T and B cells, eosinophils and mast cells, the products of which influence other cell types, such as those in the lung which respond with airway remodeling and the development of asthma. In brief the allergic cascade can be summarized as a series of cellular interactions resulting in activation of the adaptive immune system in response to allergen. Allergens enter the respiratory tract by inhalation, where they are sensed and internalized by DC that form tight networks within the airway epithelium of the lung. DC then traffic to the lymph nodes where they can present the allergen directly to naïve and memory T cells, while concurrently releasing soluble factors such as cytokines and chemokines. These responding T cells are polarized towards a Th2 type response by the DC through mechanisms that are not fully understood but probably involve both direct cell-cell contact and indirectly by the release of soluble factors. T cell production of Th2 cytokines such as IL-4, IL-5, IL-9 and IL-13 then act on B cells and eosinophils leading to induce the production of IgE antibodies, mucus secretion and airway inflammation.

Even though the pathways leading to the development of allergic disease are complex and ill-defined in parts, it is clear that DC and $CD4^+$ T cells have a central role in the process. Differences in DC and T cell biology between atopic and non-atopic people indicate that defects exist in both cell compartments and these more than likely contribute to the development of allergic disease. T cell specific differences and their role in allergies are beyond the scope of this chapter, and will not be reviewed here. Hence this chapter will focus on the role of DC in the allergic response, the interaction between allergens and DC, and evidence suggesting that some allergens are more than inert proteins and have their own biological properties that can skew towards a Th2 allergic response.

12.2.3 The players: dendritic cells

DC are the most potent APC within the immune system and are a heterogenous population that reside in all peripheral tissues and are particularly evident at sites that directly interact with the external environment. These cells are constantly "on patrol", roaming through the body in search of antigens and inflammatory signals. Within the microenvironment of the lung, DC form a network above and below the basement membrane of the airway epithelium whereby they can extend their process between the epithelial cells without disrupting the integrity of the epithelium,[10] allowing them to constantly sample the environment. DC internalize and process antigen before loading it onto major histocompatibility complex (MHC) class I and II molecules in preparation for presentation to T lymphocytes. During this process DC can transform from immature cells (high capacity for antigen uptake and processing but low antigen-presenting capacity) into more mature and potent APC with the ability to polarize naïve T cells into either Th1 or Th2 effector cells, thereby initiating an adaptive immune response. It must also be noted that in the absence of an inflammatory signal, DC will not be activated and will preferentially induce the development of tolerance, a state where DC can induce $CD4^+$ T cell expansion but not T-helper cell differentiation.[11] While this will not be discussed in detail here, it has been suggested that different DC subsets may contribute to the function of T regulatory cells and the development of tolerance[12] and may involve T regulatory cells.[13, 14]

As previously stated, allergic disorders are Th2 mediated, which requires DC to capture allergen within the airways and prime naïve T cells to proliferate and acquire Th2 effector function to initiate the allergic response. DC are indeed capable of doing this and their importance in orchestrating allergic airway inflammation has been shown by a number of studies employing animal models. These are mostly based on the model antigen ovalbumin (OVA) and alum, which induces airway inflammation and some of the hallmarks of human allergic respiratory disease. Following OVA-induced airway inflammation, production of DC progenitors is increased in the bone marrow and DC traffic to the airways where their numbers are substantially increased.[15, 16] Under steady-state conditions, resident murine lung DC inherently prime a Th2 polarized response[17, 18] unless exposed to an appropriate Th1 polarizing signal,[18] and therefore it is not surprising that these lung DC prime a Th2 skewed response following allergen exposure.[17]

Furthermore, DC can present antigen to previously primed Th2 cells[19] and a subset of DC are capable of presenting allergen to allergen-specific Th2 cells within the airway for extended periods of time,[20] which further enhances the Th2 environment induced by allergen. Collectively there have been many animal studies that have highlighted the key role DC play in priming and maintaining an allergen-specific Th2 skewed response. More recent studies using both rat and mouse models are also beginning to identify distinct DC subsets present within different areas of the lung parenchyma and airway mucosa that have distinct functional roles,[22, 23] a concept that has not been thoroughly investigated in humans. This issue will be discussed in more detail later in this chapter (section 12.4.3.2).

Defining such a direct role for DC in human allergy is more challenging, but nonetheless a growing body of evidence suggests that DC are once again pivotal. The respiratory mucosa of allergic and asthmatic patients contains a greater number of DC compared to control subjects without these conditions,[23, 24] suggesting that DC may have a role in allergic and asthmatic disease. More direct evidence for this was shown by the rapid recruitment of DC subsets from the circulation into the airway mucosa following the inhalation of common inhaled allergens in allergic asthmatic subjects,[25, 26] suggesting that recruitment of DC into the airways is an important aspect of the immune response towards inhaled allergens. In addition, there is evidence to suggest that there are functional differences between DC obtained from allergic and control subjects, described in more detail later (section 12.3.1), which adds weight to the notion that DC are instrumental in driving human allergic disease.

12.2.4 How do DC prime a Th2 response?

This is an area of intense focus but our understanding is limited, as the currently identified mechanisms do not fully explain the Th2 skewing ability of DC. It appears that DC may regulate T cell responses through both membrane-bound molecules and via soluble mediators produced by DC. In terms of molecules expressed by DC, the key co-stimulatory molecules CD80 and CD86 have been investigated for their potential to regulate a Th2 response. Monocyte-derived DC from allergic subjects show increased CD86 expression following *in vitro* allergen stimulation,[8, 27] and blocking this co-stimulatory factor during allergen-challenge in murine models prevented the development of eosinophilic airway inflammation in sensitized mice,[28, 29] suggesting CD86 may play a functional role. However, other murine studies have shown a requirement for CD80[30] or both CD80 and CD86[31] co-stimulation to elicit Th2 differentiation, which suggests that while these molecules are important, other mechanisms are also involved in Th2 differentiation.

Another membrane molecule in DC suggested to have a role in the allergic response is OX40 ligand. Thymic stromal lymphopoietin is a cytokine produced by epithelial cells that can induce Th2 responses,[32] and

OX40 ligand has recently been identified as the mediator in this response.[33] In a murine allergy model, OX40 ligand was shown to have a direct role in promoting the development of allergic features following OVA-stimulation.[34] Therefore OX40 ligand on DC has been suggested to be an important molecule that could be targeted to reduce the initiation of an allergic response. Most of these studies have been based on animal models and it will be interesting to assess the importance of OX40 ligand in human allergic disease.

In relation to soluble factors produced by allergen-stimulated DC, it has been difficult to identify a particular molecule that consistently induces a Th2 skewed response. IL-12 is a key cytokine for the induction of Th1 type responses, and while some reports suggest reduced levels of this cytokine in atopic individuals,[8, 35] other studies report similar IL-12 production by DC of atopic and non-atopic donors.[36, 37] Alternatively, murine studies have suggested that IL-10, a cytokine capable of down-regulating IL-12 and Th1 differentiation, is critical for Th2 dominated responses following inhaled allergen.[17, 18] However, the data in relation to IL-10 expression by human DC is inconsistent: we have reported increased IL-10 production by DC from atopic asthmatics compared to healthy donors[37] while others have reported the reverse.[35, 38] Together these studies suggest that neither IL-12 nor IL-10 have a fundamental role in controlling Th2 differentiation in the context of human allergic disease. Finally, GM-CSF appears to play a role in Th2 sensitization and airway inflammation in mice following intranasal HDM exposure,[39] though it is not clear whether this is also true in humans.

IL-6 is another DC-secreted cytokine thought to help mediate a Th2 response by negatively regulating IL-12 production and polarising naïve T cells towards a Th2 phenotype,[40] and identified to have a role in a murine allergy model.[17] More recent data has also highlighted the importance of IL-6 by describing a pathway whereby HDM allergen induces expression of c-Kit and its ligand stem cell factor on DC which signals through phosphatidylinositol-3 kinase to induce IL-6 production, thereby enhancing Th2 responses.[41] In this regard Hammad and co-workers[8] have described higher and sustained IL-6 expression by Der p 1 stimulated DC from allergic donors compared to DC from non-allergic donors that showed low and transient levels of IL-6 in response to Der p 1. However, it is not known in humans whether allergen exposure activates c-Kit, or whether c-Kit signaling varies between DC from allergic and non-allergic subjects. Alternatively, IL-6 may have an indirect role in allergic inflammation by negating the action of T regulatory (Treg) cells.[42] Treg cells are a small population of $CD4^+$ T cells that act to control and limit immune reactions and it has been suggested that ineffective Treg cells may have a role in the allergic response. We and others have found that Treg numbers do not differ between allergic and non-allergic subjects (also in unpublished observations).[43–45] However, over and above the absolute numbers of Tregs, the balance or ratio of allergen-specific Th2 to Treg cells may be a more important determinant of whether an allergic or healthy immune response is elicited.[44, 46, and 47] The functionality of these Treg cells has been reported to be equal[43] or only slightly diminished[44] compared to healthy controls, but when this was assessed during the allergy season when patients are highly symptomatic, Treg function appears to be significantly diminished compared to healthy controls.[44, 45] Recent data also suggests that Treg cells show allergen-specificity.[48, 49]

Given the potential for DC to modulate Treg activity, it will be interesting to see if allergen-activated DC can indeed negate Treg mediated suppression. In summary, DC are instrumental in polarizing a Th2 response to common allergens by directly acting on naïve and memory T cells, or possibly by also negating Treg mediated suppression. The mechanisms by which DC achieve this are unclear and the currently identified membrane-bound and soluble mediators do not fully account for these effects, highlighting an important need to find novel molecules that promote an allergic response. It is in this regard that some C-type lectin molecules may have a role and this will be discussed in detail below (section 12.4.3).

12.3 Interactions between allergens and DC

12.3.1 Functional differences exist between DC of allergic and non-allergic individuals

While most of the population is exposed to common aeroallergens, only a percentage will go on to develop allergic disease. This raises the question as to why some people will react inappropriately to inhaled allergens and what differences exist between DC of those that develop allergies, compared to those who do not. To address this issue, most investigators have studied two sources of DC: those that have been directly isolated from peripheral blood, and DC derived *in vitro* from monocytes. DC isolated from allergic and non-allergic donors have been examined both at baseline and following *in vitro* exposure to common allergens such as HDM and pollens. This characterization has generally focused on well-characterized cell surface markers such as the co-stimulatory molecules CD80 and CD86 and secreted proteins which are involved in T cell activation or polarization such as IL-10, IL-12, IL-1β and TNFα.

These studies have shown that monocyte-derived DC from HDM sensitive patients stimulated with Der p 1 show an upregulation of CD86 and increased production of TNFα, IL-1β and IL-10 (8), while monocyte-derived DC or myeloid DC from nonatopic patients show increased CD80 expression (8, 38) and increased IL-12[18, 35] and IL-10[35, 38] production. When these Der p 1-stimulated DC from atopic patients were co-cultured with T cells, a Th2 polarized response ensued.[8, 38] Furthermore, mature DC from atopic donors can induce naïve and memory $CD4^+$ T cells to acquire Th2 effector function, a process independent of IL-12 production by DC.[36] As stated previously (section 12.2.4), these markers are not solely responsible for Th2 polarization, suggesting other molecules are important or combinations of molecules are required. In this regard chemokines may play an important role as Der p 1-stimulation of DC from HDM-sensitive patients induces synthesis of the Th2 attracting chemokines CCL17 and CCL22, whereas DC from healthy donors synthesize the Th1 cell recruiting chemokine CXCL10.[50]

These functional differences extend to mechanisms used by DC for allergen uptake. Traditionally it has been thought that allergen was most efficiently taken up by DC when bound to IgE, which permits the interaction with the high-affinity IgE receptor, FcεR1. Such allergen-loaded DC elicit a larger T cell response.[51] DC from allergic subjects express FcεR1at much higher levels than non-allergic subjects[24, 52] and this expression is correlated with increased serum IgE concentrations.[52] While DC lack the β chain of FcεR1, which is thought to be necessary for signal transduction (51), it has been determined that ligation of FcεR1 on DC activates NFκB (53). However, monocyte-derived DC have no detectable surface-bound IgE (54) and no expression FcεR1 or FcγR1,[55] so these Fc receptors may be more important on peripheral blood DC.[56, 57] A variety of mechanisms are likely to be important in allergen uptake and processing, and this will be discussed in more detail later (section 12.4.3.1).

12.3.2 Allergens have intrinsic properties that may directly influence DC function

It is now clear that DC have a central role in orchestrating a set of events that lead to chronic airway inflammation in response to innocuous inhaled allergens. Hence the question that must now be addressed is whether allergens merely induce non-specific DC activation, or whether allergens themselves can instruct DC. As stated above,[8, 35, 38, 50] allergen-stimulation *in vitro* leads to differential effects on the function of DC from allergic and non-allergic donors. These differences cover DC surface phenotypes and patterns of cytokine/chemokine synthesis and may be partly due to the allergen *per se*, with allergens no longer viewed as inert proteins but having their own biological properties that can result in skewed immune responses (as summarized in Table 12.1). Hammad et al.[8] showed that Der p 1-stimulation

Table 12.1 Interactions between allergens and DC in human studies

Cell	Allergen	Key findings showing intrinsic allergen properties	Ref
Direct effects of allergen on DC			
moDC	Der p 1	Increased CD86, CD83, TNFα, IL-1, IL10 by DC from allergic donors and effects were due to the enzymatic property of Der p 1	(8)
moDC	Der p 1	Proteolytically active Der p 1 induced less IL-12 compared to inactive Der p 1	(7)
moDC	Der p 1	Chemokine production only induced by enzymatically active Der p 1	(50)
moDC	Birch pollen	Pollen-derived E1-phytoprostanes inhibited IL-12 production	(58)
moDC	Birch pollen	Pollen-derived E1-phytoprostanes induced chemokines that preferentially attract Th2 cells	(59)
moDC	Aspergillus protease	Upregulation of co-stimulatory and cytokine production only induced by active protease	(60)
Effect of allergen-stimulated DC on $CD4^+$ T cells			
moDC	Der p 1	Increased IL-4 by DC from allergic donors and effects were due to the enzymatic property of Der p 1	(8)
moDC	Der p 1	Less IFNγ and more IL-4 produced by proteolytically Der p1 compared to inactive Der p 1	(7)
moDC	Birch pollen	Pollen-derived E1-phytoprostanes favoured Th2 polarisation	(58)
moDC	Aspergillus protease	Protease activated DC induced enhanced IL-4 and reduced IFNγ, and no responses seen when the protease activity was neutralised	(60)
Effect of allergens on other cells			
basophils	papain	Protease allergens induce basophils to produce Th2 inducing cytokines	(9)

moDC, monocyte-derived DC

had different effects on DC from allergic individuals with HDM sensitivity, compared to those with pollen but not HDM sensitivity, and these findings were shown to be dependent on the enzymatic/proteolytic properties of Der p 1. Similarly, the proteolytic activity of Der p 1 was identified as being important in the reduced IL-12p70 production by DC stimulated with Der p1 together with lipopolysaccharide (LPS), anti-CD40 and IFNγ, with proteolytic cleavage of CD40 by Der p1 being associated with less IL-12.[(7)] When these Der p 1 conditioned DC were cultured with naïve T cells, the proteolytic activity was responsible for the Th2 skewed response.

Similarly, the development of allergic airway inflammation in mice sensitised to Der p 1 via the nasal route mice appears to be dependent on the protease activity of Der p 1.[(6)] In many mouse models of allergic inflammation, priming is dependent on co-administration of adjuvant together allergen; however, fungal proteases derived from *Aspergillus* species not only negate the requirement for adjuvant to induce allergic sensitization, but can overcome airway tolerance and induce Th2 cell activation.[(61)] Taking this into the human system, these proteases induce partial maturation of monocyte-derived DC from healthy subjects, which then induce naïve T cells to produce large amounts of IL-4 and low amounts of IFNγ and IL-12,[(60)] an effect not seen when the proteolytic activity was neutralized.

A murine study by Sokol and colleagues[(9)] has also recently shown that in response to the protease allergen papain, basophils were directly activated and produced IL-4, thereby promoting Th2 differentiation. This study not only suggested and confirmed that basophils are an important intermediary cell type responsible for Th2 differentiation but showed that this was dependent on the protease activity of the allergen. In this study papain also induced the accumulation of DC in the draining lymph nodes and it will be interesting in future to ascertain if DC are an intermediary cell type in this process and are involved in preferentially stimulating IL-4 producing basophils. It will also be interesting to investigate if papain activates DC directly to induce maturation or if this is secondary to the action of papain on basophils.

Analogous to the proteolytic activity of Der p 1 and *Aspergillus* species, components of pollen extract have been shown to modulate DC function in a way that favours a Th2 outcome. Components of birch pollen extract altered the maturation and cytokine release by monocyte-derived DC and when these pollen-exposed DC were cultured with naïve T cells, pollen induced a shift from a Th1 to a Th2 phenotype.[(58)] These effects were shown with pollen from a variety of plants, suggesting it was a general effect of pollen, which was attributed to phytoprostanes found in pollen grains. In a follow-up study, pollen phytoprostanes also altered chemokine and chemokine receptor expression, demonstrating that pollen itself is capable of regulating the immune response by producing Th2 attracting chemokines that preferentially recruit Th2 cells to pollen-exposed sites.[59]

Finally, when the effects of allergen and LPS on DC have been directly compared[43, 60, 62] it appears that these two stimuli induced very distinct patterns of response, further strengthening the notion that allergens induce a defined immune response which is different to the general strong stimulatory response seen with LPS. Overall these studies suggest that allergens such as HDM, pollen and some fungal allergens have their own intrinsic properties which can modulate a DC response resulting in a Th2 skewed immune response. An individual's propensity for the development of allergic disease is therefore likely to be governed by genetic background interacting with the physical properties of particular allergens.

12.4 Pathogen recognition receptors

DC play a crucial role in pathogen recognition and inducing innate immune responses aimed at eliminating an invading pathogen from the infected host. Recognizing an invading organism is dependent on conserved pattern-recognition receptors (PRRs) that are expressed by a wide variety of cell types, but especially DC, and in this regard the Toll-like receptor (TLR) family are probably the best characterized PRRs. However, other molecules such as the membrane bound C-type lectins can also function as PRRs. These different PRR families have different but coordinated roles in pathogen recognition, phagocytosis, antigen uptake, DC maturation, cytokine production and the subsequent development of adaptive immunity. In terms of allergic immunity, it is the family of C-type lectin receptors that appear to also function as allergen uptake receptors, and recent findings suggest they may also have a role in promoting an allergen-specific Th2 skewed immune response, as discussed in greater detail later (section 12.4.3).

12.4.1 C-type lectin receptors

C-type lectins are highly conserved molecules that usually have a calcium-dependent carbohydrate-binding protein; however, this is not invariable. Therefore the C-type lectin receptor (CLR) family is defined by the presence of one or more C-type lectin domains, which is a structural motif within the carbohydrate-recognition domain. This is found in over 1,000 proteins of diverse function and includes both soluble and membrane-bound proteins.[63] This large family of CLRs is further grouped into 17 subclasses based on the number and arrangement of carbohydrate recognition domains, with some members having a broad cellular expression pattern.[64] Due to the large number of CLRs, it is not surprising that there is also a large amount of diversity not only in the structural make-up of the individual CLRs, but also in the domains they recognize and immune responses they elicit. For example, collectins belong to the group III CLR family and are serum proteins that bind microbes and activate complement, but as they are not cell associated, they do not signal and regulate gene expression. In comparison, the group V proteins are primarily encoded within the NK-gene complex and predominantly act as NK cell receptors responding to self-determinants rather than pathogens.[63]

Due to the large number of proteins that form the CLR superfamily, this chapter will focus on several members of the CLR family that are membrane bound and present on DC. These CLR family members are collectively involved in pathogen recognition, phagocytosis, antigen uptake, cellular adhesion, migration and/or signaling. In this regard, the main CLRs that will be discussed are the membrane-bound mannose receptor, DEC-205, DC-SIGN (DC-specific ICAM-3 grabbing nonintegrin), dectin-1, dectin-2, BDCA2 (blood DC antigen 2), langerin, MGL (macrophage galactose-type lectin), MDL-1, MICL-1 (myeloid inhibitory C-type lectin receptor), members of the CLEC subfamily and the not widely studied BDCA3 (also known as thrombomodulin and CD141), which we have recently shown to have a role in asthma and allergy (section 12.4.3.2). The review of the CLR area is by no means complete but the selected examples highlight the many functions of CLRs and the many diverse functions attributed to this family. As our knowledge of the CLR family increases it may become possible to subclassify members based on similar roles within an innate immune response.

12.4.2 CLRs: pathogen recognition and beyond

12.4.2.1 Pathogen recognition, phagocytosis, endocytosis and antigen processing

Many of the CLRs are capable of binding a variety of invading pathogens including bacteria, viruses and fungi. For example, the mannose receptor can bind yeasts, human immunodeficiency virus and *Mycobacterium tuberculosis*, dectin-1 also binds to yeasts, while MGL binds to *Schistosoma mansoni* and filoviruses and DC-SIGN shows a broad pattern of recognition by binding to a variety of pathogens including fungi, viruses, bacteria, protozoa and parasites. Similar to other PRRs like the TLRs, a variety of different recognition profiles are used by each lectin. This means that some pathogens will interact with several members of the CLR family and this diversity allows a broad spectrum of bacterial and viral pathogens and antigens to be recognized and immune responses elicited. While the recognition motifs of the more widely studied CLRs have been described and include specificity for mannose structures, Lewis antigens, GlcNAc, GalNAc and β-glucans, the carbohydrate and pathogen structures recognized by other CLR family members have yet to be described.

This ability to bind pathogens has led to classification of CLRs as PRR, akin to but independent from the TLR family, which act to protect the host from invading pathogens. However, some host detrimental effects have been linked to CLRs, which questions the notion that all CLRs are conserved PRR (63). As an example, the human immunodeficiency virus uses the CLR DC-SIGN to enter DC, but uptake of the virus through this receptor actually protects the virus from degradation, allowing transmission to T cells.[65] Similarly, uptake of *M. tuberculosis* by the mannose receptor actually aids pathogen survival.[66] There are several similar reports along this line to suggest that some CLR mediated pathogen binding might be more of a reflection of exploitation of the CLR by the pathogen rather than conserved pattern recognition by the host aimed at removing the invading organisms. Further research into pathogen recognition and identification of the pathogen-associated molecular patterns recognized by the CLRs will help to identify which CLR members are true PRR. Nonetheless, many CLRs bind to invading pathogens and, as detailed below, are capable of internalizing them and initiating an immune response.

Many C-type lectins also act as phagocytic receptors on myeloid cells and it is the acidic amino acids, dileucine and tyrosine-based motifs within their cytoplasmic tail that can direct the antigen uptake and trafficking within the cell. The intracellular tail of the mannose receptor has a tyrosine-based motif which can facilitate the delivery of mannosylated ligands to early endosomes, while DEC-205, which also has an additional triacidic motif, can deliver the receptor to late-endosomes-lysosomes.[67] In comparison, dectin-1, which recognises β-glucan and hence can phagocytose yeast and yeast particles such as zymosan, uses both triacidic and tyrosine motifs for endocytosis.[68–70] The intracellular route taken by the CLR is dependent not only on the receptor motifs but also on the nature of the activating agent as shown with DC-SIGN, which can traffic to either early or late endocytic and lysosomal compartments when cross-linked either with antibodies[71] or human immunodeficiency virus[65] respectively. The fate of the CLR once internalized is also varied depending on the processes employed. Following phagocytosis of zymosan by dectin-1 the complex traffics to phagolysosomes where the receptor is degraded and new receptor synthesis occurs, whereas endocytosis of soluble ligands by dectin-1 results in either recycling of the receptor or retention of the receptor intracellularly.[68]

Indeed it is the ability of CLRs to endocytose ligands that results in the generation of antigenic peptides that can be presented to T cells. In this regard, the CLRs DEC-205, DC-SIGN, BDCA2 and the mannose receptor all have internalization motifs that can deliver antigen to late endosomal-lysosomal compartments of antigen-presenting cells like DC, whereby antigenic peptides and major histocompatilibility complexes can be formed and recycled to the cellular surface ready for antigen presentation to T cells[67, 71–74] The extent to which these processes might be relevant to allergy pathogenesis will be described in detail in section 12.4.3.

12.4.2.2 Intracellular CLR signaling and gene expression

An important feature of any PRR is not just the ability to recognize specific pathogen-associated molecular patterns but also the capacity to signal downstream to innate immunity genes. Once again dectin-1 is one of the better characterized CLRs in this respect and has been reviewed in detail elsewhere.[75] Briefly, TLR2 was one of the first PRR identified to recognise zymosan,[69] though it appears that dectin-1 may also be important in this respect. Dectin-1 engagement results in signaling through Syk with downstream activation of the mitogen-activated protein kinases p39, Erk and Jnk and NFκB and the activation of innate immune genes.[63] Syk may be an important signaling molecule for several CLRs, either through direct activation or via immunoreceptor tyrosine-based activation motif (ITAM)-containing adaptor proteins. The downstream result of these activation pathways generally results in cytokine production such as IL-2, IL-10, IL-12 and TNFα.[69] DCIR and MICL have also been shown to have an immunoreceptor tyrosine-based inhibitory motif (ITIM), but it is unknown if these ITIM-containing lectins can deliver negative signals to DC.[76, 77]

Some CLRs may also modify the responses induced by other receptors. In this regard, BDCA-2 cross-linking on plasmacytoid DC suppresses TLR-induced production of IFNα/β.[72] DC immunoreceptor (DCIR) can also suppress TLR9-induced IFNα production by plasmacytoid DC while not affecting the upregulation of co-stimulatory molecules.[78] One important aspect of this study was the efficient presentation of antigens targeted through the DCIR to T cells. Similarly, DC-SIGN ligation amplifies the LPS-stimulated IL-10 response mediated by TLR4 while concurrently preventing DC maturation.[79, 80] Dectin-1 can also synergize with both TLR2 and TLR4 ligands to increase TNFα production.[81] Overall a complex picture is emerging whereby CLRs play an important role in mediating the innate immune response to pathogens either directly or by altering the response of other PRR such as the TLRs. As described below (section 12.4.3), CLRs are also starting to be linked with allergen recognition and subsequent immune activation.

12.4.2.3 CLR mediated cellular interactions and directed immunity

There is accumulating evidence to also suggest that the CLRs are not only involved in pathogen recognition and uptake, but also have roles in adhesion and can induce immune responses of other cells. DC-SIGN is a DC-specific adhesion molecule on human DC that can mediate the interaction with other cell types such as endothelial cells, T cells and neutrophils through their expression of ICAM-2, ICAM-3 and CEACAM-1/Mac-1 respectively.[82–84] DC-SIGN therefore has a role in the adhesion and rolling of DC-SIGN positive cells along blood vessel linings of ICAM-2 positive endothelium resulting in the migration of DC from blood into tissues. It is also possible that tissue specific restriction may regulate and direct the migration of DC to specific sites, as has been shown by the mannose receptor and selectin-mediated migration of leukocytes along lymphatic endothelial cells.[85, 86] In contrast, a recent report has described hampered migration of immature DC expressing MGL and it is not until DC maturation takes place, where MGL expression is abolished, that DC regain the capacity to migrate.[87] Further work is required to assess the reasoning for this response, but it does highlight the need for a much greater understanding of CLR function.

This adhesive property of DC-SIGN not only aids in cellular trafficking but also permits interactions between DC and T cells through DC-SIGN and ICAM-3, and therefore has a role in initiating a T cell response by stabilizing the interaction and permitting the initial engagement of the TCR. Similarly, the CLR MGL is expressed on immature DC and can interact with CD45 on effector T cells which then has a direct signaling effect and prevents the action of the phosphatase, resulting in decreased Lck activity and T cell activation.[88] Another example involves DCAL-1, which can bind to a subset of $CD4^{+}CD45RA^{+}$ T cells and enhances CD3-induced proliferation with increased IL-4 secretion.[89] Dectin-2 expression on APC mediates the interaction with $CD4^{+}CD25^{+}$ regulatory T cells and mediates ultraviolet-induced tolerance to contact hypersensitivity.[90] Together this limited data does suggest that some CLRs are capable of inducing and modulating T cell responses, and as the field of study increases and the natural T cell ligands that are stimulated by CLRs on APC are identified, a more complete picture will emerge in this area.

In summary, the CLR family is a large and diverse family of proteins that, to date, are grouped together and defined by the structural motif that is the C-type lectin domain. While some members of the family do appear to act as classical PRRs and can capture antigen into the antigen processing compartments within DC allowing MHC class II restricted presentation, other CLRs may be involved in transmitting signals to responding T cells. Increased understanding of this family will come from further identifying the various pathogens, their ligands and sequence motifs used to bind to the various CLRs and by also identifying the signaling pathways elicited following engagement of the CLR, which may lead to better groupings and classification of this diverse group of CLRs. The CLR family plays an important role in innate immunity and the identification of how the CLRs interact with T cells will ultimately provide insight into how innate and adaptive immunity are regulated through the CLRs. It is in this regard that CLRs may have a role in the allergic response, and this is discussed below.

12.4.3 CLRs: their role in allergic immunity

12.4.3.1 CLRs facilitate HDM uptake by DC

DC need to be activated by allergen to instigate the allergic inflammatory cascade and it is therefore important to know by what mechanisms allergen is taken up. Immature DC can use several pathways for antigen uptake. These include macropinocytosis, a mechanism whereby antigen is endocytosed by membrane ruffling,[91] and phagocytosis.[92, 93] Other receptor-mediated mechanisms for antigen uptake include the mannose receptor.[91] DEC205,[67] langerin,[94] DC-SIGN[95] and the Fc receptors such as FcεR1[96] and FcγR1.[56] The pathway utilized varies according to the type of antigen and the type of DC. As previously stated (section 12.3.1), IgE receptors have been identified as important mediators in the uptake if allergens; however, as they are not uniformly expressed among all DC subsets, so other mechanisms must also be important to allow allergen uptake and processing of these antigens ready for T cell presentation. It is in this regard that the mannose receptor, a CLR, has been identified as a HDM receptor.

In relation to the pollen allergens Bet v 1 and Ph1 p 1, both macropinocytosis[97] and receptor-mediated mechanisms appear to be involved in allergen uptake. In this regard, the mannose receptor is used by monocyte-derived DC for uptake of both the allergenic components of yeast (54) and Der p 1.[55] Interestingly, DC from allergic donors show a greater level of mannose receptor expression and are much more efficient in Der p 1 uptake than DC from non-allergic healthy controls.[55] Based on the blocking studies reported in this study, it is likely that other mechanisms also act in concert with the mannose receptor in HDM uptake, including not just FcεR1, but perhaps other unidentified CLR are also capable of acting as allergen uptake receptors.

12.4.3.2 Can CLRs induce a Th2 skewed response?

The question that now must be asked is whether CLR signaling can directly instruct Th polarization and activation. Data is now emerging that this is indeed a possibility, as signaling via dectin-1 or antigen uptake via dectin-1 can induce a more IL-12 dominated response,[69, 98] whereas DCAL-1 may act as a co-stimulatory molecule skewing towards a Th2 response with increased IL-4 production.[89] Another example of a CLR skewing a Th response is shown with variants of *Helicobacter pylori* which bind to DC-SIGN on gastric DC and this interaction blocks skewing of naïve T cells to Th1 type cells.[99] Interestingly, the protease activity of Der p 1 can cleave DC-SIGN and DC-SIGNR on DC, which leads to reduced binding of ICAM-3, a DC-SIGN ligand that is thought to be involved in Th1 signaling in naïve cells.[100] Peanut glycoallergens are also recognized by DC through DC-SIGN and when these peanut-stimulated DC were co-cultured with naïve T cells, increased IL-4 and IL-13 production was observed, highlighting the ability of this allergen to promote a Th2 skewed response.[101] All these studies suggest that several CLRs can influence Th activation and studies into DC-SIGN suggest that it may inhibit Th1 production and therefore may increase Th2 activation, as seen in response to peanut. Some novel data from our group suggests that another CLR can directly induce a Th2 skewed response to HDM and provides a new mechanism for the maintenance of allergic respiratory disease.

The CLRs BDCA-2, -3 and -4 are all used to define subsets of DC in peripheral blood and tissues.[102] BDCA2 and BDCA4 are used to identify plasmacytoid DC, while BDCA3 defines a minor subset of myeloid DC.

It is this later C-type lectin that has caught our attention as it was one of the most differentially regulated genes identified in a microarray screen of HDM-stimulated DC showing enhanced expression on DC from allergic donors and down-regulated expression on DC from non-allergic donors.[103] The enhanced expression of BDCA3 (often referred to as thrombomodulin or CD141 in other fields of study) on HDM-stimulated monocyte-derived DC from allergic compared to non-allergic donors was confirmed in independent cohorts of study subjects at both the mRNA and protein levels. Furthermore, this discordant response between allergic and non-allergic donors was not seen following LPS stimulation. *In vivo*, these BDCA3 expressing DC were more prevalent in peripheral blood of subjects with asthmatic and allergic disease compared to healthy controls, and the level of expression per cell was also increased with allergic asthma. While our study was done in the blood, a similar response has also been seen when DC were enumerated in sputum of asthmatic and controls subjects (104). Finally, when monocyte-derived DC were FACS sorted based on BDCA3 expression, the $BDCA3^+$ cells induced a Th2 skewed HDM response while $BDCA3^-$ DC induced a mixed Th1/Th2 response to HDM.[103]

This is the first study to identify BDCA3 as having a role in the allergic response and, more importantly, as it defines a population of myeloid DC that is found in blood and lung, it could have an important role in asthma pathogenesis. Interestingly this subset (also described as mDC2 for myeloid DC subset 2) shows an approximately tenfold reduction in numbers in peripheral blood compared to the more abundant myeloid DC1 subset (mDC1). However, when DC numbers in lung sections[12] and bronchoalveolar lavage fluid[105] have been enumerated, the 2 myeloid DC subsets appear in equal numbers, suggesting that the BDCA3 expressing DC may preferentially traffic to the lung, adding more weight to the notion that this DC subset is important in the allergic response. This finding complements animal studies which suggest that different DC subsets have an important role in promoting allergic disease.[21, 22]

How does BDCA3 promote a Th2 HDM response? There is no precedent in the literature for this, or hints at what T cell ligands it might interact with, though an emerging literature is now beginning to highlight molecules that are exclusively expressed on the $BDCA3^+$ DC subset. In this regard, CLEC9A is only detected on the $BDCA3^+$ DC subset, can mediate endocytosis, may function as an activation receptor due to its cytoplasmic ITAM motif, and can induce the production of proinflammatory cytokines (106). In light of this it will be interesting to determine whether CLEC proteins can interact with allergens. Finally, several studies[102, 107–110] have partially characterized the $BDCA3^+$ DC subset in comparison to the other

CD1c$^+$ myeloid DC subset (mDC1) in order to better understand the role of this DC subset in allergies. It will be interesting in the future to confirm if BDCA3 can directly modify a T cell response. Of note here, thrombin is a natural ligand of BDCA3 and as it has proteolytic activity, this may be an important feature of HDM in the response described above.

BDCA3 is a CLR that may have a role in mediating allergic responses and this can be seen as a detrimental effect to the host; however, it is perhaps the cell type and context of the response that is most important. As previously stated, BDCA3 is also known as thrombomodulin, which is expressed by virtually all endothelial cells, and in this context it is a major component of the anti-coagulation pathway and can therefore be seen as a highly advantageous process to the host. This is yet another example of how CLRs need to be more clearly defined and ligands identified to fully understand their activity in different systems, and to better understand how therapeutic targets could be selectively designed to down-regulate some functions.

12.4.4 TLRs and CLRs: Could they be used to reduce allergic disease?

TLR biology will not be covered in great detail here, as there are many excellent reviews on the subject, but they are expressed on a wide variety of cells, including DC. In humans ten TLRs have been identified and these are classified into subfamilies based on the ligands they recognize and their cellular location. The TLR field is much more advanced than the CLR field, with most of the ligands and specificities already described. In general, TLR1, TLR2, TLR4 and TLR6 recognize lipids and are expressed on the cell surface while TLR3, TLR7, TLR8 and TLR9 recognize nucleic acids and are expressed intracellularly, typically in the late endosomes-lysosomes. Interest in the role of TLRs in allergy has coincided with emergence of the hygiene hypothesis, which suggests that one of the mechanisms by which allergic disease has rapidly increased over recent years is due to the cleaner environment in which people now live. This includes more urban living, less exposure to natural infections and changes in the bacterial flora of the gut, all of which impact on the developing immune system. Indeed, some studies have suggested that indoor endotoxin exposure early in life may protect against allergic sensitization by enhancing Th1 mediated immunity.[(111)] However, microbial infections are frequently implicated in asthma exacerbations.[(112)] Therefore there is intense interest in the interaction between exposure to microbial products and human allergic disease, and whether these microbial components could be used to down-regulate established allergic disease. In animal models, administration of lipopolypeptides immediately prior to airway challenge inhibits Th2 type responses and IgE production.[(113)] TLR2 stimulation has also been shown to inhibit established allergic airway inflammation in mice by augmenting the Th1 response.[(114)] In this regard, our research group investigated this in humans and used components of Gram-positive bacteria in combination with HDM in peripheral blood mononuclear cell cultures from allergic individuals with HDM sensitivity.[(115)] This study showed that different TLR2 ligands could all down-regulate the HDM induced production of IL-5 and IL-13, and some showed reduced IFNγ production as well. The effect was not associated with changes in antigen presentation or processing by antigen presenting cells, but did appear to be mediated through DC.

It would be interesting to investigate the potential role of mediating immune-modulation as many of the TLR ligands can also stimulate CLRs. It is possible that the CLRs may be more potent than the TLRs in regulating allergic responses due to the direct nature of the interaction, i.e. stimulating through a TLR may only indirectly regulate the allergen response, whereas CLRs might have a more direct effect on allergen uptake (e.g. HDM and the mannose receptor) in addition to modulating allergen-induced Th2 skewing (e.g. BDCA3). Future studies will need to directly compare the effects of CLRs and TLRs in mediating immune-modulation, and whether CLRs might be an important therapeutic target in allergic diseases. Time will tell if CLRs are as successful as TLRs in limiting human allergic immune responses *in vitro* and if both of these can then be used as a therapeutic tool to treat/limit established human allergic disease.

12.5 Conclusions

In conclusion, HDM and pollen allergy is globally a growing concern and a much greater understanding is needed to fully comprehend the mechanisms contributing to the exponentially increasing burden of allergic disease. Animal models have highlighted the important and fundamental role DC have in priming and maintaining an allergic response. Human studies, while limited in their scope and ability to tease apart the various aspects of sensitization and maintenance of an allergic response, have also confirmed the critical role DC play. When DC are compared between allergic and non-allergic donors, different patterns of response are observed and some of this may be due to the allergen itself, as HDM, pollen and many other allergens are now viewed as biologically active molecules that have intrinsic abilities allowing them to regulate DC function. The innate PRRs, such as the large and diverse family known as the CLRs, are beginning to be identified as having a role in allergic disease. Some members of this family have been identified as allergen uptake receptors, while others have the capacity to modify a T cell response and induce Th2 skewing. Further research into this area will be able to define this family better and identify those CLRs that have true PRR capabilities and those that are hijacked by a pathogen with detrimental host effects. In this regard, further research will also more clearly define the CLR family in the allergic response. It may be possible to work out which CLRs are pro-allergic and then target them to potentially subvert the Th2 skew or to use CLR or TLR ligands to down-regulate allergen induced Th2 responses. In this way, we may be better able to understand how respiratory allergic disease develops and how to try and limit the impact it has on human health.

References

1 Arlian, L.G. and Platts-Mills, T.A. 2001. The biology of dust mites and the remediation of mite allergens in allergic disease. *J Allergy Clin Immunol* 107: S406–413.
2 Thomas, W.R., Heinrich, T.K., Smith, W.A. and Hales, B.J. 2007. Pyroglyphid house dust mite allergens. *Protein Pept Lett* 14: 943–53.
3 Hales, B.J., Martin, A.C., Pearce, L.J., Laing, I.A., Hayden, C.M., Goldblatt, J., Le Souef, P.N. and Thomas, W.R. 2006. IgE and IgG anti-house dust mite specificities in allergic disease. *J Allergy Clin Immunol* 118: 361–7.
4 Thomas, W.R., Smith, W.A., Hales, B.J., Mills, K.L. and O'Brien, R.M. 2002. Characterization and immunobiology of house dust mite allergens. *Int Arch Allergy Immunol* 129: 1–18.
5 Hales, B.J., Chu, N.N.R., Bosco, A., Smith, W.A., Heinrich, T.K. and Thomas, W.R. 2006. Determinants of House Dust Mite Allergenicity. *Allergy and Clinical Immunology International – Journal of the World Allergy Organization* 18: 65–70.
6 Gough, L., Campbell, E., Bayley, D., Van Heeke, G. and Shakib, F. 2003. Proteolytic activity of the house dust mite allergen Der p 1 enhances allergenicity in a mouse inhalation model. *Clin Exp Allergy* 33: 1159–63.
7 Ghaemmaghami, A.M., Gough, L., Sewell, H.F. and Shakib, F. 2002. The proteolytic activity of the major dust mite allergen Der p 1 conditions dendritic cells to produce less interleukin-12: allergen-induced Th2 bias determined at the dendritic cell level. *Clin Exp Allergy* 32: 1468–75.
8 Hammad, H., Charbonnier, A.S., Duez, C., Jacquet, A., Stewart, G.A., Tonnel, A.B. and Pestel, J. 2001. Th2 polarization by Der p 1-pulsed monocyte-derived dendritic cells is due to the allergic status of the donors. *Blood* 98: 1135–41.

9 Sokol, C.L., Barton, G.M., Farr, A.G. and Medzhitov, R. 2008. A mechanism for the initiation of allergen-induced T helper type 2 responses. *Nat Immunol* 9: 310–8.
10 Jahnsen, F.L., Strickland, D.H., Thomas, J.A., Tobagus, I.T., Napoli, S., Zosky, G.R., Turner, D.J., Sly, P.D., Stumbles, P.A. and Holt, P.G. 2006. Accelerated antigen sampling and transport by airway mucosal dendritic cells following inhalation of a bacterial stimulus. *J Immunol* 177: 5861–7.
11 Sporri, R. and Reis e Sousa, C. 2005. Inflammatory mediators are insufficient for full dendritic cell activation and promote expansion of CD4+ T cell populations lacking helper function. *Nat Immunol* 6: 163–70.
12 de Heer, H.J., Hammad, H., Kool, M. and Lambrecht, B.N. 2005. Dendritic cell subsets and immune regulation in the lung. *Semin Immunol* 17: 295–303.
13 Akbari, O., DeKruyff, R.H. and Umetsu, D.T. 2001. Pulmonary dendritic cells producing IL-10 mediate tolerance induced by respiratory exposure to antigen. *Nat Immunol* 2: 725–31.
14 Akbari, O., Freeman, G.J., Meyer, E.H., Greenfield, E.A., Chang, T.T., Sharpe, A.H., Berry, G., DeKruyff, R.H. and Umetsu, D.T. 2002. Antigen-specific regulatory T cells develop via the ICOS-ICOS-ligand pathway and inhibit allergen-induced airway hyperreactivity. *Nat Med* 8: 1024–32.
15 Lambrecht, B.N., Carro-Muino, I., Vermaelen, K. and Pauwels, R.A. 1999. Allergen-induced changes in bone-marrow progenitor and airway dendritic cells in sensitized rats. *Am J Respir Cell Mol Biol* 20: 1165–74.
16 van Rijt, L.S., Prins, J.B., Leenen, P.J., Thielemans, K., de Vries, V.C., Hoogsteden, H.C. and Lambrecht, B.N. 2002. Allergen-induced accumulation of airway dendritic cells is supported by an increase in CD31(hi)Ly-6C(neg) bone marrow precursors in a mouse model of asthma. *Blood* 100: 3663–71.
17 Constant, S.L., Brogdon, J.L., Piggott, D.A., Herrick, C.A., Visintin, I., Ruddle, N.H. and Bottomly, K. 2002. Resident lung antigen-presenting cells have the capacity to promote Th2 T cell differentiation in situ. *J Clin Invest* 110: 1441–8.
18 Stumbles, P.A., Thomas, J.A., Pimm, C.L., Lee, P.T., Venaille, T.J., Proksch, S. and Holt, P.G. 1998. Resting respiratory tract dendritic cells preferentially stimulate T helper cell type 2 (Th2) responses and require obligatory cytokine signals for induction of Th1 immunity. *J Exp Med* 188: 2019–31.
19 Lambrecht, B.N., Salomon, B., Klatzmann, D. and Pauwels, R.A. 1998. Dendritic cells are required for the development of chronic eosinophilic airway inflammation in response to inhaled antigen in sensitized mice. *J Immunol* 160: 4090–4097.
20 Julia, V., Hessel, E.M., Malherbe, L., Glaichenhaus, N., O'Garra, A. and Coffman, R.L. 2002. A restricted subset of dendritic cells captures airborne antigens and remains able to activate specific T cells long after antigen exposure. *Immunity* 16: 271–83.
21 Huh, J.C., Strickland, D.H., Jahnsen, F.L., Turner, D.J., Thomas, J.A., Napoli, S., Tobagus, I., Stumbles, P.A., Sly, P.D. and Holt, P.G. 2003. Bidirectional interactions between antigen-bearing respiratory tract dendritic cells (DCs) and T cells precede the late phase reaction in experimental asthma: DC activation occurs in the airway mucosa but not in the lung parenchyma. *J Exp Med* 198: 19–30.
22 von Garnier, C., Filgueira, L., Wikstrom, M., Smith, M., Thomas, J.A., Strickland, D.H., Holt, P.G. and Stumbles, P.A. 2005. Anatomical location determines the

distribution and function of dendritic cells and other APCs in the respiratory tract. *J Immunol* 175: 1609–18.
23 Moller, G.M., Overbeek, S.E., Van Helden-Meeuwsen, C.G., Van Haarst, J.M., Prens, E. P., Mulder, P.G., Postma, D.S. and Hoogsteden, H.C. 1996. Increased numbers of dendritic cells in the bronchial mucosa of atopic asthmatic patients: downregulation by inhaled corticosteroids. *Clin Exp Allergy* 26: 517–24.
24 Tunon-De-Lara, J.M., Redington, A.E., Bradding, P., Church, M.K., Hartley, J. A., Semper, A.E. and Holgate, S.T. 1996. Dendritic cells in normal and asthmatic airways: expression of the alpha subunit of the high affinity immunoglobulin E receptor (Fc epsilon RI -alpha). *Clin Exp Allergy* 26: 648–55.
25 Jahnsen, F.L., Moloney, E.D., Hogan, T., Upham, J.W., Burke, C.M. and Holt, P. G. 2001. Rapid dendritic cell recruitment to the bronchial mucosa of patients with atopic asthma in response to local allergen challenge. *Thorax* 56: 823–6.
26 Upham, J.W., Denburg, J.A. and O'Byrne, P.M. 2002. Rapid response of circulating myeloid dendritic cells to inhaled allergen in asthmatic subjects. *Clin Exp Allergy* 32: 818–23.
27 Chen, X.Q., Yang, J., Hu, S.P., Nie, H.X., Mao, G.Y. and Chen, H.B. 2006. Increased expression of CD86 and reduced production of IL-12 and IL-10 by monocyte-derived dendritic cells from allergic asthmatics and their effects on Th1- and Th2-type cytokine balance. *Respiration* 73: 34–40.
28 Keane-Myers, A.M., Gause, W.C., Finkelman, F.D., Xhou, X.D. and Wills-Karp, M. 1998. Development of murine allergic asthma is dependent upon B7–2 costimulation. *J Immunol* 160: 1036–43.
29 Tsuyuki, S., Tsuyuki, J., Einsle, K., Kopf, M. and Coyle, A.J. 1997. Costimulation through B7–2 (CD86) is required for the induction of a lung mucosal T helper cell 2 (TH2) immune response and altered airway responsiveness. *J Exp Med* 185: 1671–9.
30 Harris, N.L., Prout, M., Peach, R.J., Fazekas de St Groth, B. and Ronchese, F. 2001. CD80 costimulation is required for Th2 cell cytokine production but not for antigen-specific accumulation and migration into the lung. *J Immunol* 166: 4908–14.
31 Schweitzer, A.N. and Sharpe, A.H. 1998. Studies using antigen-presenting cells lacking expression of both B7–1 (CD80) and B7–2 (CD86) show distinct requirements for B7 molecules during priming versus restimulation of Th2 but not Th1 cytokine production. *J Immunol* 161: 2762–71.
32 Liu, Y.J. 2007. Thymic stromal lymphopoietin and OX40 ligand pathway in the initiation of dendritic cell-mediated allergic inflammation. *J Allergy Clin Immunol* 120: 238–44.
33 Seshasayee, D., Lee, W.P., Zhou, M., Shu, J., Suto, E., Zhang, J., Diehl, L., Austin, C.D., Meng, Y.G., Tan, M., Bullens, S.L., Seeber, S., Fuentes, M.E., Labrijn, A.F., Graus, Y.M., Miller, L.A., Schelegle, E.S., Hyde, D.M., Wu, L.C., Hymowitz, S.G. and Martin, F. 2007. In vivo blockade of OX40 ligand inhibits thymic stromal lymphopoietin driven atopic inflammation. *J Clin Invest* 117: 3868–78.
34 Hoshino, A., Tanaka, Y., Akiba, H., Asakura, Y., Mita, Y., Sakurai, T., Takaoka, A., Nakaike, S., Ishii, N., Sugamura, K., Yagita, H. and Okumura, K. 2003. Critical role for OX40 ligand in the development of pathogenic Th2 cells in a murine model of asthma. *Eur J Immunol* 33: 861–9.

35 Reider, N., Reider, D., Ebner, S., Holzmann, S., Herold, M., Fritsch, P. and Romani, N. 2002. Dendritic cells contribute to the development of atopy by an insufficiency in IL-12 production. *J Allergy Clin Immunol* 109: 89–95.
36 Bellinghausen, I., Brand, U., Knop, J. and Saloga, J. 2000. Comparison of allergen-stimulated dendritic cells from atopic and nonatopic donors dissecting their effect on autologous naive and memory T helper cells of such donors. *J Allergy Clin Immunol* 105: 988–96.
37 Long, J.A., Fogel-Petrovic, M., Knight, D.A., Thompson, P.J. and Upham, J.W. 2004. Higher prostaglandin e2 production by dendritic cells from subjects with asthma compared with normal subjects. *Am J Respir Crit Care Med* 170: 485–91.
38 Charbonnier, A.S., Hammad, H., Gosset, P., Stewart, G.A., Alkan, S., Tonnel, A. B. and Pestel, J. 2003. Der p 1-pulsed myeloid and plasmacytoid dendritic cells from house dust mite-sensitized allergic patients dysregulate the T cell response. *J Leukoc Biol* 73: 91–9.
39 Cates, E.C., Fattouh, R., Wattie, J., Inman, M.D., Goncharova, S., Coyle, A.J., Gutierrez-Ramos, J.C. and Jordana, M. 2004. Intranasal exposure of mice to house dust mite elicits allergic airway inflammation via a GM-CSF-mediated mechanism. *J Immunol* 173: 6384–92.
40 Dodge, I.L., Carr, M.W., Cernadas, M. and Brenner, M.B. 2003. IL-6 production by pulmonary dendritic cells impedes Th1 immune responses. *J Immunol* 170: 4457–64.
41 Krishnamoorthy, N., Oriss, T.B., Paglia, M., Fei, M., Yarlagadda, M., Vanhaesebroeck, B., Ray, A. and Ray, P. 2008. Activation of c-Kit in dendritic cells regulates T helper cell differentiation and allergic asthma. *Nat Med* 14: 565–73.
42 Pasare, C. and Medzhitov, R. 2003. Toll pathway-dependent blockade of CD4+CD25+ T cell-mediated suppression by dendritic cells. *Science* 299: 1033–6.
43 Bellinghausen, I., Klostermann, B., Knop, J. and Saloga, J. 2003. Human CD4+CD25+ T cells derived from the majority of atopic donors are able to suppress TH1 and TH2 cytokine production. *J Allergy Clin Immunol* 111: 862–8.
44 Ling, E.M., Smith, T., Nguyen, X.D., Pridgeon, C., Dallman, M., Arbery, J., Carr, V.A. and Robinson, D.S. 2004. Relation of CD4+CD25+ regulatory T-cell suppression of allergen-driven T-cell activation to atopic status and expression of allergic disease. *Lancet* 363: 608–15.
45 Grindebacke, H., Wing, K., Andersson, A.C., Suri-Payer, E., Rak, S. and Rudin, A. 2004. Defective suppression of Th2 cytokines by CD4CD25 regulatory T cells in birch allergics during birch pollen season. *Clin Exp Allergy* 34: 1364–72.
46 Akdis, M., Verhagen, J., Taylor, A., Karamloo, F., Karagiannidis, C., Crameri, R., Thunberg, S., Deniz, G., Valenta, R., Fiebig, H., Kegel, C., Disch, R., Schmidt-Weber, C.B., Blaser, K. and Akdis, C.A. 2004. Immune responses in healthy and allergic individuals are characterized by a fine balance between allergen-specific T regulatory 1 and T helper 2 cells. *J Exp Med* 199: 1567–75.
47 Orihara, K., Narita, M., Tobe, T., Akasawa, A., Ohya, Y., Matsumoto, K. and Saito, H. 2007. Circulating Foxp3+CD4+ cell numbers in atopic patients and healthy control subjects. *J Allergy Clin Immunol* 120: 960–2.

48 Maggi, L., Santarlasci, V., Liotta, F., Frosali, F., Angeli, R., Cosmi, L., Maggi, E., Romagnani, S. and Annunziato, F. 2007. Demonstration of circulating allergen-specific CD4+CD25highFoxp3+ T-regulatory cells in both nonatopic and atopic individuals. *J Allergy Clin Immunol* 120: 429–36.
49 Thunberg, S., Akdis, M., Akdis, C.A., Gronneberg, R., Malmstrom, V., Trollmo, C., van Hage, M. and Gafvelin, G. 2007. Immune regulation by CD4+CD25+ T cells and interleukin-10 in birch pollen-allergic patients and non-allergic controls. *Clin Exp Allergy* 37: 1127–36.
50 Hammad, H., Smits, H.H., Ratajczak, C., Nithiananthan, A., Wierenga, E.A., Stewart, G.A., Jacquet, A., Tonnel, A.B. and Pestel, J. 2003. Monocyte-derived dendritic cells exposed to Der p 1 allergen enhance the recruitment of Th2 cells: major involvement of the chemokines TARC/CCL17 and MDC/CCL22. *Eur Cytokine Netw* 14: 219–28.
51 Maurer, D., Fiebiger, S., Ebner, C., Reininger, B., Fischer, G.F., Wichlas, S., Jouvin, M.H., Schmitt-Egenolf, M., Kraft, D., Kinet, J.P. and Stingl, G. 1996. Peripheral blood dendritic cells express Fc epsilon RI as a complex composed of Fc epsilon RI alpha- and Fc epsilon RI gamma-chains and can use this receptor for IgE-mediated allergen presentation. *J Immunol* 157: 607–16.
52 Foster, B., Metcalfe, D.D. and Prussin, C. 2003. Human dendritic cell 1 and dendritic cell 2 subsets express FcepsilonRI: correlation with serum IgE and allergic asthma. *J Allergy Clin Immunol* 112: 1132–8.
53 Kraft, S., Novak, N., Katoh, N., Bieber, T. and Rupec, R.A. 2002. Aggregation of the high-affinity IgE receptor Fc(epsilon)RI on human monocytes and dendritic cells induces NF-kappaB activation. *J Invest Dermatol* 118: 830–7.
54 Buentke, E., Zargari, A., Heffler, L.C., Avila-Carino, J., Savolainen, J. and Scheynius, A. 2000. Uptake of the yeast Malassezia furfur and its allergenic components by human immature CD1a+ dendritic cells. *Clin Exp Allergy* 30: 1759–70.
55 Deslee, G., Charbonnier, A.S., Hammad, H., Angyalosi, G., Tillie-Leblond, I., Mantovani, A., Tonnel, A.B. and Pestel, J. 2002. Involvement of the mannose receptor in the uptake of Der p 1, a major mite allergen, by human dendritic cells. *J Allergy Clin Immunol* 110: 763–70.
56 Fanger, N.A., Voigtlaender, D., Liu, C., Swink, S., Wardwell, K., Fisher, J., Graziano, R.F., Pfefferkorn, L.C. and Guyre, P.M. 1997. Characterization of expression, cytokine regulation, and effector function of the high affinity IgG receptor Fc gamma RI (CD64) expressed on human blood dendritic cells. *J Immunol* 158: 3090–8.
57 Reich, K., Heine, A., Hugo, S., Blaschke, V., Middel, P., Kaser, A., Tilg, H., Blaschke, S., Gutgesell, C. and Neumann, C. 2001. Engagement of the Fc epsilon RI stimulates the production of IL-16 in Langerhans cell-like dendritic cells. *J Immunol* 167: 6321–9.
58 Traidl-Hoffmann, C., Mariani, V., Hochrein, H., Karg, K., Wagner, H., Ring, J., Mueller, M. J., Jakob, T. and Behrendt, H. 2005. Pollen-associated phytoprostanes inhibit dendritic cell interleukin-12 production and augment T helper type 2 cell polarization. *J Exp Med* 201: 627–36.
59 Mariani, V., Gilles, S., Jakob, T., Thiel, M., Mueller, M.J., Ring, J., Behrendt, H. and Traidl-Hoffmann, C. 2007. Immunomodulatory mediators from pollen enhance the migratory capacity of dendritic cells and license them for Th2 attraction. *J Immunol* 178: 7623–31.

60 Lamhamedi-Cherradi, S.E., Martin, R.E., Ito, T., Kheradmand, F., Corry, D.B., Liu, Y.J. and Moyle, M. 2008. Fungal proteases induce Th2 polarization through limited dendritic cell maturation and reduced production of IL-12. *J Immunol* 180: 6000–9.

61 Kheradmand, F., Kiss, A., Xu, J., Lee, S.H., Kolattukudy, P.E. and Corry, D.B. 2002. A protease-activated pathway underlying Th cell type 2 activation and allergic lung disease. *J Immunol* 169: 5904–11.

62 Allakhverdi, Z., Bouguermouh, S., Rubio, M. and Delespesse, G. 2005. Adjuvant activity of pollen grains. *Allergy* 60: 1157–64.

63 Robinson, M.J., Sancho, D., Slack, E.C., LeibundGut-Landmann, S. and Reis e Sousa, C. 2006. Myeloid C-type lectins in innate immunity. *Nat Immunol* 7: 1258–65.

64 Zelensky, A.N. and Gready, J.E. 2005. The C-type lectin-like domain superfamily. *FEBS J* 272: 6179–217.

65 Kwon, D.S., Gregorio, G., Bitton, N., Hendrickson, W.A. and Littman, D.R. 2002. DC-SIGN-mediated internalization of HIV is required for trans-enhancement of T cell infection. *Immunity* 16: 135–44.

66 Kang, P.B., Azad, A.K., Torrelles, J.B., Kaufman, T.M., Beharka, A., Tibesar, E., DesJardin, L.E. and Schlesinger, L.S. 2005. The human macrophage mannose receptor directs Mycobacterium tuberculosis lipoarabinomannan-mediated phagosome biogenesis. *J Exp Med* 202: 987–99.

67 Mahnke, K., Guo, M., Lee, S., Sepulveda, H., Swain, S.L., Nussenzweig, M. and Steinman, R.M. 2000. The dendritic cell receptor for endocytosis, DEC-205, can recycle and enhance antigen presentation via major histocompatibility complex class II-positive lysosomal compartments. *J Cell Biol* 151: 673–84.

68 Herre, J., Marshall, A.S., Caron, E., Edwards, A.D., Williams, D.L., Schweighoffer, E., Tybulewicz, V., Reis e Sousa, C., Gordon, S. and Brown, G.D. 2004. Dectin-1 uses novel mechanisms for yeast phagocytosis in macrophages. *Blood* 104: 4038–45.

69 Rogers, N.C., Slack, E.C., Edwards, A.D., Nolte, M.A., Schulz, O., Schweighoffer, E., Williams, D.L., Gordon, S., Tybulewicz, V.L., Brown, G.D. and Reis e Sousa, C. 2005. Syk-dependent cytokine induction by Dectin-1 reveals a novel pattern recognition pathway for C type lectins. *Immunity* 22: 507–17.

70 Underhill, D.M., Rossnagle, E., Lowell, C.A. and Simmons, R.M. 2005. Dectin-1 activates Syk tyrosine kinase in a dynamic subset of macrophages for reactive oxygen production. *Blood* 106: 2543–50.

71 Engering, A., Geijtenbeek, T.B., van Vliet, S.J., Wijers, M., van Liempt, E., Demaurex, N., Lanzavecchia, A., Fransen, J., Figdor, C.G., Piguet, V. and van Kooyk, Y. 2002. The dendritic cell-specific adhesion receptor DC-SIGN internalizes antigen for presentation to T cells. *J Immunol* 168: 2118–26.

72 Dzionek, A., Sohma, Y., Nagafune, J., Cella, M., Colonna, M., Facchetti, F., Gunther, G., Johnston, I., Lanzavecchia, A., Nagasaka, T., Okada, T., Vermi, W., Winkels, G., Yamamoto, T., Zysk, M., Yamaguchi, Y. and Schmitz, J. 2001. BDCA-2, a novel plasmacytoid dendritic cell-specific type II C-type lectin, mediates antigen capture and is a potent inhibitor of interferon alpha/beta induction. *J Exp Med* 194: 1823–34.

73 Engering, A.J., Cella, M., Fluitsma, D.M., Hoefsmit, E.C., Lanzavecchia, A. and Pieters, J. 1997. Mannose receptor mediated antigen uptake and presentation in human dendritic cells. *Adv Exp Med Biol* 417: 183–7.

74 Tacken, P.J., Torensma, R. and Figdor, C.G. 2006. Targeting antigens to dendritic cells in vivo. *Immunobiology* 211: 599–608.

75 Brown, G.D. 2006. Dectin-1: a signalling non-TLR pattern-recognition receptor. *Nat Rev Immunol* 6: 33–43.

76 Bates, E.E., Fournier, N., Garcia, E., Valladeau, J., Durand, I., Pin, J.J., Zurawski, S.M., Patel, S., Abrams, J.S., Lebecque, S., Garrone, P. and Saeland, S. 1999. APCs express DCIR, a novel C-type lectin surface receptor containing an immunoreceptor tyrosine-based inhibitory motif. *J Immunol* 163: 1973–83.

77 Marshall, A.S., Willment, J.A., Lin, H.H., Williams, D.L., Gordon, S. and Brown, G.D. 2004. Identification and characterization of a novel human myeloid inhibitory C-type lectin-like receptor (MICL) that is predominantly expressed on granulocytes and monocytes. *J Biol Chem* 279: 14792–802.

78 Meyer-Wentrup, F., Benitez-Ribas, D., Tacken, P.J., Punt, C.J., Figdor, C.G., de Vries, I.J. and Adema, G.J. 2008. Targeting DCIR on human plasmacytoid dendritic cells results in antigen presentation and inhibits IFN-alpha production. *Blood* 111: 4245–53.

79 Caparros, E., Munoz, P., Sierra-Filardi, E., Serrano-Gomez, D., Puig-Kroger, A., Rodriguez-Fernandez, J.L., Mellado, M., Sancho, J., Zubiaur, M. and Corbi, A. L. 2006. DC-SIGN ligation on dendritic cells results in ERK and PI3K activation and modulates cytokine production. *Blood* 107: 3950–8.

80 Geijtenbeek, T.B., Van Vliet, S.J., Koppel, E.A., Sanchez-Hernandez, M., Vandenbroucke-Grauls, C.M., Appelmelk, B. and Van Kooyk, Y. 2003. Mycobacteria target DC-SIGN to suppress dendritic cell function. *J Exp Med* 197: 7–17.

81 Ferwerda, G., Meyer-Wentrup, F., Kullberg, B.J., Netea, M.G. and Adema, G.J. 2008. Dectin-1 synergizes with TLR2 and TLR4 for cytokine production in human primary monocytes and macrophages. *Cell Microbiol* 10(10): 2058–66.

82 van Gisbergen, K.P., Ludwig, I.S., Geijtenbeek, T.B. and van Kooyk, Y. 2005. Interactions of DC-SIGN with Mac-1 and CEACAM1 regulate contact between dendritic cells and neutrophils. *FEBS Lett* 579: 6159–68.

83 van Gisbergen, K.P., Paessens, L.C., Geijtenbeek, T.B. and van Kooyk, Y. 2005. Molecular mechanisms that set the stage for DC-T cell engagement. *Immunol Lett* 97: 199–208.

84 van Gisbergen, K.P., Sanchez-Hernandez, M., Geijtenbeek, T.B. and van Kooyk, Y. 2005. Neutrophils mediate immune modulation of dendritic cells through glycosylation-dependent interactions between Mac-1 and DC-SIGN. *J Exp Med* 201: 1281–92.

85 Hemmerich, S., Bistrup, A., Singer, M.S., van Zante, A., Lee, J.K., Tsay, D., Peters, M., Carminati, J.L., Brennan, T.J., Carver-Moore, K., Leviten, M., Fuentes, M.E., Ruddle, N.H. and Rosen, S.D. 2001. Sulfation of L-selectin ligands by an HEV-restricted sulfotransferase regulates lymphocyte homing to lymph nodes. *Immunity* 15: 237–47.

86 Irjala, H., Johansson, E.L., Grenman, R., Alanen, K., Salmi, M. and Jalkanen, S. 2001. Mannose receptor is a novel ligand for L-selectin and mediates lymphocyte binding to lymphatic endothelium. *J Exp Med* 194: 1033–42.

87 van Vliet, S.J., Paessens, L.C., Broks-van den Berg, V.C., Geijtenbeek, T.B. and van Kooyk, Y. 2008. The C-type lectin macrophage galactose-type lectin impedes migration of immature APCs. *J Immunol* 181: 3148–55.

88 van Vliet, S.J., Gringhuis, S.I., Geijtenbeek, T.B. and van Kooyk, Y. 2006. Regulation of effector T cells by antigen-presenting cells via interaction of the C-type lectin MGL with CD45. *Nat Immunol* 7: 1200–8.
89 Ryan, E.J., Marshall, A.J., Magaletti, D., Floyd, H., Draves, K.E., Olson, N.E. and Clark, E.A. 2002. Dendritic cell-associated lectin-1: a novel dendritic cell-associated, C-type lectin-like molecule enhances T cell secretion of IL-4. *J Immunol* 169: 5638–48.
90 Aragane, Y., Maeda, A., Schwarz, A., Tezuka, T., Ariizumi, K. and Schwarz, T. 2003. Involvement of dectin-2 in ultraviolet radiation-induced tolerance. *J Immunol* 171: 3801–7.
91 Sallusto, F., Cella, M., Danieli, C. and Lanzavecchia, A. 1995. Dendritic cells use macropinocytosis and the mannose receptor to concentrate macromolecules in the major histocompatibility complex class II compartment: downregulation by cytokines and bacterial products. *J Exp Med* 182: 389–400.
92 Inaba, K., Inaba, M., Naito, M. and Steinman, R.M. 1993. Dendritic cell progenitors phagocytose particulates, including bacillus Calmette-Guerin organisms, and sensitize mice to mycobacterial antigens in vivo. *J Exp Med* 178: 479–88.
93 Svensson, M., Stockinger, B. and Wick, M.J. 1997. Bone marrow-derived dendritic cells can process bacteria for MHC-I and MHC-II presentation to T cells. *J Immunol* 158: 4229–36.
94 Valladeau, J., Ravel, O., Dezutter-Dambuyant, C., Moore, K., Kleijmeer, M., Liu, Y., Duvert-Frances, V., Vincent, C., Schmitt, D., Davoust, J., Caux, C., Lebecque, S. and Saeland, S. 2000. Langerin, a novel C-type lectin specific to Langerhans cells, is an endocytic receptor that induces the formation of Birbeck granules. *Immunity* 12: 71–81.
95 Geijtenbeek, T.B., Torensma, R., van Vliet, S.J., van Duijnhoven, G.C., Adema, G.J., van Kooyk, Y. and Figdor, C.G. 2000. Identification of DC-SIGN, a novel dendritic cell-specific ICAM-3 receptor that supports primary immune responses. *Cell* 100: 575–85.
96 Maurer, D., Fiebiger, E., Reininger, B., Ebner, C., Petzelbauer, P., Shi, G.P., Chapman, H.A. and Stingl, G. 1998. Fc epsilon receptor I on dendritic cells delivers IgE-bound multivalent antigens into a cathepsin S-dependent pathway of MHC class II presentation. *J Immunol* 161: 2731–9.
97 Noirey, N., Rougier, N., Andre, C., Schmitt, D. and Vincent, C. 2000. Langerhans-like dendritic cells generated from cord blood progenitors internalize pollen allergens by macropinocytosis, and part of the molecules are processed and can activate autologous naive T lymphocytes. *J Allergy Clin Immunol* 105: 1194–201.
98 Gross, O., Gewies, A., Finger, K., Schafer, M., Sparwasser, T., Peschel, C., Forster, I. and Ruland, J. 2006. Card9 controls a non-TLR signalling pathway for innate anti-fungal immunity. *Nature* 442: 651–6.
99 Bergman, M.P., Engering, A., Smits, H.H., van Vliet, S.J., van Bodegraven, A.A., Wirth, H.P., Kapsenberg, M.L., Vandenbroucke-Grauls, C.M., van Kooyk, Y. and Appelmelk, B.J. 2004. Helicobacter pylori modulates the T helper cell 1/T helper cell 2 balance through phase-variable interaction between lipopolysaccharide and DC-SIGN. *J Exp Med* 200: 979–90.

100 Furmonaviciene, R., Ghaemmaghami, A.M., Boyd, S.E., Jones, N.S., Bailey, K., Willis, A.C., Sewell, H.F., Mitchell, D.A. and Shakib, F. 2007. The protease allergen Der p 1 cleaves cell surface DC-SIGN and DC-SIGNR: experimental analysis of in silico substrate identification and implications in allergic responses. *Clin Exp Allergy* 37: 231–42.
101 Shreffler, W.G., Castro, R.R., Kucuk, Z.Y., Charlop-Powers, Z., Grishina, G., Yoo, S., Burks, A.W. and Sampson, H.A. 2006. The major glycoprotein allergen from Arachis hypogaea, Ara h 1, is a ligand of dendritic cell-specific ICAM-grabbing nonintegrin and acts as a Th2 adjuvant in vitro. *J Immunol* 177: 3677–85.
102 Dzionek, A., Fuchs, A., Schmidt, P., Cremer, S., Zysk, M., Miltenyi, S., Buck, D.W. and Schmitz, J. 2000. BDCA-2, BDCA-3, and BDCA-4: three markers for distinct subsets of dendritic cells in human peripheral blood. *J Immunol* 165: 6037–46.
103 Yerkovich, S.T., Roponen, M., Smith, M.E., McKenna, K., Bosco, A., Subrata, L.S., Mamessier, E., Wikstrom, M.E., Le Souef, P., Sly, P.D., Holt, P.G. and Upham, J.W. 2009. Allergen-enhanced thrombomodulin (blood dendritic cell antigen 3, CD141) expression on dendritic cells is associated with a TH2-skewed immune response. *J Allergy Clin Immunol* 123(1): 209–16.
104 McCarthy, N.E., Jones, H.A., Marks, N.A., Shiner, R.J., Ind, P.W., Al-Hassi, H.O., English, N.R., Murray, C.M., Lambert, J.R., Knight, S.C. and Stagg, A.J. 2007. Inhaled allergen-driven CD1c up-regulation and enhanced antigen uptake by activated human respiratory-tract dendritic cells in atopic asthma. *Clin Exp Allergy* 37: 72–82.
105 Tsoumakidou, M., Tzanakis, N., Papadaki, H.A., Koutala, H. and Siafakas, N.M. 2006. Isolation of myeloid and plasmacytoid dendritic cells from human bronchoalveolar lavage fluid. *Immunol Cell Biol* 84: 267–73.
106 Huysamen, C., Willment, J.A., Dennehy, K.M. and Brown, G.D. 2008. CLEC9A is a novel activation C-type lectin-like receptor expressed on BDCA3+ dendritic cells and a subset of monocytes. *J Biol Chem* 283: 16693–701.
107 Demedts, I.K., Bracke, K.R., Maes, T., Joos, G.F. and Brusselle, G.G. 2006. Different roles for human lung dendritic cell subsets in pulmonary immune defense mechanisms. *Am J Respir Cell Mol Biol* 35: 387–93.
108 Demedts, I.K., Brusselle, G.G., Vermaelen, K.Y. and Pauwels, R.A. 2005. Identification and characterization of human pulmonary dendritic cells. *Am J Respir Cell Mol Biol* 32: 177–84.
109 Lindstedt, M., Lundberg, K. and Borrebaeck, C.A. 2005. Gene family clustering identifies functionally associated subsets of human in vivo blood and tonsillar dendritic cells. *J Immunol* 175: 4839–46.
110 MacDonald, K.P., Munster, D.J., Clark, G.J., Dzionek, A., Schmitz, J. and Hart, D.N. 2002. Characterization of human blood dendritic cell subsets. *Blood* 100: 4512–20.
111 Gereda, J.E., Leung, D.Y., Thatayatikom, A., Streib, J.E., Price, M.R., Klinnert, M.D. and Liu, A.H. 2000. Relation between house-dust endotoxin exposure, type 1 T-cell development, and allergen sensitisation in infants at high risk of asthma. *Lancet* 355: 1680–3.
112 Gern, J.E. and Busse, W.W. 2002. Relationship of viral infections to wheezing illnesses and asthma. *Nat Rev Immunol* 2: 132–8.

113 Akdis, C.A., Kussebi, F., Pulendran, B., Akdis, M., Lauener, R.P., Schmidt-Weber, C.B., Klunker, S., Isitmangil, G., Hansjee, N., Wynn, T.A., Dillon, S., Erb, P., Baschang, G., Blaser, K. and Alkan, S.S. 2003. Inhibition of T helper 2-type responses, IgE production and eosinophilia by synthetic lipopeptides. *Eur J Immunol* 33: 2717–26.
114 Patel, M., Xu, D., Kewin, P., Choo-Kang, B., McSharry, C., Thomson, N.C. and Liew, F.Y. 2005. TLR2 agonist ameliorates established allergic airway inflammation by promoting Th1 response and not via regulatory T cells. *J Immunol* 174: 7558–63.
115 Taylor, R.C., Richmond, P. and Upham, J.W. 2006. Toll-like receptor 2 ligands inhibit TH2 responses to mite allergen. *J Allergy Clin Immunol* 117: 1148–54.

Index

FSC
www.fsc.org
MIX
Papier | Fördert
gute Waldnutzung
FSC® C083411

Kolibri 360 GmbH
Ferdinand-Jühlke-Straße 7
99095 Erfurt, Deutschland
produktsicherheit@kolibri360.de